# The Neuroimaging of Brain Diseases

# The Neuroimaging of Brain Diseases

Editor: Miles Scott

FOSTER ACADEMICS
www.fosteracademics.com

www.fosteracademics.com

FOSTER ACADEMICS

**Cataloging-in-publication Data**

The neuroimaging of brain diseases / edited by Miles Scott.
p. cm.
Includes bibliographical references and index.
ISBN 978-1-64646-614-6
1. Brain--Diseases--Imaging. 2. Nervous system--Diseases--Imaging.
3. Medical radiology. 4. Diagnostic imaging. 5. Imaging systems in medicine.
I. Scott, Miles.
RC349.D52 N48 2023
616.804 754--dc23



Foster Academics,
118-35 Queens Blvd., Suite 400,
Forest Hills, NY 11375, USA

ISBN 978-1-64646-614-6 (Hardback)

# Contents


**Preface** ..... VII

Chapter 1 **Using fMRI to Study Valuation and Choice** ..... 1
P. Read Montague, Ann H. Harvey and Ulrich Kirk

Chapter 2 **Application of Diffusion- and Perfusion-Weighted Imaging in Acute Ischemic Stroke** ..... 15
Vincent Lai

Chapter 3 **Social Neuroscience Tasks: Employing fMRI to Understand the Social Mind** ..... 34
D.Y. Phua and G.I. Christopoulos

Chapter 4 **Social Pain and the Brain: How Insights from Neuroimaging Advance the Study of Social Rejection and Variants of Normal** ..... 60
Richard S. Pond, Jr., Stephanie B. Richman, David S. Chester and C. Nathan DeWall

Chapter 5 **The Brain is not "as-if" — Taking Stock of the Neuroscientific Approach on Decision Making** ..... 93
Kirsten G. Volz and Gerd Gigerenzer

Chapter 6 **Active and Passive fMRI for Presurgical Mapping of Motor and Language Cortex** ..... 124
Victoria A.L. Mosher, Einat Liebenthal and Bradley G. Goodyear

Chapter 7 **Structural and Functional Magnetic Resonance Imaging in Hepatic Encephalopathy** ..... 149
Long Jiang Zhang, Guang Ming Lu and Hui Mao

Chapter 8 **Neuroimaging of Epilepsy: EEG-fMRI in the Presurgical Evaluation of Focal Epilepsy** ..... 167
Mirko Avesani, Silvia Giacopuzzi and Antonio Fiaschi

Chapter 9 **Brain Mapping of Language Processing Using Functional MRI Connectivity and Diffusion Tensor Imaging** ..... 203
Todd L. Richards and Virginia W. Berninger

Chapter 10 **FDG-PET Imaging in Neurodegenerative Brain Diseases..........220**
L. K. Teune, A. L. Bartels and K. L. Leenders

**Permissions**

**List of Contributors**

**Index**

# Preface

This book has been an outcome of determined endeavour from a group of educationists in the field. The primary objective was to involve a broad spectrum of professionals from diverse cultural background involved in the field for developing new researches. The book not only targets students but also scholars pursuing higher research for further enhancement of the theoretical and practical applications of the subject.

Neuroimaging is a sub-field of medical imaging that focuses on the entire central nervous system (CNS) including the brain and the spinal cord. Neuroimaging studies help in describing how the brain functions and how diverse activities affect the brain. It is majorly used to diagnose diseases and monitor brain health. Some of the important neuroimaging techniques include electroencephalography (EEG), positron emission tomography (PET), functional magnetic resonance imaging (fMRI), computerized tomography (CT), magnetoencephalography (MEG), single photon emission computed tomography (SPECT), diffusion tensor imaging (DTI), and diffuse optical tomography (DOT). These techniques are essential tools in investigating nervous system diseases and disorders such as Alzheimer's disease, brain tumors, stroke, Parkinson's disease, epilepsy, schizophrenia (SZ), and bipolar disorder (BP). Recent advancements in neuroimaging enable more accurate diagnosis, monitoring and prognosis of neurological, neuropsychological and psychiatric disorders. This book brings forth some of the most recent developments and research in neuroimaging and elucidates the unexplored aspects of diagnosing brain diseases. It is a vital tool for individuals associated with neuroimaging of brain diseases.

It was an honour to edit such a profound book and also a challenging task to compile and examine all the relevant data for accuracy and originality. I wish to acknowledge the efforts of the contributors for submitting such brilliant and diverse chapters in the field and for endlessly working for the completion of the book. Last, but not the least; I thank my family for being a constant source of support in all my research endeavours.

**Editor**

1

# Using fMRI to Study Valuation and Choice

P. Read Montague, Ann H. Harvey and Ulrich Kirk

## 1. Introduction

The ability to make decisions relies on brain mechanisms designed to value our environment and elicit appropriate actions based on those values. These mechanisms allow an agent to predict the value of a potential action both immediately and into the future, and then execute the chosen action. Because the ability to find food or choose a mate directly impacts the survival of a species, it is easy to see how these goal-seeking behaviors would acquire reward value in the brain. But what is the internal value of a piece of art, a label on a bottle, an idea, or a social gesture by another person? Humans use resources (both energy and money) to acquire these types of abstract rewards, and they affect decision-making behavior in a manner similar to primary rewards such as food, water, and sex. In fact, abstract rewards can be powerful motivators: pursuit of these rewards can even cause humans to forego basic needs to acquire them. In this chapter we review experiments in the field of neuroimaging that explore how value is constructed in the human brain across a variety of domains. We then focus on a series of experiments conducted to probe the brain responses underlying preference decisions for art, and how these preferences can be altered by external variables in the environment. These experiments combine neuroscience, psychology, and economics to probe the underlying neurobiology of valuation and choice behavior in humans.

## 2. The study of valuation and choice in the human brain

Like all mobile creatures, a variety of human decisions requires the ability to differentially value choices and their potential outcomes. Many of these decisions relates to the acquisition of food, water, and sex, choices that allow us to survive as a species. In the learning literature, these types of appetitive stimuli are known as primary rewards. Early work on reward processing in alert monkeys demonstrated that midbrain dopaminergic neurons track the delivery of such primary rewards (Romo and Schultz, 1990). Since that time, a large body of ongoing research in this area has provided evidence that dopaminergic target structures are a key component in the brain's reward circuit, and they subsequently respond to an array of primary rewards (Schultz et al, 1997, Breiter et al, 1997, Berns et al, 2001).

However, we make many decisions in our everyday life that have little or no connection to such primary rewards. We make decisions about which brand of paper towels to buy, what to wear, how to spend our afternoon, etc. These types of decisions have components beyond simply meeting our basic needs, and there is often no clear best answer. And yet we routinely make preference judgments and choices for these types of stimuli. Furthermore, we get satisfaction from making these decisions, even in the absence of receiving any primary reward for our efforts. Neuroimaging experiments over the last several years have shed light on the neural mechanisms associated with valuation of abstract rewards. One area that has been shown repeatedly to be activated by diverse rewarding stimuli is the ventromedial prefrontal cortex (VMPFC). This brain region has been shown in several neuroimaging studies to be active for a variety of primary and abstract rewards including sports cars (Erk et al, 2002), cola preference (McClure et al, 2004), pleasant odors (Rolls et al, 2003), wine price (Plassmann et al, 2008), facial attractiveness (O'Doherty et al 2003) and money (Knutson et al, 2003). Mounting evidence in these studies and others supports the idea that this region is involved in converting the value of these diverse stimuli to a common scale for action selection (Montague and Berns, 2002).

### 2.1. Current research on valuation and choice

The overall goal of this research is to use fMRI to understand how value is constructed for abstract rewards in the human brain. Are value mechanisms for abstract rewards plugging into the same mechanisms dedicated to primary rewards? And if valuation is dynamic, how do context changes modulate responses in these brain areas and subsequently alter the value of an abstract reward? Such a mechanism for comparing value across a set of choices must fit into the existing data on valuation mechanisms for primary rewards, but also extend to the broader context of choices that do not involve primary reward feedback. The series of experiments herein elucidate the neural correlates of valuation for abstract rewards and begin to parameterize ways in which the signal can be modulated by external influences including familiarity and social gestures.

### 2.2. Using art to study valuation

In this chapter we summarize a series of experiments to study subjective decision-making by looking at how humans value visual art. Art represents an interesting category of rewards because they maintain their value even when separated from a primary reinforcer. Despite the fact that that value is a complex variable that depends largely on a person's current internal and external states, humans are incredibly efficient at assigning value to abstract rewards and making appropriate decisions. For our experiments, we assume that expressed behavioral preference for a piece of art represents its internal value. Expressed preference is a common tool used in marketing, psychological, behavioral economics, and imaging experiments to assess the value of rewards. While this is just one example of a subjective decision, it is well-suited to study using fMRI for several reasons. The first reason is simply a practical one: visual art is an easy stimulus to deliver to subjects while inside an MRI scanner. Secondly, people can fairly easily evaluate their preference for art. Even subjects with very little exposure to art can find pieces that they enjoy and pieces that they dislike without having a working knowledge of the art or artist. Third, painting preferences are very unique to the individual. For a given set of paintings, the art that you like/dislike will be different from the art that I like/dislike. This makes the stimulus set more robust for analysis, since we will be unlikely to accidentally bias our analysis toward certain features of the stimuli.

In the first set of experiments, we examined neural responses to abstract rewards using images of paintings as stimuli. Human subjects viewed paintings passively in an fMRI experiment, and were asked to rate their subjective preference and familiarity for every painting after the scanning session (Figure 1). 80 paintings were chosen to represent a wide array of abstract and representational art from the Western tradition.

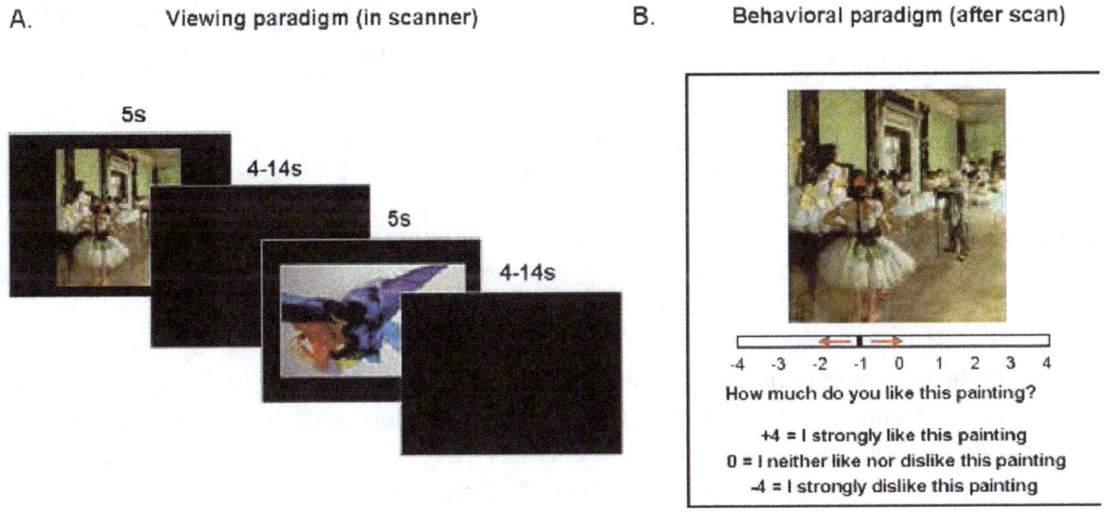


**Figure 1.** Experiment paradigm for (A) passive viewing of paintings during fMRI task and (B) behavioral ratings after fMRI session

We first examined the behavioral relationship between preference and familiarity for the paintings (Figure 2A). When we compared the subjective ratings for the two parameters for each painting, we found a striking, positive correlation (Figure 3.2A, $y = 1.04x + 0.086$, $R^2 = 0.976$). Preference varied linearly with familiarity, although of course it is not known if these scales themselves are linear with respect to internal states of preference or familiarity. BOLD responses in several brain regions were found to vary significantly with subjective preference and with familiarity (Figure 2B). Considerable overlap was found to exist between the two groups, including activation in the ventromedial prefrontal cortex, the bilateral caudate, retrosplenial cortex, and bilateral parahippocampal gyrus, further supporting the relationship between these parameters found behaviorally.

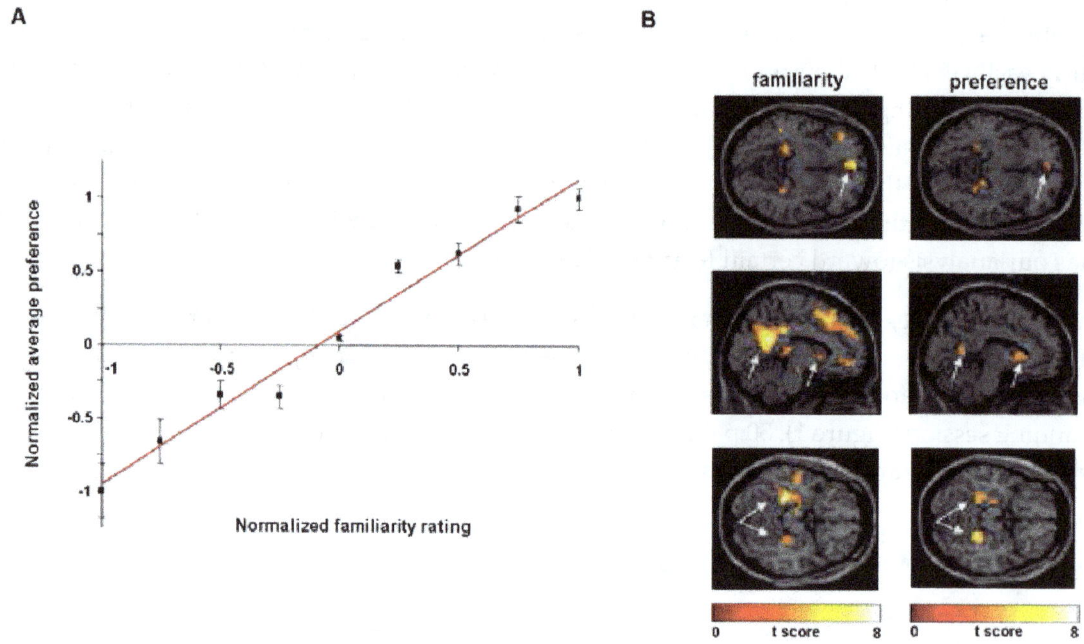


**Figure 2.** Behavioral correlation between average preference and familiarity (A) and BOLD responses during passive viewing of paintings that correlate with preference and familiarity (B).

The results of the art viewing experiment provide evidence that BOLD responses correlated with painting preference overlap with brain regions known to process a variety of rewarding stimuli. We also demonstrate a strong behavioral and neural correlation between preference and familiarity, suggesting that familiarity is a key factor in the valuation of abstract rewards. These results demonstrate that BOLD responses in several overlapping brain regions encode expressed preference and familiarity for artwork. The region of the vmpfc overlaps with a region previously found to encode preference for colas (McClure et al 2004). This work provides evidence that preferences for abstract stimuli such as art can generate reward responses in the brain similar to primary rewards. The second important finding is that familiarity for these stimuli is encoded in similar brain regions, and may play an important role in determining preferences for art. Notably, we located these neural signatures while subjects passively viewed the artwork in the scanner and were not asked to evaluate the paintings at the time of the viewing. The fact that neural responses during passive viewing correlate with behavioral ratings after the presentation suggest that our brains are doing continuous valuation of stimuli in our environment even in the absence of explicit decisions.

### 2.3. The influence of favors on valuation and decision-making

Subjective decisions may include simple aesthetic choices, but many of our most important decisions are subtle and complex value choices, as in the case of medical decisions and prescribing behavior in the medical and biomedical device industries. Every year, physicians prescribe millions of dollars worth of prescription drugs to treat their patients' illnesses. Often there are comparable drug treatment strategies for a given disease, with slight variations in side effects, cost, etc. How does a physician decide between drug A and drug B? Perhaps in her experience she has found that drug A is more easily tolerated by her patients, or the cost of drug A is lower. But we know that there are other factors at work as well. Each year the pharmaceutical industry directs approximately 90% of its $21 billion marketing budget toward physicians (Brennan et al 2006). This includes sponsored events, lunches, gifts, conferences, and other physician-industry interactions. The effect of such gifts on physician decision-making behavior is unmistakable. In several reports on such issues, while physicians routinely deny that gifts could influence their prescribing behavior, and yet receiving samples, industry-paid meals, funding for travel and paid speaking engagements from a pharmaceutical company for a certain drug have all been found to result in more favorable viewpoints and increased prescribing of the particular drug (Wazana, 2000). The fact that physicians are largely unaware of the potential biasing effects of these gestures suggests that external influences are acting in ways that subvert cognitive awareness or control. While biases can be self-serving (Dana and Loewenstein, 2003), they may also be rooted in biological mechanisms that subvert cognitive control. For example, social gestures from a sender to a receiver are known to bias decisions made by the recipient, especially when the decision relates to the sender – a feature of social exchange known as reciprocity. Recent experiments have begun to shed light on the neural mechanisms of reciprocity-eliciting gestures (King-Casas et al, 2005, Rilling et al, 2002, Li et al, 2009, van den Bos et al, 2009); however, almost nothing is known about the influence of an 'open-loop' favor where there is no possibility for reciprocating interactions between the sender and the receiver.

We next investigated how external social value can manipulate value judgments for abstract rewards. In the same way that familiarity and preference were tightly linked, perhaps preference judgments depend on other contextual factors. A particularly salient real-world example is the use of monetary favors to influence preferences. We hypothesized that social favors can bias subjective preferences, even for objects unrelated to the favor itself. We have addressed this hypothesis by employing a collection of monetary favor and preference experiments. A monetary favor is sent from an agent to a subject and we tested the influence of this favor on subjects' preference for art, a domain where there is no objectively 'correct' answer and no economic relationship exists between the favor and the preference judgment.

During functional brain imaging sessions, subjects passively viewed images of artwork paired with company logos; one of the companies sponsored the subjects' participation in the experiment (Figure 3). After scanning, the subjects provided preference ratings for all the paintings.

The behavioral results showed that preference for paintings paired with the sponsoring company's logo was higher than those paired with the non-sponsor logo (Harvey et al 2010). The functional imaging results revealed that activity in the ventromedial prefrontal cortex tracked the sponsorship category of the painting (Figure 4, Harvey et al 2010). This imaging study is the first to indicate that a monetary favor transfers value to a proxy and influences judgment of objects in spatial proximity, with corresponding changes in neural activity as measured by fMRI. Furthermore, the experiment was designed with no reciprocal interaction

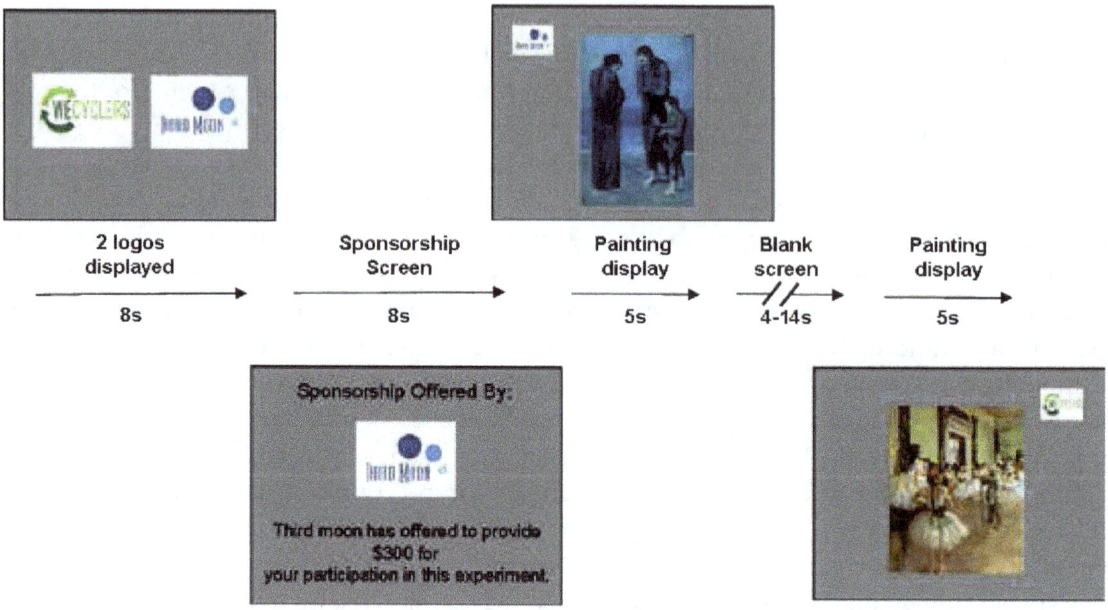


**Figure 3.** Experiment paradigm for the favor task (Harvey et al. 2010). Subjects are shown 2 logos, and one of the companies represented by the logo is indicated as the sponsor company. Subjects then viewed a series of paintings paired with either the sponsor company logo, or another non-sponsor logo. After the MRI session subjects rated each of the paintings based on their preference.

between the company and the receiver, suggesting that the favor is capable of influencing behavior even when the receiver has no explicit stake in the outcome of the interaction.

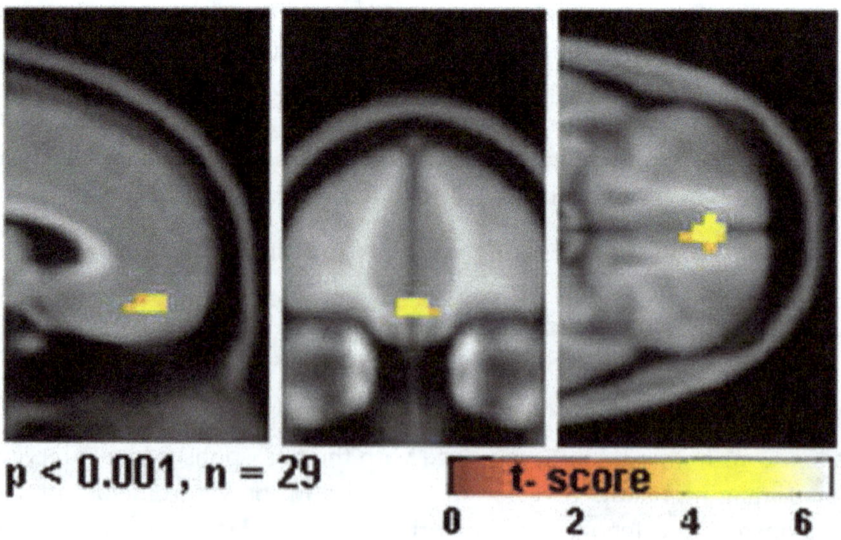


**Figure 4.** Region of the VMPFC that differentially responds to sponsor and non-sponsor paintings in the favor task (Harvey et al 2010). The voxels displayed show BOLD activity for linearly increasing painting preference.

We hypothesized that social favors can bias subjective preferences, even for objects unrelated to the favor itself. We addressed this hypothesis by employing a collection of monetary favor and revealed preference experiments. Using an art-viewing paradigm possessing no objectively correct answer for preferring one piece of art over another in conjunction with fMRI, we show that sponsorship of the experiment by a company endows the company's logo with the capacity to bias revealed preference for art displayed next to the logo. These sponsorship effects do not possess a special collection of brain responses, but instead modulate responses in neural networks normally activated by a wide range of preference judgments. The results raise the important possibility that monetary favors bias judgments by acting through existing valuation mechanisms, and individuals may therefore have difficulty detecting the gesture's influence over their subjective preferences even for objects seemingly unrelated to the favor.

## 2.4. Mitigation of the effects of favors using domain expertise

In the last series of experiments we examined whether the biasing effects of the social gesture on valuation judgments could be mitigated. In the case of medical professionals, biases from monetary gifts or other favors from pharmaceutical companies is thought to be mitigated through a variety of mechanisms. These include disclosing potential conflicts of interest, not accepting large gifts or favors, and oversight from the institution regarding biases in prescribing behavior. In addition, the fact that medical professionals have expertise in their domain of decision-making is taken as an argument that they should be more objective in their judgment than the average person making a similar decision. To test this directly, we recruited a group of participants with expertise in the domain of art to perform the favor task outlined in the previous section. The hypothesis was that these subjects have training in assessing art that may insulate them against the biasing gesture of the sponsoring company. And if so, there should be neurobiological correlates to the difference in behavior between art experts and non-experts.

Art experts with a minimum of 5 years of experience working in a visual art-related field were asked to undergo an fMRI scan while they viewed images of artwork, paired either with a sponsor company logo or another non-sponsor company logo. After the fMRI session, each subject rated their preference for the art that was displayed in the scanner. The setup was identical to the previously discussed experiments, except that student art was used rather than well known paintings to eliminate the possibility that differences in results between art experts and non-experts was due solely to familiarity with the paintings.

In the behavioral results, there was no difference in preference for the sponsor paintings compared to the non-sponsor paintings, in contrast to the control subjects who showed a significantly higher preference for sponsor paintings. We hypothesized that if the experts did not show an effect of the sponsorship on preference ratings for paintings, BOLD activity in the VMPFC should not be sensitive to the sponsorship in the expert group as originally seen in the control subjects whose behavior reflected the bias toward preferring sponsor paintings. This was indeed the case: while both the controls and art experts had activity in the VMPFC that correlated linearly with painting preference for all paintings, the experts did not show differential activity in this region for sponsor compared to non-sponsor paintings.

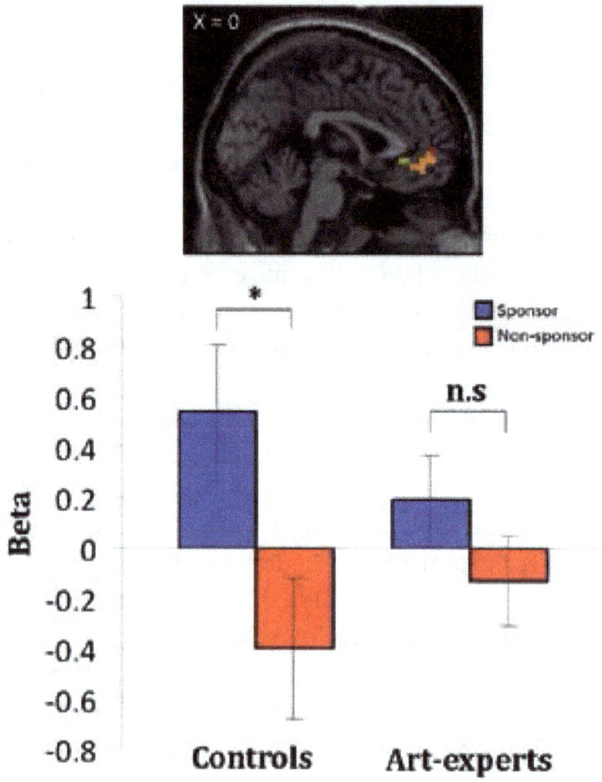


**Figure 5.** Activity in the VMPFC (top panel) increases linearly for painting preference in both control subjects and art experts. However, while control subjects showed differential activity in this area for sponsor compared to non-sponsor paintings (bottom panel), the VMPFC of the art experts did not discriminate between the two types of paintings (Kirk et al. 2011).

The next natural question based on the behavioral results was: if art experts do not show an effect of sponsorship on their behavior or activity in the ventromedial prefrontal cortex, which region of the brain might be involved in the mitigation of this effect? To explore this further, we examined activity in the dorsolateral prefrontal cortex (DLPFC), a region known to be involved in executive control (Wagner et al. 2011) and modulation of valuation in other experiments (Hare et al. 2009, Li et al. 2011).

We generated a contrast to look for differences in BOLD response between art experts and controls in the DLPFC for linearly increases preferences for paintings. This region was significantly more active in a linear preference regressor for art experts than controls (Figure 6). No other brain region showed differential activity for this contrast.

We also found that activity in this region of the DLPFC was functionally connected to the VMPFC, and the coupling of these two regions was stronger during presentation of sponsor paintings than during presentation of non-sponsor paintings. Thus the DLPFC may be a region through which modulation of activity in the VMPFC may occur. Furthermore, we repeated the same functional connectivity analysis in a group of controls that were selected because

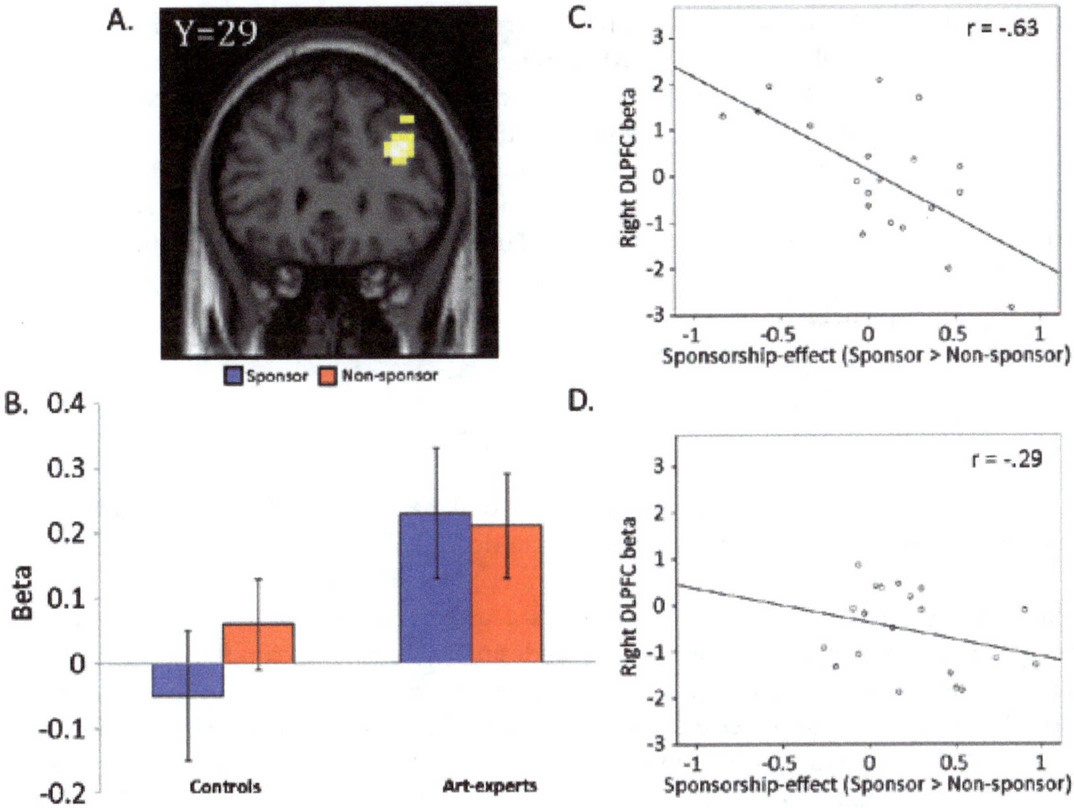


**Figure 6.** (A) BOLD responses in the DLPFC are greater for linear correlations with preference in the art experts compared to control subjects. (B) Beta responses in this region for sponsor and non-sponsor paintings in both controls and art-experts (from Kirk et al. 2011).

they did not show a behavioral sponsorship bias. In these participants, we replicated the functional connectivity result between the VMPFC and the DLPFC (Kirk et al 2011). The result indicates that the modulation of the VMPFC by DLPFC may be a more general mechanism by which a person could be insulated by biasing maneuvers, rather than being specific to the individuals with specific domain expertise such as the art experts used in this study.

## 2.5. Future research

In future experiments, we plan to further explore the neurobiology underlying human valuation and behavioral bias, and the ways in which values may be altered with external influences, training, or intervention. There are several lines of questions that lend themselves to the types of experimental manipulations described in this chapter. For example, it may be possible to teach people to train their responses either behaviorally or with real-time feedback during fMRI sessions to become less sensitive to bias. This could be extremely useful for professions where expertise and decision-making should be immune to external influence. One particular profession would be physicians and prescribing behavior: if it is possible to assess bias and make changes to their behavior, such intervention may be a much better option than current methods of disclosing conflicts of interest as a method of mitigating bias. Additionally, it is possible that there exist subtypes of people within the population that may be more or less susceptible to bias. Paradigms such as these could be used to parametrically evaluate susceptibility and the effects of intervention. And finally, if a person is biased in one domain are they necessarily biased in another domain as well? Perhaps art experts are not only insulated from bias within the domain of art viewing but across multiple domains that require evaluation without being susceptible to bias. Future research in the areas described will hopefully lead to the discovery of strategies to improve decision-making behavior and knowledge of potential bias across a range of domains.

## 3. Conclusion

We have used fMRI in conjunction with behavioral paradigms to investigate the neural correlates of subjective decision-making. Our metric for subjective decisions was behavioral preference for visual art. While this is just one example of a subjective decision, it is well-suited to study using fMRI for several reasons. The first reason is simply a practical one: visual art is an easy stimulus to deliver to subjects while inside an MRI scanner. Secondly, people can fairly easily evaluate their preference for art. Even subjects with very little exposure to art can find pieces that they enjoy and pieces that they dislike without having a working knowledge of the art or artist. Third, painting preferences are very unique to the individual. For a given set of paintings, the art that you like/dislike will be different from the art that I like/dislike. This makes the stimulus set more robust for analysis, since we will be unlikely to accidentally bias our analysis toward certain features of the stimuli. In the first experiment, visual art was passively presented to subjects while they underwent an fMRI scan. We showed that subjects' stated preference for the paintings, made *after* the scanning session was complete, correlated linearly with the neural responses in several brain regions. The regions with increased BOLD activity included the ventral striatum and the ventromedial prefrontal cortex, regions that are activated by a wide range of rewarding stimuli. In our experiments, however, subjects were not asked to make judgments and were unaware that they would be rating the paintings after the scanner session. This manipulation provides evidence that the brain is likely making continuous valuation judgments even without any explicit query. The results provide further support to the idea that the mechanisms that encode value for primary rewards largely overlap with those for subjective assessments of stimuli with little or no link to such rewards.

In the second set of experiments, we were interested in whether or not external social influences could alter preferences for art. Previous studies have shown that other external factors can alter perception and preferences, with corresponding changes in neural responses. People perceive art as more beautiful when they believe it to be created by an artist compared to a computer (Kirk et al, 2008), the taste of wine is more pleasant (Plassmann et al, 2008) and the perceived efficacy of analgesics is improved if the product is believed to be more expensive (Waber et al 2008). Rather than price or perceived quality, we designed an experiment to test the effect of a monetary favor on subjects' preference judgments. Favors are a particular type of open-loop social gesture whereby an agent provides a gift with no explicit expectation of reciprocity. Recent neurobiological experiments have sought to explore the neural underpinnings of reciprocity (King-Casas et al, 2005, Rilling et al, 2002), but to date no fMRI experiments have addressed the influence of monetary favors on decision-making. In our experiment we used subjective preferences for artwork as a tool for measuring the influence of a monetary favor. When a company paid the subject for their participation in the experiment, the visual juxtaposition of the "sponsor" logo made individuals more likely to like those paintings as compared to paintings paired with another, non-sponsor logo. We ran the experiment at three levels of monetary compensation; while there was a trend toward preferring sponsor paintings in all conditions, only the $300 effect was significant. Despite the fact that it took the largest sum of money to influence preferences in this task, it is unlikely that small favors have no biasing effect on behavior. This task, compared to real-world examples of biasing gestures, was relatively mild. The subjects had no option to pay back the company; the gesture was a single-shot interaction rather than a repeated encounter, as is typical of most social gestures. Furthermore, there was absolutely *no incentive* for subjects to change their preference ratings based on the sponsorship; they were paid exactly the same amount no matter how they answered. The fact that such a mild gesture influences preference judgments completely unrelated to the favor suggests that favors are plugging into reciprocity mechanisms without the individual being aware of the effect. The neural results showed that, rather than a global effect of sponsorship on any brain region, the influence of the sponsor adds linearly to brain responses that more generally encode painting preference.

And finally, we examined the ways in which valuation bias from a favor can be mitigated with domain expertise. We chose art experts for the study because of their experience with the type of stimuli used in the study. We hypothesized that expertise within a domain is one way in which an individual might be insulated by biasing maneuvers such as a monetary favor or other social gesture. While a monetary favor was capable of biasing behavior for a group of control subjects in the previous experiments, the art experts in this study did not show a behavioral preference for sponsor compared to non-sponsor paintings. In the fMRI data, we showed that the VMPFC, a region of the brain known to respond during valuation experiments, was responsive to increasing painting preference for both controls and art experts. However, this region was not differentially sensitive to sponsorship in the art experts, suggesting that the biasing maneuver of the monetary favor was somehow mitigated in this group. We found a candidate region of the dorsolateral prefrontal cortex that may play a role in the mitigation of bias. This region was functionally connected to the VMPFC in the art experts, and also in a group of controls that did not show the sponsorship effect. The results suggest that domain expertise may be one way in which individuals may insulate themselves from bias, but other strategies may be involved for control subjects who show similar effects.

## Acknowledgements

We would like to thank the members of the Human Neuroimaging Laboratory for assistance in conducting the studies discussed in this chapter. In particular we thank the MRI technologists who assisted in collecting the fMRI data, the software development team that assisted in coding the task stimuli and development of the Hyperscan technology and NEMO experiment environment. We thank Ron Fisher for early work and collaboration on the art experiment paradigm. We would also like to thank George Denfield for co-author contributions to the published experiments discussed in the chapter (Harvey et al 2010).

## Author details

P. Read Montague, Ann H. Harvey and Ulrich Kirk

Virginia Tech Carilion Research Institute, Virginia, USA

## References

[1] Berns, G.S., McClure, S.M., Pagnoni, G., Montague, P.R. (2001). Predictability modulates human brain response to reward. J Neurosci. 21, 2793-8.

[2] Breiter, H.C., Gollub, R.L., Weisskoff, R.M., Kennedy, D.N., Makris, N., Berke, J.D., Goodman, J.M., Kantor, H.L., Gastfriend, D.R., Riorden, J.P., Mathew, R.T., Rosen, B.R., Hyman, S.E. (1997). Acute effects of cocaine on human brain activity and emotion. Neuron 19, 591-611.

[3] Breiter, H.C., Aharon, I., Kahneman, D., Dale, A., Shizgal, P. (2001). Functional imaging of neural responses to expectancy and experience of monetary gains and losses. Neuron 30, 619-39.

[4] Brennan, TA, Rothman, DJ, Blank, L, Blumenthal, D, Chimonas, SC, Cohen, JJ, Goldman, J, Kassirer, JP, Kimball, H, Naughton, J, Smelser, N. (2006). Health industry practices that create conflicts of interest. JAMA 295, 429-433.

[5] van den Bos, W, van Dijk, E, Westenberg, M, Rombouts, S A R B, & Crone, E A (2009) What motivates repayment? Neural correlates of reciprocity in the Trust Game. Soc Cogn Affect Neurosci 4:294-304.

[6] Dana, J., Loewenstein, G. (2003). A social science perspective on gifts to physicians from industry. JAMA 290, 252-255.

[7] Erk, S., Spitzer, M., Wunderlich, A.P., Galley, L., Walter, H. (2002). Cultural objects modulate reward circuitry. NeuroReport 13, 2499-2503.

[8] Hare TA, Camerer CF, Rangel A (2009) Self-control in decision-making involves modulation of the VMPFC valuation system. Science 324:646-648.

[9] Harvey, A.H., Kirk, U., Denfield, G.H., Montague, P.R. (2010). Monetary favors and their influence on neural responses and revealed preference. J Neurosci 30, 9597-9602.

[10] King-Casas, B., Tomlin, D.A., Anen, C., Camerer, C.F., Quartz, S.R., Montague, P.R. (2005). Getting to know you: reputation and trust in a two-person economic exchange. Science 308, 78-83.

[11] Kirk, U, Skov, M, Hulme, O, Christensen, MS, & Zeki, S (2009) Modulation of aesthetic value by semantic context: an fMRI study. Neuroimage 44:1125-1132.

[12] Kirk, U., Harvey, A.H., Montague, P.R. (2011). Domain expertise insulates against judgment bias by monetary favors through a modulation of ventromedial prefrontal cortex. PNAS 108, 10332-10336.

[13] Li, J, Xiao, E, Houser, D, & Montague, PR (2009) Neural responses to sanction threats in two-party economic exchange. Proc Natl Acad Sci U S A 106:16835-16840.

[14] Li J, Delgado MR, Phelps EA (2011) How instructed knowledge modulates the neural systems of reward learning. Proc Natl Acad Sci U S A. 108:55-60.

[15] Knutson, B., Fong, G.W., Bennett, S.M., Adams, C.M., Hommer, D. (2003). A region of mesial prefrontal cortex tracks monetarily rewarding outcomes: characterization with rapid event-related fMRI. Neuroimage 18: 263-272.

[16] McClure, S.M., Li, J., Tomlin, D., Cypert, K.S., Montague, L.M., Montague, R.M. (2004). Neural correlates of behavioral preference for culturally familiar drinks. Neuron 44, 379-387.

[17] Montague, P.R., Berns, G.S. (2002). Neural Economics and the biological substrates of valuation. Neuron 36, 265-284.

[18] O'Doherty, J, Winston, J, Critchley, H, Perrett, D, Burt, DM, & Dolan, RJ (2003) Beauty in a smile: the role of medial orbitofrontal cortex in facial attractiveness. Neuropsychologia 41:147-155.

[19] Rilling, J.K., Gutman, D.A., Zeh, T.R., Pagnoni, G., Berns, G.S., Kilts, C.D. (2002). A neural basis for social cooperation. Neuron 35, 395-405.

[20] Rolls, E.T., Kringelbach, M.L., de Araujo, I.E. (2003). Different representations of pleasant and unpleasant odours in the human brain. Eur J Neurosci 18, 695-703.

[21] Romo, R, Schultz, W (1990). Dopamine neurons of the monkey midbrain: contingencies of responses to active touch during self-initiated arm movements. J. Neurophysiology 63(3):592-606.

[22] Schultz W, Dayan P, Montague PR. (1997). A neural substrate of prediction and reward. Science 14, 1593-9.

[23] Schultz, W, Romo, R (1990). Dopamine neurons of the monkey midbrain: contingencies of responses to stimuli eliciting immediate behavioral reactions. J. Neurophysiology 63, 607-624.

[24] Wagner AD, Maril A, Bjork RA, Schacter DL (2001) Prefrontal contributions to executive control: fMRI evidence for functional distinctions within lateral prefrontal cortex. Neuroimage 14(6):1337-1347.

[25] Wazana, A. (2000). Physicians and the pharmaceutical industry: is a gift ever just a gift? JAMA 283, 373-380.

# 2

# Application of Diffusion- and Perfusion-Weighted Imaging in Acute Ischemic Stroke

Vincent Lai

## 1. Introduction

Stroke is one leading cause of morbidity and mortality worldwide, with acute ischemia constituting approximately 80% of all cases (Srinivasan et al. 2006). In the past imaging was primarily used to exclude hemorrhage and other causes. Yet diagnostic classification and clinical prognosis are major challenges in acute stroke. This is of particular importance since the approval of intravenous tissue plasminogen activator therapy for acute ischemic stroke within a narrow therapeutic window of 4.5 hours (Hacke et al. 2008; Wahlgren et al. 2008). It then becomes clear that advance imaging techniques would be much needed to identify this subgroup of patient who could be beneficial for thrombolytic therapy.

Computed tomography (CT) scan has been the traditional method for acute stroke imaging with excellent sensitivity for acute intracerebral hemorrhage, but demonstrates limited sensitivity for detection of ischemic infarction, with a reported sensitivity of 40-60% only within 6 hours of onset, and a negative predictive valve of 17% (von Kummer et al. 2001). Magnetic resonance (MR) imaging has no doubt superior spatial and contrast resolution as compared with CT, achieving higher sensitivity and accuracy. It has even emerged over last few years to become as sensitive as CT in depiction of acute intracranial hemorrhage (Fiebach et al. 2004; Kidwell et al. 2004). Perfusion-weighted imaging (PWI) and diffusion-weight imaging (DWI) had played an influencing role since their introduction in late 1980s. Application DWI and PWI offer complex information regarding infarction and perfusion deficits, significantly improving the diagnostic yield. In a recent meta-analysis, Schellinger et al. (2010) found that the ability to correctly diagnose acute ischemic stroke on MR was significantly higher than CT, demonstrating an odds ratio of 25 ($p$<0.0001; confidence interval: 8-79). It also brings forward the concept of salvageable brain tissue as indicated by penumbra which is a rather dynamic entity that exists within a narrow range of perfusion pressures, carrying significant implication on therapy selection and prediction of clinical outcome. The goal is to salvage the ischemic but viable penumbral tissue from progression into infarction.

## 2. Diffusion-weighted imaging

In DWI, the random motion or diffusion pulse of water molecules in a tissue compartment through a magnetic field gradient causes phase shifting leading to intravoxel dephasing and hence loss of signal intensity (Poustchi-Amin et al. 2001). In region of acute infarct or irreversible ischemia, the decreased diffusion of water molecules due to presence of cytotoxic edema (neuronal and glial cell swelling) from intracellular water accumulation and disruption of membrane ionic homeostasis will manifest as an increase in signal intensity, reflecting a decrease in apparent diffusion coefficient (ADC). ADC is "apparent" only because the actual measurement cannot be obtained by DWI due to presence of unmeasured variables that influence the rate of diffusion, such as temperature of the tissue and actual route of the diffusing molecule. Images are acquired sequentially with the axis of diffusion sensitization in three orthogonal planes, with their average yielding an image with minimal anisotropy-related hyperintensity. As a result, infracted tissue appears bright in comparison with normal bran tissue. This has significant impact in helping to identify area of acute ischemia from chronic ischemic, and hence stratify treatment plan.

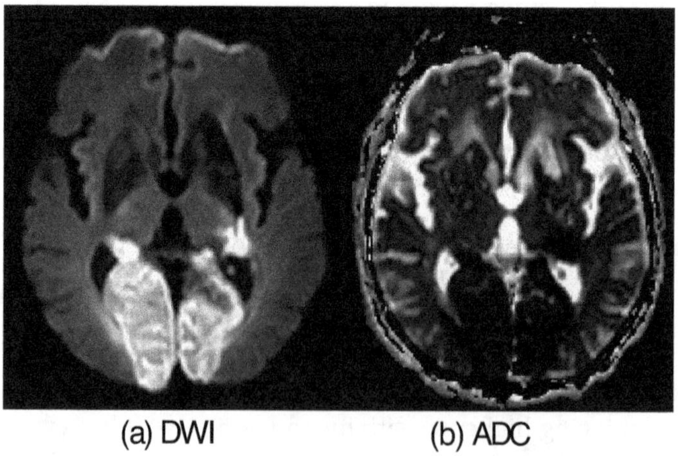


**Figure 1.** a) DWI shows hyperintense signal along bilateral posterior cerebral arterial territories. b) corresponding ADC map demonstrates hypointense signal.

In human, restricted diffusion showing increased DWI signal with reduced ADC value (Figure 1) have been observed as early as 30 minutes after onset of ischemia (Srinivasan et al. 2006). ADC continues to decrease for 3-5 days, reaching its minimum value of about 50% between 24-48 hours after symptoms onset before returning to baseline at approximately 1-4 weeks, so called pseudonormalization. At this stage, mildly hyperintense DWI signal with normalized ADC value will be seen. ADC increases afterwards with value higher than normal value associated with variable DWI signal (from T2 effect) for upto months, presumably related to increased quantity of extracellular water. It is important to note that DWI signal can remain hyperintense for a long period (initially due to restricted diffusion but latter due to T2 shine-through effect) and cannot reliably estimate infarct age alone, while reduced ADC value almost always point to acute infarction. Yet, tissue with very low ADC value may recover and no single threshold can distinguish salvageable from unsalvageable tissue (Fiehler et al. 2002). Therefore we must interpret DWI with ADC maps together cautiously.

DWI-ADC carries high sensitivity (88-100%) and specificity (86-100%) in depiction of acute ischemia (Beaulieu et al. 1999; Gonzalez et al. 1999; Lövblad et al. 1997, 1998). However, with increasing cases of DWI-negative stroke reported and bearing in mind the existence of patient selection bias in the reported series, the true sensitivity probably lies between 80%-90% in general (Schellinger et al. 2010). In a prospective randomized study comparing between DWI and CT scan in evaluation of acute ischemic stroke, Fiebach et al. (2002) reported that the sensitivity of infarct detection was significantly better based on DWI (91%) than on CT (61%), achieving good interrater homogeneity and better accuracy even for readers with limited experience. This is due to relative insensitivity of CT for ischemia beyond 10ml per 100/min. as compared with DWI (Barber et al. 1999). False negative is unusual but is generally more common in posterior fossa stroke (Oppenheim et al. 2000) due to the presence of susceptibility artifacts from basal skull. Risk of hemorrhagic transformation is one feared complication and frequently asked question, especially when thrombolysis is contemplated. It had been postulated that a DWI lesion volume > $100cm^3$ was highly associated with hemorrhagic transformation, in particular when there was no associated DWI-PWI mismatch, hence contraindication to thrombolysis. However this would require further study for confirmation. Mixed results had been shown regarding the accuracy of baseline DWI in determination of final infarct volume. While it was widely thought that it would underestimate the final size of infarction (Yamada et al. 2002), Warach et al. (2000) in his double-blinded placebo-controlled study involving patients suffering from anterior-circulation stroke syndromes, found that baseline DWI lesion volume significantly correlated with baseline National Institute of Health Stroke Scale (NIHSS) scores and follow-up lesion volume at 12 weeks. Therefore, it is well established that DWI is accurate and superior to CT for diagnosis of acute ischemic stroke and can probably predict baseline clinical stroke severity as well as final lesion volume.

## 3. Perfusion-weighted imaging

PWI provides information on hypoperfused area and momentary hemodynamic state of the brain tissue before structural brain tissue damage, therefore to identify areas of reversible ischemia early before it progresses to permanent infarction. It can be performed by exogenous method (dynamic or steady state susceptibility contrast-enhanced MR imaging by injection of MR contrast) or by endogenous method (arterial spin labeling by magnetically tagging water protons in arterial blood).

### 3.1. Mechanism

Dynamic susceptibility contrast-enhanced MR perfusion imaging involves rapid imaging with gradient echo or spin echo echo-planar imaging during the first passage of a paramagnetic contrast agent through the entire brain. 10 to 20 brain slices are usually repeatedly imaged immediately before and for 70 to 80 seconds after contrast injection, with 20 to 40 images per slice obtained. It makes use of the tissue signal changes caused by susceptibility (T2*) effects to generate signal drop (shortening of T2 and T2*) and creates a hemodynamic time-signal intensity curve for each voxel, which in turns depends on cerebral blood volume and cerebral blood flow (Seevinck et al. 2010). It is through the dynamic monitoring of these signal changes in perfused tissue that hemodynamic parameters can be estimated. In contrary, steady state susceptibility contrast-enhanced MR perfusion allows estimation of blood volume, micro-vessel density and vessel size from the contrast-induced signal changes. Spin echo and gradient echo transverse relaxation rates are measured before and after contrast injection, typically with use of ultrasmall superparamagnetic iron oxide particles (longer half-life and higher suscept-ibility difference) from which parameters are derived (Wu EX et al. 2004). This method however is mainly of use in research level only.

Quantification depends on measuring the signal intensity change within tissues which itself is the susceptibility effect of the contrast agent. The ram images are processed on a pixel-by-pixel basis to generate perfusion maps of different parameters. Time-to-peak (TTP) can be readily obtained by simple data processing from the tissue response curve. Cerebral blood flow (CBF), cerebral blood volume (CBV) and mean transit time (MTT) are time dependent parameters requiring utilization of computational deconvolution methods (such as singular value decomposition, circular value decomposition, Fourier transformation) with knowledge of arterial input function for quantification. The arterial input function is defined under visual control by drawing 5-10 intravascular voxels within the proximal & distal segments of the concerned artery of the unaffected hemisphere (Zaro-Weber et al. 2010a). Point to note is that these are relative values only due to variable confounding factors which will be discussed in later section.

Arterial spin labeling is a non-invasive method exploiting the spins of endogenous water protons to measure perfusion without the need of gadolinium. An inversion radiofrequency pulse is used to tag & invert the spin polarity of the flowing arterial protons with respect to stationary arterial proton, at a level proximal to the imaging slab (Deibler et al. 2008). The tagged spins then enter the imaging plane and exchange with tissue, allowing pair-wise subtraction to yield the perfusion map after acquisition of multiple runs for signal intensity averaging. The detected MR signals would be analyzed and perfusion parameters can be obtained. However, it has a low signal-to-noise ratio requiring longer imaging time.

### 3.2. Image analysis

Perfusion imaging is the method of choice for demonstrating ischemic brain tissue in hyper-acute stage of stroke. The central portion with maximal perfusion abnormality will progress irreversibly to infarction while the outer area with only slight perfusion abnormality may recover (Hossmann 1994; Rohl et al. 2001). No single threshold has thus far been able to reliably discriminate salvageable from unsalvageable tissue definitely (Wu O et al. 2006) since absolute quantification of cerebral perfusion is not really possible and perfusion thresholds change with time (Butcher et al. 2003). Interpretation is based on the concept that as CBF falls, CBV is initially unchanged or increased (from vasodilatation due to autoregulation) in conjunction with prolonged MTT and TTP. If such autoregulatory mechanism is exhausted, CBV will then decrease and CBF continues to fall to a level of irreversible ischemia with eventual infarction. Therefore a mismatch between MTT/TTP and CBV or CBF map indicates presence of potentially salvageable tissue (Figure 2).

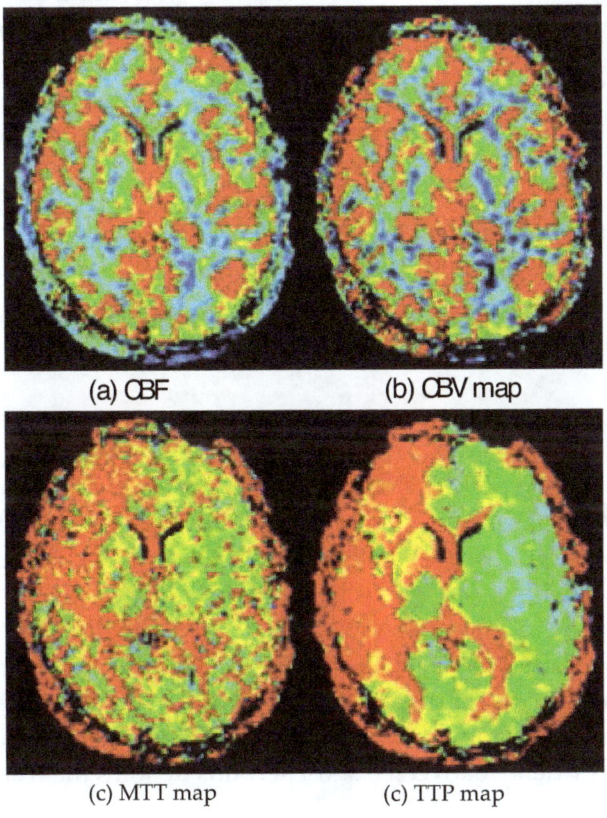


**Figure 2.** Patient with right internal carotid artery (ICA) occlusion shows mild reduced a) CBF & b) CBV; but marked elevated c) MTT & d) TTP along right ICA territory.

### 3.3. Parameters threshold

Depending on different processing methods, differing results regarding the reliability and threshold of each parameter resulted. MTT or TTP delay relative to the contralateral hemisphere has been used in preference to CBF & CBV because of the more conspicuous changes and better correlation with initial stroke severity and change in infarct size, hence final functional outcomes in individual patient (Kane et al. 2007; Muir et al. 2006). In the contrary, pre-treatment lesions on DWI and ADC maps were non-discriminative.

### *3.3.1. Time-to-peak (TTP)*

Restrepo et al. (2004) found that TTP map was most useful in demonstrating perfusion changes, showing good signal-to-noise ratio facilitating identification of lesion boundary, rendering it a parametric surrogate marker for efficacy of acute stroke treatment. A perfusion delay of 6 seconds relative to the non-affected hemisphere on TTP maps acquired before the initiation of stroke treatment helped predict the lesion size on T2-weighted images on day 8 irrespective of the treatment regimen (Kidwell et al. 2002; Nighoghossian et al. 2003; Seitz et al. 2005). Neumann-Haefelin et al. (1999) reported a TTP delay of >6 seconds best predicted final infarct volume while a TTP delay >4 seconds correlated best with acute stage neurologic deficit, signifying the true penumbra lies between 4 to 6 seconds. Kajimoto et al. (2003) depicted same result with a TTP delay of >4 seconds (sensitivity 79%, specificity 96%) in his study evaluating patients with chronic stroke. Sobesky et al. (2004 & 2005) validated these threshold values in patients with acute stroke, and demonstrated matched results when comparing with PET-derived data, also showing a TTP delay threshold of >4 seconds with sensitivity of 84% & specificity of 77%, and a penumbral volume threshold of >6 seconds. Takasawa et al. (2008) later reported a TTP delay threshold of >4.8 seconds which is also similar, as supported more recently, by Zaro-Weber et al. (2010a) showing a TTP delay threshold of >4.2 seconds best predicted penumbral flow, with a sensitivity of 91% and specificity of 82%. These consistent findings strengthen the TTP delay threshold to lie between >4-5 seconds.

### *3.3.2. Mean transit time (MTT)*

Grandin et al. (2001 & 2003) reported a MTT delay of 8.1 seconds best predicted infarct growth whereas a MTT delay of 5.3 seconds defined the hypoperfused area that did not progress to infarction, to indicate oligemic tissue. Yamada et al (2002) supported the accuracy of MTT maps showing a sensitivity of 85-94% and positive predictive value of 54-61% for final infarct volume. Such results were in coherent with other studies, with Parsons et al. (2002) depicting a >6 seconds threshold, Bristow et al. (2005) depicting a >7seconds threshold, Takasawa et al. (2008) depicting a> 6-7 seconds threshold, and more recently, Zaro-Weber (2010a) demonstrating a >5.3 seconds threshold with a sensitivity of 88% & specificity of 78%. Therefore, we can conclude that a MTT delay between 5.3 -8.1 seconds denotes the true penumbra.

### *3.3.3. Cerebral blood flow (CBF)*

CBF has found to be a good indicator of penumbral flow. Early study by Liu et al. (2000) revealed a cut off value of 48% of the unaffected hemisphere for depiction of penumbral flow. From positron emission tomography (PET) scan, it was found that neurological dysfunction occurred after CBF dropped below 20mL/100g of brain tissue per minute while infarction occured shortly after CBF dropped below 10mL/100g of brain tissue per minute (Latchaw et al. 2003). Zaro-Weber et al. confirmed in two of his recent trials (2009 & 2010a) that threshold values of <20mL/100g/min (sensitivity 76%, specificity 96%) and <21.7mL/100g/min (sensitivity 89%, specificity 87%) respectively were of best estimate of penumbral flow, adding to its consistency and strength in validation. Therefore, a CBF between 10 -20mL/100g of brain tissue per minute becomes the intermediate zone and represents penumbral flow.

#### *3.3.4. Cerebral blood volume (CBV)*

CBV shows the least correlation with penumbral flow with limited studies validating its penumbral threshold level in past literatures, especially in comparison with PET. Liu et al. (2000) depicted the threshold level to be 87% of the unaffected hemisphere while Hatazawa et al. (1999) found the threshold level to be 85% in their studies comparing with single photon emission CT (SPECT). Zaro-Weber et al. (2010a) recently, in the only study comparing with PET, found the penumbral threshold flow at <1.5mL/100g with a sensitivity of 82% and specificity of 79%.

## 4. Diffusion-weighted — Perfusion-weighted imaging

Ischemia is a complex and multifactorial process. Its clinical severity on initial presentation is a major determinant of clinical outcome, correlating strongly with the extent of the lesion. Proportion of patients with diffusion/perfusion mismatch and its size will depend on the severity of stroke and time delay to imaging. Based on the heterogeneity of the ADC and PWI values in depiction of ischemic lesion (Bandera et al. 2006), as well as occasional recovery of DWI-abnormal tissue (Davis & Donnan 2005), it becomes clear that it is unlikely any single DWI or PWI parameters or threshold values will reliably predict the degree of ischemia or infarct. Combination of diffusion- and perfusion-weighted imaging has revolutionized acute stroke imaging, allowing early & accurate delineation of the actual ischemic lesion or penumbra. Diffusion-perfusion mismatch is a quantitative and reliable measure with important pathophysiologic & therapeutic implications, becoming the surrogate of ischemic penumbra that provides valuable information for neurointervention planning, especially within the crucial therapeutic window. The Desmoteplase for Acute Ischemic Stroke and Dose Escalation of Desmoteplase for Acute Ischemic Stroke studies demonstrated that patients with PWI-DWI mismatchs who were treated with desmoteplase experienced higher rate of reperfusion and better clinical outcome (Furlan et al. 2006; Hacke et al. 2005). Earlier studies by Parsons et al. (2001 & 2002) demonstrated greater recanalization, reperfusion and penumbral salvage in a group of patients with DWI-PWI mismatch compared with the control group in acute stroke patients treated with intravenous tissue plasminogen activator. Luby & Warach (2007) also found that mismatch volumes can provide highly reliable and consistent results with improved sensitivity. Early PWI lesions are typically larger than early DWI lesions. Finding of normal diffusion-weighted images and altered perfusion parameters (mismatch) is a simple and practical mean to define the tissue at risk, which correlates with poor clinical outcome (Derex et al. 2004; Parsons et al. 2002). If untreated or reperfusion does not occur, progressive enlargement of the DWI lesion over time is expected, signifying progressive infarction of the initial PWI lesion. This can be rapid in patient with poor collateral circulation. Conversely, a pattern of DWI lesion equaling the volume of PWI lesion indicates absence of penumbra or no salvageable tissue.

## 5. Reliability and pitfalls

The reliability of mismatch volume and percentage of measurements had been discussed though not extensively investigated. Obtaining precise parameters is one major problem as only the "relative" but not absolute perfusion changes can be measured due to presence of significant confounding factors, hence nowadays we mostly rely on the relative maps of perfusion. So, exactly how precise can the penumbral threshold be quantitatively estimated by CBF, CBV, TTP and MTT? What are the overall accuracy, reproducibility and reliability?

Firstly, perfusion imaging is sensitive to vascular delays (tracer arrival delay and tissue transit time) and dispersion effects (Calamante et al. 2002), especially in the derivation of the nondeconvoluted TTP map. Any minor physiologic change such as heart rate and cardiac output can potentially change the mismatch zone. Lack of standardization between MR machines, measurement technique or associated errors from pulse sequence parameters, image processing and analytic software are other major concerns. Measurement of arterial input function is particularly problematic with lack of standardized protocol in measurement of signal intensity around the artery. Besides, the tissue signal intensity does not demonstrate a linear relationship to tissue contrast concentration (Latchaw et al. 2003). Past studies attempted to optimize perfusion maps by venous output function (Knutsson et al. 2007), separated measurement of CBV (Newman et al. 2003), advanced mathematical correction (van Osch et al. 2003), partial volume artifact correction, and bulk-blood correction (Zaharchuk et al. 2009) but were found technically difficult requiring further validation.

We have to understand that considerable individual variation regarding the penumbral flow exists and absolute quantification of the perfusion maps is difficult. So far, perfusion maps had been mainly validated with respect to infarct delineation on follow-up MR imaging but with uncertainty of perfusion changes during the time interval in between (Zaro-Weber et al. 2010a). Improved validation had been made by direct comparison with PET for in vivo perfusion measurement in normal subjects and chronic cerebrovascular dusease, but with only few in acute stroke setting (Grandin et al. 2005; Ibaraki et al. 2007; Lin et al. 2001; Ostergaard et al. 1998; Tanaka et al. 2006), raising uncertainty that such values may not precisely demonstrate the exact tissue at greatest risk of infarction, hence leading to misleading & unreliable interpretation (Keir & Wardlaw 2000). Despite so, PET-based calibration of perfusion imaging demonstrated superior result with best correction of the absolute perfusion values. Nevertheless, different post-processing algorithms differ, producing variations in lesion size and measured parameters. Indeed, ideal technique of perfusion imaging and its post-processing have not yet established. Zaro-Weber et al. (2010b) found that the variation of penumbral flow for each patient was high and hence with great error, emphasizing the need for an individual correction procedure or calibration with independent cohort. In a later study, he also found that the mean flow rate on contralateral hemisphere well explained the variability of individual perfusion thresholds such that it could be used to yield the best estimate of penumbral threshold. Based on these, a PET-validated look-up table was derived to calibrate the best individual penumbral threshold from the values of the contralateral hemispheric reference, allowing a much improved volumetric congruence. Linear regression analysis demonstrated best agreement for TTP and good agreement for CBF and MMT while that for CBV was less pronounced. Despite this seemingly advantage, further validation (especially in an independent cohort) will be needed before its implementation in clinical use. In the meantime, standardization in both the data processing methods and software is also much needed. A consensus on which parameter is best to be used for prediction should also be made.

Arterial spin labeling has additional limitation regarding its own method, in that assumptions on tagging efficiency, delay time to imaging and flow quantification are based on normal population. Whether the same setting can be translated to various disease states has yet to be tested properly (Deibler et al. 2008). Besides, it has a relatively low signal-to-noise ratio, further adding to uncertainty in its accuracy. Therefore dynamic contrast enhanced susceptibility MR imaging technique is still the preferred method for quantitative perfusion imaging.

## 6. Transient ischemic attack

Transient ischemic attack should not be taken lightly as it carries a subsequent risk of ischemic stroke of 10% within 7 days and 30% within 90 days of symptoms onset, in particularly during the first 48 hours (Johnston et al. 2000; Mlynash et al. 2009). Subsequent risk of myocardial infarction, arrhythmia and congestive heart failure are increased. Hence appropriate prevention strategy is important in reducing the risk.

Establishment of the diagnosis of transient ischemic attack has been a major challenge since most patient present normal neurologically with resolution of the clinical deficit at the time of consultation and imaging, resulting in negative finding on conventional MR brain imaging. DWI & PWI can provide objective measurement of brain ischemia, even better than angiography as lesions are mostly small and may reflect occlusion of distal intracranial vessels that is angiographically occulted. Past studies demonstrated variable lesion depiction rate from 16 to 67% on DWI in patients with TIA (Crisostomo et al. 2003; Kastrup et al. 2002; Kidwell et al. 1999; Krol et al. 2005; Redgrave et al. 2007; Restrepo et al. 2004; Rovira et al. 2002) but it had been argued that these patients should be labeled as ischemic stroke with infarction rather, regardless of the duration of symptoms with a clinical implication of potential poorer clinical outcome. This was still much debatable as report had described complete resolution of both DWI and PWI abnormalities on follow-up images (Kidwell et al. 1999; Neumann-Haefelin et al. 2000; Rovira et al. 2002). Initial studies had also found that approximately one-thirds of the DWI lesions would normalized to a certain degree if they were imaged within a 3 hour time window (Fiehler et al. 2002; Kidwell et al. 2000). PWI should substantiate the yield given its ability to reveal hypoperfusion accompanying or preceding development of DWI abnormalities. Nevertheless, the occurrence of patients with positive PWI and negative DWI was variable, reported to be 3 to 33% (Krol et al. 2005; Mlynash et al. 2009; Restrepo et al. 2004). Ma et al. (2009) explained in his study model that the classical mismatch pattern would fragment with time due to a number of more random events such as variable ages & composition of the clots, random locations of vessel occlusion with consequent differences in vulnerability of tissue, and variable degree of collateralization from neighboring vessels.

Therefore, the yield is expected to be >50% if such patients are scanned urgently after symptom onset. It is useful in helping to identify a subset of patients with diffusion-perfusion mismatch who would require close observation, and possible further investigation such as angiography assessment which would then have a high yield (>50%) for detection of potentially relevant lesion, hence to assist in subsequent management. It helps to differentiate those that who are likely to improve or reverse spontaneously from those who are likely to progress.

## 7. Clinical impact

There is no true imaging gold standard in acute stroke. DWI has a well established role in depiction of acute infarction while it is also clear that perfusion imaging can provide information that cannot be depicted in other techniques, thus seemingly superior. After all, is there a role for perfusion imaging in affecting clinical decision making and hence, influencing patient outcomes? Previously, we have already discussed that perfusion-diffusion mismatch correlates with poor clinical outcome and that treatment of large perfusion-diffusion mismatch can result in improved clinical outcome. Such can lead to the attracting prospect of expanding the narrow therapeutic time window by selecting eligible patients via DWI-PWI mismatch, as demonstrated in various series & trials (Albers et al. 2006; Davis et al. 2008; Furlan et al. 2006; Hacke et al. 2005 & 2009; Parsons et al. 2002; Schellinger et al. 2007), but with lack of proper prospective study or strong evidence-based validation so far to support its role in alteration of patient outcomes. Beside, the exact role of perfusion imaging was often vague and its benefits in decision making were usually under-evaluated or retrospectively compared with clinical parameters only (Provenzale et al. 2008). Further, it is not yet established that patients without mismatch will be unresponsive to thrombolysis, since DWI lesions can potentially resolve as discussed previously. More importantly, nowadays in most stroke centers, decisions for administration of thrombolytic agents in patients suffering from acute ischemic stroke are often made without prior perfusion imaging, nor even diffusion imaging. Decisions are routinely made on clinical ground in particular for those presenting at <4.5 hours, raising doubts over its added value. This is perhaps the main reason for lack of literature addressing the influencing role of perfusion imaging in decision making of thrombolysis. In addition, the feasibility and practicality of MR imaging in acute stroke assessment are always in doubt. Cleary, time is an important factor. The whole process of perfusion imaging together with subsequent data analysis can be time-consuming especially in less experience hands. After all, routine use of PWI to assess acute ischemic stroke is open to dispute. Until we have a compelling randomized prospective blinded study assessing the efficacy of perfusion imaging in decision making in assessment of acute ischemic stroke, perhaps the most convincing role at present is prediction of final infarct volume which demonstrates strong correlation, and hence helping to predict the clinical outcome in individual patient. On the other hand, it can also be of great use in monitoring of evolution of ischemia and subsequent therapeutic response. Despite these seemingly limitations and arguments on methodical issues, many believe that the accumulated evidence of the importance of DWI-PWI mismatch is already good enough to establish a role in daily practice if allow.

## 8. Conclusion

With advances in imaging technology, there is substantial evidence and data to support the feasibility & superiority of MR imaging in acute ischemic stroke. PWI is complementary to DWI in acute stroke assessment. DWI-PWI mismatch provides a good, rapid & reliable estimation of the penumbra, helping to select suitable candidate for acute thrombolytic therapy, especially for patients presenting with unknown onset time or beyond the 4.5 hours therapeutic window. PWI lesion can resolve rapidly after successful thrombolysis or reperfusion, leading to improved clinical outcome. Only then will we know for every individual patient, at certain time after stroke, with particular clinical features and parameters on DWI/ PWI, which will be the best clinical management.

## Author details

Vincent Lai

The University of Hong Kong, Hong Kong

## References

[1] Albers GW, Thijs VN, Wechsler L, Kemp S, Schlaug G, Skalabrin E, Bammer R, Kakuda W, Lansberg MG, Shuaib A, Coplin W, Hamilton S, Moseley M & Marks MP; DEFUSE Investigators. (2006). Magnetic resonance imaging profiles predict clinical response to early reperfusion: the diffusion and perfusion imaging evaluation for understanding stroke evolution (DEFUSE) study. *Ann Neurol*, Vol.60, No.5, pp. 508-517

[2] Bandera E, Botteri M, Minelli C, Sutton A, Abrams KR & Latronico N. (2006). Cerebral blood flow threshold of ischemic penumbra and infarct core in acute ischemic stroke. A systemic review. *Stroke*, Vol.37, No.5, pp. 1334-1339

[3] Barber PA, Darby DG, Desmond PM, Gerraty RP, Yang Q, Li T, Jolley D, Donnan GA, Tress BM & Davis SM. (1999). Identification of major ischemic change. Diffusion-weighted imaging versus computed tomography. *Stroke*, Vol.30, No.10, pp. 2059-2065

[4] Beaulieu C, de Crespigny A, Tong DC, Moseley ME, Albers GW & Marks MP. (1999). Longitudinal magnetic resonance imaging study of perfusion and diffusion in stroke: evolution of lesion volume and correlation with clinical outcome. *Ann Neurol*, Vol.46, No.4, pp. 568-578

[5] Bristow MS, Simon JE, Brown RA, Eliasziw M, Hill MD, Coutts SB, Frayne R, Demchuk AM & Mitchell JR. (2005). MR perfusion and diffusion in acute ischemic stroke:

human gray and white matter have different thresholds for infarction. *J Cereb Blood Flow Metab,* Vol.25, No.10, pp. 1280-1287

[6] Butcher K, Parsons M, Baird T, Barber A, Donnan G, Desmond P, Tress B & Davis S. (2003). Perfusion thresholds in acute stroke thrombolysis. *Stroke,* Vol.34, No.9, pp. 2159-2164

[7] Calamante F, Gadian DG & Connelly A. (2002). Quantification of perfusion using bolus tracking magnetic resonance imaging in stroke: assumptions, limitations, and potential implications for clinical use. *Stroke,* Vol.33, No.4, pp. 1146-1151

[8] Crisostomo RA, Garcia MM & Tong DC. (2003). Detection of diffusion-weighted MRI abnormalities in patients with transient ischemic attack: correlation with clinical characteristics. *Stroke,* Vol.34, No.4, pp. 932-937

[9] Davis SM & Donnan GA. (2005). Using mismatch on MRI to select thrombolytic responders: an attractive hypothesis awaiting confirmation. *Stroke,* Vol.36, No.5, pp. 1106-1107

[10] Davis SM, Donnan GA, Parsons MW, Levi C, Butcher KS, Peeters A, Barber PA, Bladin C, De Silva DA, Byrnes G, Chalk JB, Fink JN, Kimber TE, Schultz D, Hand PJ, Hankey G, Muir K, Gerraty R, Tress BM & Desmond PM; EPITHET investigators. (2008). Effects of alteplase beyond 3 h after stroke in the Echoplanar Imaging Thrombolytic Evaluation Trial (EPITHET): a placebo-controlled randomized trial. *Lancet Neurol,* Vol.7, No.4, pp. 299-309

[11] Deibler AR, Pollock JM, Kraft RA, Tan H, Burdette JH & Maldjian JA. (2008). Arterial spina-labeling in routine clinical practice, part 1: Technique and artifacts. *AJNR Am J Neuroradiol,* Vol.29, No.7, pp. 1228-1234

[12] Derex L, Nighoghossian N, Hermier M, Adeleine P, Berthezene Y, Philippeau F, Honnorat J, Froment JC & Trouillas P. (2004). Influence of pretreatment MRI parameters on clinical outcome, recanalization and infarct size in 49 stroke patients treated by intravenous tissue plasminogen activator. *J Neurol Sci,* Vol.225, No.1-2, pp. 3-9

[13] Fiebach JB, Schellinger PD, Jansen O, Meyer M, Wilde P, Bender J, Schramm P, Jüttler E, Oehler J, Hartmann M, Hähnel S, Knauth M, Hacke W & Sartor K. (2002). CT and diffusion-weighted MR imaging results in higher accuracy and lower interrater variability in the diagnosis of hyperacute ischemic stroke. *Stroke,* Vol.33, No.9, pp. 2206-2210

[14] Fiebach JB, Schellinger PD, Gass A, Kucinski T, Siebler M, Villringer A, Olkers P, Hirsch JG, Heilnd S, Wilde P, Jansen O, Röther J, Hacke W & Sartor K. (2004). Stroke magnetic resonance imaging is accurate in hyperacute intracerebral hemorrhage: a multicenter study on the validity of stroke imaging. *Stroke,* Vol.35, No.2, pp. 502-506

[15] Fiehler J, Foth M, Kucinski T, Knab R, von Bezold M, Weiller C, Zeumer H & Röther J. (2002). Severe ADC decreases do not predict irreversible tissue damage in humans. *Stroke,* Vol.33, No.1, pp. 79-86

[16] Furlan AJ, Eyding D, Albers GW, Al-Rawi Y, Lees KR, Rowley HA, Sachara C, Soehngen M, Warach S & Hacke W; DEDAS Investigators. (2006). Dose Escalation of Desmoteplase for Acute Ischemic Stroke (DEDAS): evidence of safety and efficacy 3 to 9 hours after stroke onset. *Stroke,* Vol.37, No.5, pp. 1227-1231

[17] Gonzalez RG, Schaefer PW, Buonanno FS, Schwamm LH, Budzik RF, Rordorf G, Wang B, Sorensen AG & Koroshetz WJ. (1999). Diffusion-weighted MR imaging: diagnostic accuracy in patients imaged within 6 hours of stroke symptom onset. *Radiology,* Vol.210, No.1, pp. 155-162

[18] Grandin CB, Duprez TP, Smith AM, Mataigne F, Peeters A, Oppenheim C & Cosnard G. (2001). Usefulness of magnetic resonance-derived quantitative measurements of cerebral blood flow and volume prediction of infarct growth in hyperacute stroke. *Stroke,* Vol.32, No.5, pp. 1147-1153

[19] Grandin CB. (2003). Assessment of brain perfusion with MRI: methodology and application to acute stroke. *Neuroradiology,* Vol.45, No.11, pp. 755-766

[20] Grandin CB, Bol A, Smith AM, Michel C & Cosnard G. (2005). Absolute CBF and CBV measurements by MRI bolus tracking before and after acetazolamide challenge: repeatability and comparison with PET in humans. *Neuroimage,* Vol.26, No.2, pp. 525-535

[21] Hacke W, Albers G, Al-Rawi Y, Boqousslavsky J, Davalos A, Eliasziw M, Fischer M, Furlan A, Kaste M, Lees KR, Soehngen M & Warach S; DIAS Study Group. (2005). The Desmoteplase in Acute Ischemic Stroke Trial (DIAS): a phase II MRI-based 9-hour window acute stroke thrombolysis trial with intravenous desmoteplase. *Stroke,* Vol.36, No.1, pp. 66-73

[22] Hacke W, Kaste M, Bluhmki E, Brozman M, Dávalos A, Guidetti D, Larrue V, Lees KR, Medeghri Z, Machnig T, Schneider D, von Kummer R, Wahlgren N, Toni D & ECASS investigators. (2008). Thrombolysis with alteplase 3 to 4.5 hours after acute ischemic stroke. *N Engl J Med,* Vol.359, No.13, pp. 1317-1329

[23] Hacke W, Furlan AJ, Al-Rawi Y, Davalos A, Fiebach JB, Gruber F, Kaste M, Lipka LJ, Pedraza S, Ringleb PA, Rowley HA, Schneider D, Schwamm LH, Leal JS, Söhngen M, Teal PA, Wilhelm-Ogunbiyi K, Wintermark M & Warach S. (2009). Intravenous desmoteplase in patients with acute ischemic stroke selected by MRI perfusion-diffusion weighted imaging or perfusion CT (DIAS-2): a prospective, randomized, double-blind, placebo-controlled study. *Lancet Neurol,* Vol.8, No.2, pp. 141-150

[24] Hatazawa J, Shimosegawa E, Toyoshima H, Ardekani BA, Suzuki A, Okudera T & Miura Y. (1999). Cerbral blood volume in acute brain infarction : a combined study

with dynamic susceptibility contrast MRI and 99MTC-HMPAO-SPECT. *Stroke,* Vol. 30, No.4, pp. 800-806

[25] Hossmann KA. (1994) Viability thresholds and the penumbra of focal ischemia. *Ann Neurol,* Vol.36, No.4, pp. 557-565

[26] Ibaraki M, Ito H, Shimoseqawa E, Toyoshima H, Ishigame K, Takahashi K, Kanno I & Miura S. (2007). Cerebral vascular mean transit time in healthy humans: a comparative study with PET and dynamic susceptibility contrast-enhanced MRI. *J Cereb Blood Flow Metab,* Vol.27, No.2, pp. 404-413

[27] Johnston SC, Gress DR, Browner WS & Sidney S. (2000). Short-term prognosis after emergency-department diagnosis of TIA. *JAMA,* Vol.284, No.22, pp. 2901-2906

[28] Kajimoto K, Moriwaki H, Yamada N, Hayashida K, Kobayashi J, Miyashita K & Naitomi H. (2003). Cerebral hemodynamic evaluation using perfusion-weighted magnetic resonance imaging : comparison with positron emision tomography values in chronic occlusive carotid disease. *Stroke,* Vol.34, No.7, pp. 1662-1666

[29] Kane I, Carpenter T, Chappell F, Rivers C, Armitage P, Sandercock P & Wardlaw J. (2007). Comparison of 10 different magnetic resonance imaging processing methods in acute ischemic stroke: Effect on lesion size, proportion of patients with diffusion/ perfusion match, clinical scores, and radiologic outcomes. *Stroke,* Vol.38, No.12, pp. 3158-3164

[30] Kastrup A, Schulz JB, Mader I, Dichqans J & Küker W. (2002). Diffusion-weighted MRI in patients with symptomatic internal carotid artery disease. *J Neurol,* Vol.249, No.9, pp. 1168-1174

[31] Keir SL & Wardlaw JM. (2000). Systemic review of diffusion and perfusion imaging in acute ischemic stroke. *Stroke,* Vol.31, No.11, pp. 2723-2731

[32] Kidwell CS, Alger JR, Di Salle F, Starkman S, Villablanca P, Bentson J & Saver JL. (1999). Diffusion MRI in patients with transient ischemic attacks. *Stroke,* Vol.30, No.6, pp. 1174-1180

[33] Kidwell CS, Saver JL, Mattiello J, Starkman S, Vinuela F, Duckwiler G, Gobin YP, Jahan R, Vespa P, Kalafut M & Alger JR. (2000). Thrombolytic reversal of acute human cerebrak ischemic injury shown by diffusion/perfusion magnetic resonance imaging. *Ann Neurol,* Vol.47, No.4, pp. 462-469

[34] Kidwell CS, Saver JL, Starkman S, Duckwiler G, Jahan R, Vespa P, Villablanca JP, Liebeskind DS, Gobin YP, Vinuela F & Alger JR. (2002). Late secondary ischemic injury in patients receiving intraarterial thrombolysis. *Ann Neurol,* Vol.52, No.6, pp. 698-703

[35] Kidwell CS, Chalela JA, Saver JL, Starkman S, Hill MD, Demchuk AM, Butman JA, Patronas N, Alger JR, Latour LL, Luby ML, Baird AE, Leary MC, Tremwel M, Ovbiagele B, Fredieu A, Suzuki S, Villablanca JP, Davis S, Dunn B, Todd JW, Ezzeddine

MA, Haymore J, Lynch JK, Davis L & Warach S. (2004). Comparison of MRI and CT for detection of acute intracerebral hemorrhage. *JAMA*, Vol.292, No.15, pp. 1823-1830

[36] Knutsson L, Borjesson S, Larsson EM, Risberg J, Gustafson L, Passant U, Stahlberg F & Wirestam R. (2007). Absolute quantification of cerebral blood flow in normal volunteers : correlation betwen Xe-133 SPECT and dynamic susceptibility contrast MRI. *J Magn Reson Imaging*, Vol.26, No.4, pp. 913-920

[37] Krol AL, Coutts SB, Simon JE, Hill MD, Sohn CH & Demchuk AM; VISION Study Group. (2005). Perfusion MRI abnormalities in speech or motor transient ischemic attack patients. *Stroke*, Vol.36, No.11, pp. 2487-2489

[38] Latchaw RE, Yonas H, Hunter GJ, Yuh WT, Ueda T, Sorensen AG, Sunshine JL, Biller J, Wechsler L, Higashida R & Hademenos G. (2003). Guidelines and recommendations for perfusion imaging in cerebral ischemia: a scientific statement for healthcare professionals by the writing group on perfusion imaging, from the Council on Cardiovascular Radiology of the American Heart Association. *Stroke*, Vol.34, No.4, pp. 1084–1104

[39] Lin W, Celik A, Derdeyn C, An H, Lee Y, Videen T, Ostergaard L & Powers WJ. (2001). Quantitative measurements of cerebral blood flow in patients with unilateral carotid artery occlusion: a PET and MR study. *J Magn Reson Imaging*, Vol.14, No.6, pp. 659-667

[40] Liu Y, Karonen JO, Vanninen RL, Ostergaard L, Roivainen R, Nuutinen J, Perkio J, Kononen M, Hamalainen A, Vanninen EJ, Soimakallio S, Kuikka JT & Aronen HJ. (2000). Cerebral hemodynamics in human acute ischemic stroke : a study with diffusion- and perfusion-weighted magnetic resonance imaging an SPECT. *J Cereb Blood Flow Metab*, Vol.20, No.6, pp. 910-920

[41] Lövblad KO, Baird AE, Schlaug G, Benfield A, Siewert B, Voetsch B, Conner A, Burzynski C, Edelman RR & Warach S. (1997). Ischemic lesion volumes in acute stroke by diffusion-weighted magnetic resonance imaging correlate with clinical outcome. *Ann Neurol*, Vol.42, No.2, pp. 164-170

[42] Lövblad KO, Laubach HJ, Baird AE, Curtin F, Schlaug G, Edelman RR & Warach S. (1998). Clinical experience with diffusion-weighted MR in patients with acute stroke. *AJNR Am J Neuroradiol*, Vol.19, No.6, pp. 1061-1066

[43] Luby M & Warach S. (2007). Reliability of MR perfusion-weighted and diffusion-weighted imaging mismatch measurement methods. *AJNR Am J Neuroradiol*, Vol.28, No.9, pp. 1674-1678

[44] Ma H, Zavala JA, Teoh H, Churilov L, Gunawan M, Ly J, Wright P, Phan T, Arakawa S, Davis SM & Donnan GA. (2009). Fragmentation of the classical magnetic resonance mismatch "penumbral" pattern with time. *Stroke*, Vol.40, No.12, pp. 3752-3757

[45] Mlynash M, Olivot JM, Tong DC, Lansberg MG, Eyngorn I, Kemp S, Moseley ME & Albers GW. (2009). Yield of combined perfusion and diffusion MR imaging in hemispheric TIA. *Neurology,* Vol.72, No.13, pp. 1127-1133

[46] Muir KW, Buchan A, von Kummer R, Rother J & Baron JC. (2006). Imaging of acute stroke. *Lancet Neurol,* Vol.5, No.9, pp. 755-768

[47] Newman GC, Delucia-Deranja E, Tudorica A, Hospod FE & Patlak CS. (2003). Cerebral blood volume measurements by T*2-weighted MRI and contrast infusion. *Magn Reson Med,* Vol.50, No.4, pp. 844-855

[48] Neumann-Haefelin T, Wittsack HJ, Wenserski F, Siebler M, Seitz RJ, Modder U & Freund HJ. (1999). Diffusion- and perfusion-weighted MRI: the DWI/PWI mismatch region in acute stroke. *Stroke,* Vol.30, No.8, pp. 1591-1597

[49] Neumann-Haefelin T, Wittsack HJ, Wenserski F, Li TQ, Moseley ME, Siebler M & Freund HJ. (2000). Diffusion- and perfusion-weighted MRI in a patient with a prolonged reversible ischemic neurological deficit. *Neuroradiology,* Vol.42, No.6, pp. 444-447

[50] Nighoghossian N, Hermier M, Adeleine P, Derex L, Dugor JF, Philippeau F, Ylmaz H, Honnorat J, Dardel P, Berthezène Y, Froment JC & Trouillas P. (2003). Baseline magnetic resonance imaging parameters and stroke outcome in patients treated by intravenous tissue plasminogen activator. *Stroke,* Vol.34, No.2, pp. 458-463

[51] Oppenheim C, Logak M, Dormont D, Lehericy S, Manai R, Samson Y, Marsault C & Rancurel G. (2000). Diagnosis of acute ischemic stroke with fluid-attenuated inversion recovery and diffusion-weighted sequences. *Neuroradiology,* Vol.42, No.8, pp. 602-607

[52] Ostergaard L, Johannsen P, Host-Poulsen P, Vestergaard-Poulsen P, Asboe H, Gee AD, Hansen SB, Cold GE, Gjedde A & Gyldensted C. (1998). Cerebral blood flow measurements by magnetic resonance imaging bolus tracking: comparison with $[^{15}O]H_2O$ positron emission tomography in humans. *J Cereb Blood Flow Metab,* Vol.18, No.9, pp. 935-940

[53] Parsons MW, Yang Q, Barber PA, Darby DG, Desmond PM, Gerraty RP, Tress BM & Davis SM. (2001). Perfusion magnetic resonance imaging maps in hyperacute stroke: relative cerebral blood flow most accurately identifies tissue destined to infarct. *Stroke,* Vol.32, No.7, pp. 1581-1587

[54] Parsons MW, Barber PA, Chalk J, Darby DG, Rose S, Desmond PM, Gerraty RP, Tress BM, Wright PM, Donnan GA & Davis SM. (2002). Diffusion- and perfusion-weighted MRI response to thrombolysis in stroke. *Ann Neurol,* Vol.51, No.1, pp. 28-37

[55] Poustchi-Amin M, Mirowitz SA, Brown JJ, McKinstry RC & Li T. (2001) Principles and applications of echo-planar imaging: a review for the general radiologist. *Radiographics,* Vol.21, No.3, pp. 767-779

[56] Provenzale JM, Shah K, Patel U & McCrory DC. (2008). Systemic review of CT and MR perfusion imaging for assessment of acute cerebrovascular disease. *AJNR Am J Neuroradiol,* Vol.29, No.8, pp. 1476-1482

[57] Redgrave JN, Coutts SB, Schulz UG, Briley D & Rothwell PM. (2007). Systemic review of associations between the presence of acute ischemic lesions on diffusion-weighted imaging and clinical predictors of early stroke risk after transient ischemic attack. *Stroke,* Vol.38, No.5, pp. 1482-1488

[58] Restrepo L, Jacobs MA, Barker PB & Wityk RJ. (2004). Assessment of transient ischemic attack with diffusion- and perfusion-weighted imaging. *AJNR Am J Neuroradiol,* Vol.25, No.10, pp. 1645-1652

[59] Røhl L, Ostergaard L, Simonsen CZ, Vestergaard-Poulsen P, Andersen G, Sakoh M, Le Bihan D & Gyldensted C. (2001) Viability thresholds of ischemic penumbra of hyperacute stroke defined by perfusion-weighted MEI and apparent diffusion coefficient. *Stroke,* Vol.32, No.5, pp. 1140-1146

[60] Rovira A, Rovira-Gols A, Pedraza S, Grivé E, Molina C & Alvarez-Sabin J. (2002). Diffusion-weighted MR imaging in the acute phase of transient ischemic attacks. *AJNR Am J Neuroradiol,* Vol.23, No.1, pp. 77-83

[61] Schellinger PD, Thomalla G, Fiehler JF, Köhrmann M, Molina CA, Neumann-Haefelin T, Ribo M, Singer OC, Zaro-Weber O & Sobesky J. (2007). MRI-based and CT-based thrombolytic therapy in acute stroke within and beyond established time windows: an analysis of 1210 patients. *Stroke,* Vol.38, No.10, pp. 2640-2645

[62] Schellinger PD, Bryan RN, Caplan LR, Detre JA, Edelman RR, Jaigobin C, Kidwell CS, Mohr JP, Sloan M, Sorensen AG & Warach S. (2010). Evidence-based guideline: The role of diffusion and perfusion MRI for the diagnosis of acute ischemic stroke: report of the Therapeutics and Technology Assessment Subcommittee of the American Academy of Neurology. *Neurology,* Vol.75, No.2, pp. 177-185

[63] Seevinck PR, Deddens LH & Dijkhuizen RM. (2010). Magnetic resonance imaging of brain angiogenesis after stroke. *Angiogenesis,* Vol.13, No.2, pp. 101-111

[64] Seitz RJ, Meisel S, Weller P, Junghans U, Wittsack HJ & Siebler M. (2005). Initial ischemic event: perfusion-weighted MR imaging and apparent diffusion coefficient for stroke evaluation. *Radiology,* Vol.237, No.3, pp. 1020-1028

[65] Sobesky J, Zaro Weber O, Lehnhardt FG, Hesselmann V, Thiel A, Dohmen C, Jacobs A, Neveling M & Heiss WD. (2004). Which time-to-peak threshold best identifies penumbral flow? A comparison of perfusion-weighted magnetic resonance imaging and positron emission tomography in acute ischemic stroke. *Stroke,* Vol.35, No.12, pp. 2843-2847

[66] Sobesky J, Zaro Weber O, Lehnhardt FG, Hesselmann V, Neveling M, Jacobs A & Heiss WD. (2005). Does the mismatch match the penumbra? Magnetic resonance

imaging and positron emission tomography in early ischemic stroke. *Stroke,* Vol.36, No.5, pp. 980-985

[67] Srinivasan A, Goyal M, Azri FA & Lum C. (2006). State-of-the-art imaging of acute stroke. *Radiographics,* Vol.26, Suppl 1, pp. s75-s95

[68] Takasawa M, Jones PS, Guadagno JV, Christensen S, Fryer TD, Harding S, Gillard JH, Williams GB, Aigbirhio FI, Warburton WA, Ostergaard L & Baron JC. (2008). How reliable is perfusion MR in acute stroke?: validation and determination of the penumbra threshold against quantitative PET. *Stroke,* Vol.39, No.3, pp. 870-877

[69] Tanaka Y, Nariai T, Nagaoka T, Akimoto H, Ishiwata K, Ishii K, Matsushima Y & Ohno K. (2006). Quantitative evaluation of cerebral hemodynamics in patients with moyamoya disease by dynamic susceptibility contrast magnetic resonance imaging-comparison with positron emission tomography. *J Cereb Blood Flow Metab,* Vol.26, No.2, pp. 291-300

[70] Tissue plasminogen activator for acute ischemic stroke. The National Institute of Neurological Disorders and Stroke rt-PA Stroke Study Group. (1995). *N Engl J Med,* Vol.333, No. 24, pp. 1581-1587

[71] van Osch MJ, Vonken EJ, Viergever MA, van der Grond J & Bakker CJ. (2003). Measuring the arterial input function with gradient echo sequences. *Magn Reson Med,* Vol. 49, No.6, pp. 1067-1076

[72] von Kummer R, Bourquain H, Bastianello S, Bozzao L, Manelfe C, Meier D & Hacke W. (2001). Early prediction of irreversible brain damage after ischemic stroke at CT. *Radiology,* Vol.219, No.1, pp. 95-100.

[73] Wahlgren N, Ahmed N, Dávalos A, Hacke W, Millán M, Muir K, Roine RO, Toni D, Lees KR & SITS investigators. (2008). Thrombolysis with alteplase 3-4.5 h after acute ischemic stroke (SITS-ISTR) : an observational study. *Lancet,* Vol.372, No.9646, pp. 1303-1309

[74] Warach S, Pettigrew LC, Dashe JF, Pullicino P, Lefkowitz DM, Sabounjian L, Harnett K, Schwiderski U & Gammans R. (2000). Effect of citicoline on ischemic lesions as measured by diffusion-weighted magnetic resonance imaging. Citicoline 010 Investigators. *Ann Neurol,* Vol.48, No.5, pp. 713-722

[75] Wu EX, Tang H & Jensen JH. (2004). Applications of ultrasmall superparamagnetic iron oxide contrast agents in the MR study of animal models. *NMR Bomed,* Vol.17, No.7, pp. 478-483

[76] Wu O, Christensen S, Hjort N, Dijkhuizen RM, Kucinski T, Fiehler J, Thomalla G, Röther J & Ostergaard L. (2006). Characterizing physiological heterogeneity of infarction risk in acute human ischemic stroke using MRI. *Brain,* Vol.129, No.9, pp. 2384-2393

[77] Yamada K, Wu O, Gonzalez RG, Bakker D, Ostergaard L, Copen WA, Weisskoff RM, Rosen BR, Yagi K, Nishimura T & Sorensen AG. (2002). Magnetic resonance perfu-

sion-weighted imaging of acute cerebral infarction: effect of the calculation methods and underlying vasculopathy. *Stroke*, Vol.33, No.1, pp. 87-94

[78] Zaharchuk G, Bammer R, Straka M, Newbould RD, Rosenberg J, Olivot JM, Mlynash M, Lansberg MG, Schwartz NE, Marks MM, Albers GW & Moseley ME. (2009). Improving dynamic susceptibility contrast MRI measurement of quantitative cerebral blood flow using corrections for partial volume and nonlinear contrast relaxivity : a Xenon computed tomographic comparative study. *J Magn Reson Imaging,* Vol.30, No. 4, pp. 743-752

[79] Zaro-Weber O, Moeller-Hartmann W, Heiss WD & Sobesky J. (2009). The performance of MRI-based cerebral blood flow measurements in acute and subacute stroke compared with 15O-water positron emission tomography : identification of penumbral flow. *Stroke,* Vol.40, No.7, pp. 2413-2421

[80] Zaro-Weber O, Moeller-Hartmann W, Heiss WD & Sobesky J. (2010a). MRI perfusion maps in acute stroke validated with 15o-water positron emission tomography. *Stroke,* Vol.41, No.3, pp. 443-449

[81] Zaro-Weber O, Moeller-Hartmann W, Heiss WD & Sobesky J. (2010b). A simple positron emission tomography-based calibration for perfusion-weighted magnetic resonance maps to optimize penumbral flow detection in acute stroke. *Stroke,* Vol.41, No. 9, pp. 1939-1945

# 3

# Social Neuroscience Tasks: Employing fMRI to Understand the Social Mind

D.Y. Phua and G.I. Christopoulos

## 1. Introduction

The purpose of the present chapter is to introduce and describe some fMRI-compatible tasks that social scientists can employ to study various social phenomena. fMRI (functional Magnetic Resonance Imaging) is one of the principal methods for studying *in vivo* human brain-related responses associated with cognitive functions. Given the increasing availability of brain imaging scanners, the less complicated analysis methods, and the lower costs of using fMRI, more social scientists (from e.g., social psychology, political science, business, economics, philosophy and culture science) have become interested in integrating neuroscience into their own research agenda. It is expected that this trend will continue as multidisciplinary research becomes more popular.

Crossing or mixing disciplines has always been both challenging and very rewarding. In the case of neuroscience, the unwillingness to cross disciplines is often implicated with a lack of appreciation for the potential of fMRI and neuroscience methodologies. In addition, social scientists are often overwhelmed by the complexity of neuroscience and are unsure whether it is worthwhile to invest time and energy in enriching their methodological tools with fMRI. Therefore, there is an exigency for an introductory chapter aiding non-neuroscientists (or, generally, researchers with less exposure to experimental methods of neuroscience) to understand how cognitive neuroscientists have employed fMRI in elucidating social phenomena.

As such, the general aims of this chapter are to:

i. Offer inspiration on novel approaches for studying social phenomena using neuro-science methods

ii. Help readers form and answer proper questions using an appropriate methodology

iii. Understand how neuroscience epistemologically approaches various phenomena

To achieve these aims, we here present an overview of fMRI tasks that have been successfully used to study social phenomena. Note here that we focus on the *tasks* employed and not in the social neuroscience theories or neurobiology implicated in the phenomena. We believe that this is a pedagogically more efficient way for the non-expert scientist or student to be introduced to the methodology of social neuroscience, since it approaches social neuroscience from an applied, hands-on perspective. To that end, in the following paragraphs we present tasks that are related to:

- Facial expression recognition
- Perception of biological motion
- Mimicry
- Mirror neurons system
- Mentalizing and understanding mental states of others
- Empathy
- Distinguishing self from others
- Morality
- Kinship, romantic and maternal love
- Attitudes and evaluative processes
- Race and stereotypes
- Culture
- Social interactions

We note that what follows is a brief introduction of different tasks. Most, if not all, of the tasks can be used for pure behavioral research. What makes these tasks special is that they abide to some general rules that allow for the specificities imposed by the fMRI methodology:

- The need for many repetitions (trials). Because of the large measurement error, it is advisable that each condition has a good number of trials. In other words, the design should be able to measure the same variable many times. Of course, here one needs to balance design efficiency with psychological factors such as boredom, learning and memory effects.
- The need for relatively quick presentation of stimuli. For instance, it is rather rare to have a long scenario as a stimulus, especially if one is an inexperienced researcher. Because of the temporal properties of the fMRI signal, it is also advisable, with maybe some exceptions, to present stimuli quickly, whereas the participant should be able to provide behavioral responses (if any) easily without a lot of motor or attention demands.

- Isomorphic stimuli. This is quite critical, as the brain is sensitive to a wide space of stimulus differences that could override our main targeted dimension. See below at the paragraphs about face recognition for a demonstration.
- Other needs such as good randomization and general or trial-specific time constraints.

Of course, the present text cannot cover all aspects of fMRI research and methods. We therefore strongly suggest that readers do get familiar with the nuances of an fMRI experiment (e.g., fMRI experiments typically require a large number of repetitions of the same condition). A good starting point would be Huettel, Song and McCarthy (2009). In addition, readers should be familiar with the basic tenets of experimental methodology (such as employing proper controls, separating dependent and independent variables, and avoiding confounding factors) which are typically more crucial in fMRI experiments.

Yet, we would like to emphasize three important points that are often misinterpreted:

1. **Ask 'How' and not (only) 'Where'.** It is important to form research questions that are related to specific cognitive mechanisms and, ideally, aim to test alternative/competing theoretical models of behavior. "Fishing expeditions" without concrete anatomical, function (and/or computational) hypotheses and models should be avoided. It is critical to understand how modern neuroscience aids in understanding *mechanisms* (i.e., *how* the brain processes information to produce behavioral response). Therefore, cognitive and / or computational models are essential before proceeding to fMRI experiments.

2. **Avoid reverse inference.** This is a very common error, which is elegantly described in Poldrack (2006). Imagine we find a brain area X (e.g., amygdala) that demonstrates a higher response to a stimulus A (e.g., a face with fear expression) than B (a control face with a neutral expression). The, to a great extent correct, inference is that amygdala responds to face stimuli depicting expressions of fear (A → X). Assume that in another study, a researcher employs stimulus Y (e.g., the face of an outgroup member) and finds that area X (i.e., amygdala) is activated. Often the conclusion drawn (and many times published) is that Y promotes the mental state associated with A (i.e., faces of outgroup members promote fear responses). Of course, this is a *reverse inference,* and is problematic. What we established was that A →X and that Y → X but not X → A or X→ Y. Amygdala responds to many mental states in addition to fear. Therefore, researchers should be very careful when attempting to infer the *mental state* based on *brain responses*. Proper experimental design with appropriate controls can help in alleviating these issues. Moreover, instead of approaching the variables categorically, many times it might be more appropriate to seek brain-related responses as a function of different levels of input stimulus intensity. For instance, instead of examining how the brain responds to positive and negative monetary rewards (e.g. receiving $10 vs. losing $10), one could allow for larger variation (e.g. outcome -$40, -$20, -$10, $10, $20, $30) of parameters.

3. **Deal with complexity**. Another common mistake made by researchers new to neuroscience is that they often try to solve very complex problems that introduce multiple variables and/or do not have concrete, measurable responses. Neuroscience methodology is most appropriate for straightforward questions that have few variables and very

specific responses. Remember that the neurofunctional data collected will be very complex. On average, a brain image is captured every two seconds by the scanner, equating to over 100,000 data points in 20 to 30 minutes. These time-series data points are then combined across participants, thus increasing the complexity of dataset. Fortunately, there are specialized software packages that can do such processing and analysis. However, this does not negate the need for careful experimental designs that take into consideration the complexity of the data. Lack of attention to the design may make subsequent interpretation difficult, if not meaningless.

Other neurobiological methods such as psychophysiology, EEG, fNIRS, genetics, psychopharmacology will not be covered. Readers are encouraged to further explore possibilities from other sources. Yet, many tasks and principles described here might be much related to these methods.

## 2. Facial recognition

Facial recognition goes beyond face processing; the latter refers to the mere ability to differentiate individuals. Facial recognition includes human's ability to decipher social information embedded in facial expressions. Some studies have explored the neurobiological basis for often-unconscious responses to specific facial expressions, such as emotional expressions (e.g., Harrison, Singer, Rotshtein, Dolan, & Critchley, 2006), untrustworthiness (e.g., Engell, Haxby & Todorov, 2007) or averted eye gaze (e.g., Hoffman & Haxby, 2000). In such studies, the principal methodology has been to contrast brain responses between conditions. For example, judgment studies of another's trustworthiness obtain behavioral ratings of the trustworthiness associated with different faces. These ratings were then used to regress against neural responses in order to compare brain signals when viewing faces rated as trustworthy versus viewing those rated as untrustworthy (e.g., Engell, et al., 2007; Winston, Strange, O'Doherty, & Dolan, 2002). Using a similar methodology, Hoffman and Haxby (2000) investigated the differential blood-oxygen-level-dependent (BOLD) responses [the principal signal derived from fMRI] when participants viewed photographs of faces looking directly versus away from the camera (i.e., direct versus averted eye gaze). This was to examine whether regions associated with perception of the face identity are also involved in perception of the changeable aspects of the face. Averted eye gaze redirect one's spatial attention in social communication, and thus different neural mechanisms should be involved. To better understand the different processes involved in facial processing, Narumoto and colleagues (2001) examined the differential brain responses towards faces as a function of attention focus (i.e., focus on contours, identity or emotional expressions).

Researchers have also investigated how people recognize speech from visual perception (i.e., lip-reading). Typical methodologies used include the comparison of brain responses when participants viewed videos of facial gurning (meaningless opening and closing of mouth) versus silent mouthing of random numbers (e.g., Calvert, et al., 1997; Campbell, et al., 2001). Buccino and colleagues (2004) also examined if the brain response observed when viewing human verbal communicative actions are generalizable to viewing of other species' communicative actions. Their stimuli included silent video sequences of a man speaking, a monkey lip-smacking and a dog barking.

## 3. Perceptions of biological motion

Human beings are naturally sensitive to motion. Studies on perception of motion often concentrated on biological motion. These include facial movements such as mouth or eye movements (e.g., Puce, Allison, Bentin, Gore, & McCarthy, 1998) or bodily movements (e.g., Pelphrey, Morris, Michelich, Allison, & McCarthy, 2005). Some research has also expanded into the investigation of the neuronal mechanisms involved in perception of non-human facial movements (Buccino, et al., 2004) and complex actions that are not in one's motor repertoire (Calvo-Merino, Glaser, Grèzes, Passingham, & Haggard, 2005). Another stream of research examines biological motion depicted as point-light displays; in these tasks, subjetcs have to either judge the biological plausibility of the implied motion or to discriminate between different types of biological motion (for instance moving left or right ;McKay, et al., 2012). However, more complex discrimination tasks such as agent and expression intensity recognition (Sevdalis & Keller, 2011) have not yet been adequately examined in fMRI environments.

Individuals are also capable of perceiving implied motion. Implied motions are static images that suggest there is motion involved when the image was captured. As such, while studies on perception of actual motion often use video clips as stimuli, studies on implied motion relied on static photographs (e.g., Kourtzi & Kanwisher, 2000; Senior, et al., 2000). In these studies, participants were shown photographs of an agent in action (human, animal or a natural agent such as wave). Motion was not actually present or viewed, just implied by the static images. This allows for a deeper understanding of how humans perceive motion. Results have suggested that the extrastriate cortex is not merely involved in passive perception of motion, but also critical for visual cognition that allows for interpretation of static images with implied motion.

Furthermore, Iacoboni and colleagues (1999) investigated whether the same neural substrates are responsible for perception of motion versus actual execution of the action. This is known as *direct matching hypothesis*, which suggests that observing an action stimulates the same brain regions as actually executing the action. In addition, they also looked at the neural responses of imitation, which is learning and executing an action after observing it being performed. In most of their studies, they used actions that were familiar to participants, such as simple fingers movements. Buccino and colleagues (2004) expanded this line of research into the imitation of complex hand movements that were not in participants' motor repertoire. For instance, participants who were non-guitarists observed and later executed finger movements of guitar chords.

## 4. Mimicry

While imitation involves a conscious 'copying' of actions, mimicry is defined as an unconscious copying of gestures, postures or mannerisms of another person. Mimicry often takes place in social interactions and has been found to facilitate social exchanges and enhance feelings of affiliation and liking. Some mimicry actions studied include contagious yawning (Nahab, Hattori, Saad, & Hallett, 2009), smiling (Wild, Erb, Eyb, Bartels, & Grodd, 2003) and even subtle social stimuli such as pupil dilation (Harrison, et al., 2006). Typically, participants either passively viewed images (e.g., smiling or yawning) or videos (e.g., social interaction or hand movements) or instructed to perform similar actions as shown in the videos.

The effects of mimicry in social affections have been widely reported in behavioral studies. Recently, Kühn and colleagues (2010) sought to better understand this social phenomenon. Using videos of dyadic interactions, participants were instructed to take the perspective of the person filmed from first-person perspective. When the interaction partner was mimicking, stronger activation were shown in the neural reward mechanisms, which researchers infer as partially supporting the liking effect during mimicry (notice that this interpretation could be a demonstration of reverse inference – see introduction). On another note, while mimicry is unconscious, it can be enhanced or inhibited by eye contact with the partner (Wang, Ramsey, & de C. Hamilton, 2011). Wang and colleagues tested this by instructing participants to imitate the hand actions of a person in the video who is either looking at or away from the camera.

## 5. Mirror neurons

Mirror neurons are neurons that respond to a particular action and will respond regardless if the individual is passively observing or actively executing the action (Chong, Cunnington, Williams, Kanwisher, & Mattingley, 2008; Kilner, Neal, Weiskopf, Friston, & Frith, 2009). Studies on mirror neurons often use the paradigm of *fMRI adaptation* or *repetition suppression*. fMRI adaptation is the effect of reduced BOLD responses as a result of repeated presentation of a sensory stimulus (Chong, et al., 2008). Extending this idea to mirror neurons, if mirror neurons do exist, there should be reduced neural responses when observing an action that was previously executed relative to a novel action. This effect is also known as cross-modality adaptation, as the repetition suppression effect is observed across different 'modes' of a particular action (executive versus observation).

There have been conflicting reports on the existence of brain areas that resemble the behavior of mirror neurons in humans. Using pantomimed hand actions as stimuli, Chong and colleagues (2008) found effects of cross-modality adaptation in the right inferior parietal lobe, thus suggesting the existing of the human mirror neuron system in that region. However, their studies were refuted by Lingnau and colleagues (2009) who did not find the adaptation effect when simple right-handed motor actions were first executed and subsequently observed. This null result could be due to the use of meaningless actions, as the mirror neurons may only be activated by goal-direction actions (Kilner, et al., 2009).

## 6. Mentalizing and understanding mental states of others (Theory of Mind)

The term Theory of Mind (ToM) refers to the ability to attribute mental states (e.g., attitudes, perceptions, attitudes, intentions) to others in order to predict and explain behavior of another person (Premack & Woodruff, 1978). In such studies, participants are often instructed to infer the mental states of a target, which can be a person (Mitchell, Banaji, & Macrae, 2005b), a dog (Mitchell, Banaji, & Macrae, 2005a) or a character in a fictional story (Vogeley, et al., 2001). Cartoons or comic strips have also been used as stimuli in some studies (Gallagher, et al., 2000; Walter, et al., 2004). Mason and collegues (2004) found that ToM mechanisms are also involved when participants evaluate whether certain motor actions can be performed by another individual.

### 6.1. Empathy

There are two aspects of empathy: (i) the cognitive ability to understand and predict another person's mental states, as well as (ii) the affective ability to experience an appropriate emotion in response to another person's mental state (Baron-Cohen & Wheelwright, 2004).

Studies on empathy often use emotional facial expressions as stimuli. Typically, the tasks involve either passive observation of another's emotional expression, imitate the expressions observed or to independently generate specific emotional expression (e.g., Carr, Iacoboni, Dubeau, Mazziotta, & Lenzi, 2003; Wicker, et al., 2003). Findings from these studies often suggest the involvement of ToM and mimicry mechanisms in empathy. Merely instructing participants to describe the emotion of a facial expression was sufficient to engage brain areas commonly associated with ToM, thus suggesting the involvement of unconscious mimicry in empathy (Schulte-Rüther, Markowitsch, Fink, & Piekfe, 2007). Furthermore, BOLD responses of these regions have been positively correlated with self-ratings on the Balanced Emotional Empathy Scale (Lawrence, et al., 2006; Schulte-Rüther, et al., 2007).

Many studies have also looked into the neural responses associated with empathetic responses towards others' pain. In a study by Singer and colleagues (2004), they recruited couples and examined the BOLD response of the female partners when they saw their male partners being administered painful electric stimulation. Their findings suggest that only the affective region, but not the sensory regions, of the pain matrix (areas typically activated when a participant is experiencing pain) is involved in empathetic pain. Jackson and colleagues (2006) also demonstrated both common and distinct neural activations between imagining oneself versus imagining others in painful situations. Participants were shown pictures of feet and hands in some common painful situations (e.g., toes being caught under a heavy object), and tasked to evaluate the level of pain if they were in that situation (self condition) or another individual were in that situation (other condition).

Biases in empathy between ingroup versus outgroup targets are also common research directions. Cheon and colleagues (2011) examined how culture can affect empathy (for details, see below under the section 'Culture'). Cikara and Fiske (2011) hypothesized that individuals show differential empathy responses toward different outgroup members, depending on the stereotype of the specific outgroup. To examine this phenomenon, participants saw different types of events (e.g., "had stomachache after lunch") paired with a photograph of an outgroup member (e.g., elderly person, homeless person, business person). Furthermore, they also examined empathy for positive events (e.g., "found $5 bill") instead of merely focusing on negative or emotionally painful events.

### 6.2. Distinguishing self from others

Being able to distinguish the self from others is fundamental for many higher-order abilities, such as directing goal-specific actions and self-reflection of one's mental or emotional states. One way we distinguish our actions from others' is through our intentions to move. This is also known as *self-agency*, which is the knowledge of being the source of causality. A common paradigm used to investigate this phenomenon is through the mismatch of sensory-action consequence. Typically, participants performed a simple task with periodic "interference" from the experimenter. Such tasks may involve pressing a button to produce a certain color (Spengler, von Cramon, & Brass, 2009) or directing a target down a path (Farrer & Frith, 2002). During the "interference", the action produced would be the opposite of what the participants had intended, thus producing incongruence (or mismatch) between their actions and the actual consequences.

Some tasks may also use temporal mismatch rather than consequential mismatch. In other words, there will be a time lag between their actions and the perception of their actions. For example, participants performed some simple hand movements while the same actions on a screen. They may be viewing either a visual feedback of their own actions with varying degree of temporal delay (Leube, et al., 2003), or similar actions performed by an actor (Macuga & Frey, 2011). For the latter paradigm, it is important that participants know whether they are watching a pre-recorded action or live feedback of their own action.

Another aspect of distinguishing the self is our ability to recognize our own faces and own mental or emotional states. Many neuroscience studies on self-face recognition showed participants photographs of either themselves, a close or familiar other and a stranger. The stimuli were digital morphs between these pictures (Uddin, Kaplan, Molnar-Szakacs, Zaidel, & Iacoboni, 2005) or simply the original facial photographs (e.g., Platek, Keenan, Gallup Jr, & Mohamed, 2004; Platek et al., 2006). In a study on self's emotional reflection, participants were shown photographs of people displaying different emotions and asked to evaluate their own emotional response to each photograph. This revealed a neural network in the prefrontal cortex that is specifically recruited for evaluation of own emotions (Ochsner et al., 2004). In another study on high-functioning individuals with autism, this ability to separate self from others has also been demonstrated; these individuals were impaired in representing their own social intention but not in distinguishing others' social actions from the self (Chiu et al., 2008).

### 6.3. Morality

The main focus of experimental studies of morality is the evaluation of moral judgments. Thus, participants are commonly asked to either evaluate the morality of an action (for instance, driving away after bumping another parked car) or to decide how they themselves would respond in a moral dilemma (e.g., smothering a loud crying baby in order to save oneself and fellows from enemy soldiers). Moll and colleagues (2002) compared emotionally charged pictures that either conveyed moral violations (e.g., physical assaults) or not (e.g., accidents). In a later study (Moll et al., 2005), in order to examine neurobehavioral differences between emotion with and without moral aspect, they also contrasted pictures of pure disgust with and without indignation.

Besides identifying the neural correlates, the principal goal is often to uncover the dimensions that can account for moral judgments. Often, these are in comparison with basic emotions. For instance, recent research has compared 'utilitarian' and 'non-utilitarian' choices. A classic example is the choice of whether to adopt a new vaccine that will ensure immunity to the vast majority of people but will also introduce the disease to a small minority. Adopting the vaccine is the utilitarian choice as the decision criterion is overall welfare; non-utilitarian option is not to adopt the vaccine in order to avoid harm to innocent people. Other dimensions include personal versus impersonal dilemmas (Greene, Sommerville, Nystrom, Darley, & Cohen, 2001); consequences, action (versus inaction) and intentionality (Borg, Hynes, Van Horn, Grafton, & Sinnott-Armstrong, 2006); and harm versus dishonesty versus disgust (Parkison et al., 2011; Haidt, 2002; Rozin, Lowery, Imada, & Haidt, 1999). A useful resource of condensed moral vignettes can be found at Knutson et al. (2010).

We would like to add two important words of caution with regards to the morality studies. Firstly, it is unlikely that participants have encountered the situations used in such experiments. This raises reasonable criticisms as to whether the moral judgments made during the experimental sessions are realistic or credible. Secondly, the experimental moral situations versus either (i) other moral situations or (ii) non-moral situations might be different on more than one dimension. For instance, the contrasted scenarios often also differ in the emotional reaction elicited, levels of social desirability or involvement of bodily harm (Heekeren, Wartenburger, Schmidt, Schwintowski & Williringer, 2003). Therefore, great care should be given in the development of proper controls.

### 6.4. Kinship, romantic and maternal love

The aim of this group of studies is often to examine the neuronal responses associated with positive feelings towards close others (such as romantic partners or children). The universality of both romantic and maternal love (Jankowiak & Fischer, 1992) has been associated with the involvement of a strong, evolutionary mechanism. Typically, in these studies, participants engage in passive viewing of pictures of a person they 'feel love' towards, often a romantic partner or an infant (Aron et al., 2005; Strathearn, Fonagy, Amico & Montague, 2009; Strathearn, Li, Fonagy, & Montague, 2008; Zeki, 2007). Mashek, Aron and Fisher (2000) suggested that a photograph is more effective in eliciting a positive response compared to either touch or voice of the person.

In such studies, the experimenter often has to control for familiarity. Some common controls used include pictures of familiar but emotionally neutral acquaintances, such as photographs of babies whom they have known for the same amount of time. Another important methodological issue to note is with regard to one's emotional response. Intensity of emotional response towards a pictorial stimulus often diminishes after 30 seconds of exposure (Mashek, Aron & Fisher, 2000).

## 7. Attitudes and evaluative processes

Two fundamental concepts in social psychology are attitudes (i.e., 'relatively stable ideas about whether something is good or bad'; Cunningham & Zelazo, 2007, pp. 97) and evaluation (i.e., temporally narrower appraisals). Theoretically, a major categorization of processes refers to implicit (mostly automatic) versus explicit (mostly controlled) processes (also known as Dual Attitude Theory; see Greenwald & Banaji, 1995). Implicit, automatic attitudes towards specific social constructs are often measured by the Implicit Association Test (IAT; Greenwald, McGhee, & Schwartz, 1998). Information gleaned from IAT is valuable in an fMRI context as it can be correlated with brain responses.

One common method used to study 'automatic/implicit' versus 'controlled/explicit' attitude-related responses is the manipulation of the duration of presentation of a stimulus. Stimuli can be presented to participants subliminally by carefully manipulating the duration of presentation such that presentation is so short that stimulus cannot be consciously perceived by participants but yet long enough for unconscious perception to take place. Cunningham and colleagues (2004) found higher amygdala response in participants when Afro-American faces, relative to Caucasian faces, were presented subliminally. This effect was not found when the stimuli were presented supraliminally. Another method of inducing automatic responses is to frame the task in an analogous way. For instance, Cunningham and colleagues (2003, 2004) asked participants to either evaluate a word (e.g., "murder") as a 'good' or 'bad' word, or to evaluate whether it is an abstract or concrete term. The former evaluation is more likely to elicit controlled (and thus socially desirable) responses from the participants.

## 8. Race and stereotype

The effect of controlled versus automatic responses is a major question in studies on racial stereotyping as well. Physiological measures, and in particular, neuronal responses have an advantage over traditional behavioral measures, particularly self-report, as the responses are less likely to be 'controlled' by the participants. This aids in reducing social desirability issues as well as uncovering 'hidden' temporal patterns to responses; in addition, behavioral responses can be more easily influenced by extraneous factors, such as fatigue and order effects. Thus, neuroscience is a good supplement to the more traditional behavioral methodologies. The prototypical fMRI task in such studies involves the presentation of same- and other-race face stimuli; the amygdala is often activated when out-group faces are presented (Hart et al., 2000; but see next paragraph & Phelps et al., 2000).

It is important to point out some important issues that should be taken into consideration when designing a study related to race. Firstly, neural responses to race-based stimuli might depend, to a great extent, on the duration of the presentation itself. Differences in behavioral and brain responses are likely to be related to whether the stimulus is presented subliminally or supraliminally. Differences in neural responses to ingroup and outgroup faces disappear when the stimuli are presented for a longer duration, which allows for conscious elaboration (see Phelps et al., 2000).

Secondly, the mere exposure to outgroup faces might induce cognitive depletion effect for some participants. Richeson and colleagues (2003) found that performance in a Stroop color-naming task was more impaired after interaction with an Afro-American person; however, this effect is limited to Caucasian participants who exhibited anti-Afro-American evaluative bias.

Thirdly, researchers should take extra care in the interpretation of differences in neural responses to the different faces. Differences may also result from mere increased familiarity (even to low level characteristics such as color patterns), perception exposure or social knowledge (in contrast to biases or stereotypes; Eberhardt, 2005). For example, Golarai and colleagues (2004) found that the difference in fusiform activation when perceiving Caucasian versus Afro-American faces extend to perception of scrambled faces as well.

One should also note that it might be easier to uncover the neural responses implicated in stereotyping when implicit (rather than explicit) measurements are used. For instance, in Phelps et al. (2000), no differences were found in amygdala response when Caucasian versus Afro-American faces were presented explicitly; however, differential amygdala response emerged when implicit attitudes measures (e.g., IAT or startle responses) were used instead. Furthermore, event-related responses employing EEG have been very prolific in showing implicit racial biases and their successful or unsuccessful regulation (see Amodio & Bartholow, 2011, for a review).

## 9. Culture

Behavioral evidence has demonstrated that cultural experiences can influence responses at a variety of tasks. Tasks in such cultural studies look at basic mechanisms (e.g., visual processing) as well as more complex behaviors (e.g., social cognition). One of the fundamental goals of culture neuroscience is to evaluate differences in neural responses between people with different cultural backgrounds. Below are some central phenomena that have been studied.

*Holistic versus analytic processing of visual information.* In such studies, common stimuli used are pictures with a foreground object against a background. It has been hypothesized that Caucasians will fixate to the central object while Asians also pay equal attention to the background (Chua, Boland, & Nisbett, 2005). This is likely to be related to a more general holistic (versus analytic) processing style characterizing Asian societies (as compared with North American societies; Chiao et al., 2009). Another task that has been used to study this phenomena is the "framed-line test" (Kitayama, Kawamura, & Larsen, 2003), which sustains that perceptual comparisons mechanisms are different between Japanese and US students.

Though widely used and examined, both the framed-line task and the cultural basis of the holistic/analytic dipole in perceptual terms have been challenged as their results either contradict basic visual science findings, which offers simpler explanations (see Zhou, Gotch, Zhou & Liu, 2008) or they seem to be produced by the natural (and not the cultural environment; Ueda & Komiya, 2012).

*Emotional faces recognition.* Similar to the 'racial stereotypes' experiments described in the previous section, participants in these studies are presented with emotional faces from either the same or different cultures as themselves to investigate the differences in neural activations and possible mechanisms to behaviors towards members of same versus different cultures (Chiao, et al., 2008). Adams Jr and colleagues (2009) had also used another task to study the same phenomenon. They used the 'Reading the mind in the Eyes' test (Baron-Cohen, Wheelwright, Hill, Raste, & Plumb, 2001), where participants described the mental state of a person based only on the picture of his/her eyes.

*Social elements, such as responses to status and hierarchy.* Freeman and colleagues (2009) examined how culture shapes individual's neural reward mechanisms. In their study, participants passively viewed pictures of body displays displaying dominate body posture or subordinate body posture. Cheon and colleagues (2011) also examined how cultural preferences for social hierarchy influence empathy for outgroup members, while further examining how these preferences interact with different cultural groups (Japanese / Korean vs. European / Americans). Participants viewed photographs of scenes that were emotionally painful or neutral. They also indicated their empathy level toward the person in the photograph through a button-press controller in the scanner.

Recent developments in culture science suggest that a valuable method will be to use individuals who have been acculturated into two different cultures (i.e., biculturals). This allows researchers to compare differential cultural responses within the same individuals, instead of comparing between groups of participants. Such differential responses can be elicited by priming these bicultural participants with different cultural images, hence activating the respective cultural frame (for more details see Hong, Morris, Chiu, & Benet-Martinez, 2000; Oyserman & Lee, 2008). This line of research demonstrated that priming biculturals with different cultural images is associated with differential behavioral and neuronal responses (for instance, priming with either Asian or Western images is associated with different responses in culturally sensitive tasks). This suggests that cultural experience influences brain function, which is at odds with the static and essentialistic interpretation of inherent cultural differences in neural responses.

It is important for researchers to be mindful of some major issues when engaging in cross-cultural research. In addition to the issues that are also present in cross-cultural behavioural research (e.g., matched samples across cultures, properly translated instructions), cross-cultural neuroimaging has additional caveats that researchers need to be aware of:

1. **Scanner compatibility**. Typically, neuroimaging data from different cultures are captured by different scanners. It is thus important that researchers should strive to collect data that are captured by the same, or not very highly similar, MRI machines with the same

sequences. Furthermore, interscanner reliability tests have to be carried out to ensure that any differences found that not due to scanner variability (see Sutton et al., 2008).

2. **Task selection**. Standardised, non-verbal visuospatial tasks are preferable to numerical tasks, as the potential for language-mediated cultural bias is higher in the latter. Hedden et al. (2002) have a list of useful neuropsychological tests that researchers may want to refer to.

3. **Brain templates**. Most brain templates used by major neuroimaging software are based on data collected from Caucasian samples. However, there is a demonstrated variability in brain structural anatomy across populations (Tang et al., 2010), which may make the existing templates inappropriate. Some possible solutions include either finding a more appropriate template or to use templates derived from the sampled population itself.

## 10. Social interactions

A revolutionary development in social neuroscience is the introduction of game-theoretic methods in the study of social interactions. In such experiments, participants typically play particular roles in highly-structured social exchanges (i.e., games) to stimulate real social interactions.

There are multiple advantages to this methodology. Firstly, the interactions involve real monetary outcomes, thus making available a metric of phenomena that are otherwise difficult to capture (e.g., the dilemmas involved in trust or reciprocity). In addition, incentivizing the choices participants make allows researchers to study certain social phenomena that are highly sensitive to social desirability problems. For instance, participants might self-report that they are very trusting towards other people; however, they might behave otherwise when their choices or actions have financial consequences.

Another advantage is that there is a wealth of behavioral, simulation and theoretical studies related to such social-economic games. Optimal or 'rational' behaviors (e.g., Nash equilibrium) are well-characterized and studied. The mathematical descriptions of the various choices one can make are also readily available. Furthermore, behavioral explanations and formal computational models of the different choices have also been described in sufficient details. As such, it is possible to model the underlying, hidden computations or processes that change parametrically on a trial-by-trial basis. Moreover, one can study how dynamic social interactions evolve over time. This allows social neuroscientists to move beyond mere brain mapping to the examination of brain mechanisms involved, as described in the introduction of this chapter. In other words, the research focus can thus move from social neuroscience to *social computational neuroscience*.

Social computational neuroscience should include the following steps:

1. Adopt or develop a simulated interaction (game), based on the phenomenon being studied. Ensure that the behavioral choices actually reflect the phenomenon in question.

2. Find one or more algorithms that can describe the choices available. In dynamic environments, the focus can be on how previous interactions update the representations of the self, partner and their relationship.

3. Fit the algorithm/s to actual behaviors in order to identify the optimal values for the parameters of each model.

4. Identify whether the computations implied by the models are actually taking place in the brain. This will ensure the biological plausibility of the model.

An excellent example of the social computational neuroscience approach is the study by Behrens, Hunt, Woolrich and Rushworth (2008). The authors wanted to study the behavioral and neuronal responses related to advice from a partner. In their game, participants had to choose between different cards offering rewards associated with different and unknown probabilities (step 1). At the same time, they received advice from a partner who may or may not be trustworthy. Thus, participants needed to update, on each trial, the probability that the advisor is reliable (or not). The authors hypothesized that the probability was updated using basic reinforcement learning algorithms (step 2). They then fitted their model to the behavior in order to identify the (otherwise hidden) probability associated with their partner's perceived reliability. The outcome was a time-series of updated values, on a trial-by-trial basis (step 3). Next, they fitted the time-series values to the BOLD responses, which thus allowed them to identify the brain areas that appeared to subserve the relevant calculations (step 4).

As illustrated, this approach allows the identification of individual or group differences of very subtle and hidden computations. Another example of its application is the differentiation of participants according to whether they update the value of social gestures in social interactions. This is well demonstrated in a series of studies by King-Casas and colleagues (2005, 2008). In these studies, the authors used a paradigm known as the Trust Game (see figure 1).

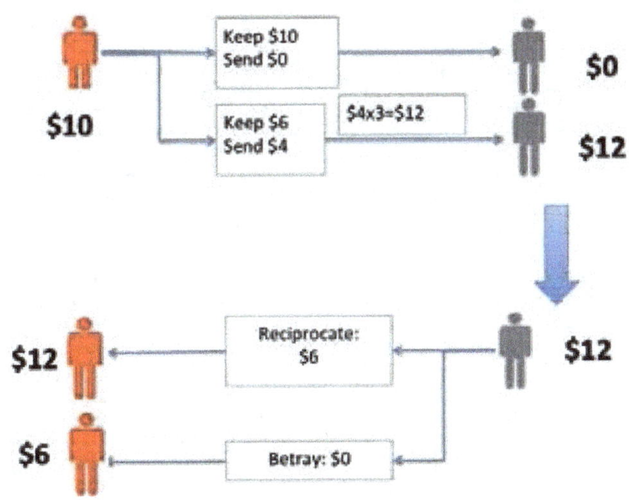


**Figure 1.** The Trust Game

In a typical trust game, player A (red in figure 1) is given an amount (e.g., $10). Player A has the choice to keep the amount, or to send ('invest') a portion of it to player B (gray in figure 1). The amount sent to the partner will then be tripled by the experimenter (as shown in our example, $4 was invested, and thus player B receives $12). Next, player B has to decide how much of the received amount (i.e., $12 in this case) to send back to player A as an indication reciprocity.

King-Casas and colleagues measured the BOLD responses as participants played the trust game. In the first study, they identified a neuronal response reflecting the computational learning signals that represented the intentions of the social partner. In the following study, they included participants who were diagnosed with Borderline Personality Disorder (BDP). This disorder is strongly characterized by inadequate and brief social relationships (see American Psychiatric Association, 2000, for more details). By analyzing behavior in the trust game, they found that participants with BDP cooperated less as the game progressed, thus indexing a breach of trust in the dyad. This was reflected in these participants' insula brain responses, which failed to represent the magnitude of offers received. This series of studies elegantly demonstrated how a simple simulated social interaction can be used to uncover social deficits.

Many similar games have been used to describe or simulate various social interactions. It is beyond the scope of the current chapter to elaborate on each game. Nevertheless, we present a list of relevant papers together with the major constructs they measured in Table 1.

| **Game / Task** | **Concept** | **References (fMRI or behavioural studies)** |
|---|---|---|
| Prisoner's Dilemma; ultimatum game | Cooperation / Competition; unfairness | Rilling et al., (2004) |
| Social allocations / social value orientation / fairness | Social predisposition | Hsu, Anen & Quartz (2008)<br>Haruno & Frith (2010)<br>Tricomi, et al. (2010) |
| Ball-tossing task (Cyberball) | Social Rejection | Williams, Cheung & Choi (2000) |
| Trust game | Trust, reciprocation | King-Casas, et al. (2005, 2008) |
| Observational learning | Learning from others | Burke, et al. (2010) |
| Altruistic punishment | Altruistic punishment | de Quervain, et al. (2004) |
| Work-or-shirk | Mentalising | Hampton, et al. (2008) |
| Beauty contest | Depth of strategic reasoning | Coricelli & Nagel (2009)<br>See also Bhatt & Camerer (2005) |
| Social comparisons, envy and Schadenfreude | Schadenfreude occurs when envied persons fall from grace | Takahashi, et al. (2009);<br>Fliessbach et al. (2007) |
| Punishment games | Parochial altruism; norm enforcement | Baumgartner, et al. (2011) |
| Promise game | Promise keeping | Baumgartner, et al. (2009) |
| Bargaining Games | Bargaining/Suspicion/Strategic Deception | Bhatt, et al. (2010) |

**Table 1.** A limited list of games employed in the study of social interactions

## 11. Criticisms, issues and the future

A common criticism to social neuroscience in general (and games in particular) is the lack of ecological validity as the tasks seem to fail to represent the complexity of actual social interactions. The same argument has been directed towards non-social decision-making studies in neuroeconomics (Volz & Gigerenzer, Chapter 22, this Book). There have been plenty of responses to this criticism.

Firstly, participants do appear to be sensitive to the experimental manipulations and thus display the behaviors that truly represent their social preference or even social pathology (see above for example of participants with BDP). This is illustrated in many neuroeconomic studies where participants demonstrated consistent risk aversion (Christopoulos, Tobler, Bossaerts, Dolan, & Schultz, 2009), even with small monetary rewards. In addition, these games can be the basis or building block of more realistic and sophisticated simulations of social interactions (see Wolf, Dziobej, & Heekeren, 2010). Furthermore, this approach allows for an understanding of basic or fundamental cognitions which can contribute to subsequent models of more complex behaviors.

Nevertheless, this criticism is not unfounded and has been constructive in bringing improvements to the field of social neuroscience. A number of recent studies have tried to relate neuroimaging results with real life behaviors. Kanai, Feilden, Firth and Rees (2011) used brain volumetric techniques to correlate neuroanatomical structural differences (i.e., size of specific brain structures) with the size of one's social networks (e.g., Facebook). In another study, Falk, Berkman, Whalen and Lieberman (2011) demonstrated that neural responses to health messages can predict whether the participant will reduce unhealthy behaviors (i.e., smoking in their study) over-and-above self-reported intentions.

In conclusion, social neuroscience is in its infancy. It can be expected that studies trying to understand basic mechanisms will eventually corroborate with studies that more closely investigate real life, out-of-the-lab behaviors.

## Acknowledgements

We thank Bobby Cheon and Mark Khei for their invaluable comments on an earlier draft of the present paper. The preparation of this article was partially supported by the Academic Research Fund (AcRF) Tier 1 (RG 1/11 M4010946.010) of the Ministry of Education, Singapore awarded to the second author.

## Author details

D.Y. Phua[1,2] and G.I. Christopoulos[1,2,3]

1 Nanyang Business School, Nanyang Technological University, Singapore

2 Culture Science Institute, Nanyang Tchnological University, Singapore

3 Virginia Tech Carilion Research Institute, VA, USA

## References

[1] Adams Jr, R. B., Rule, N. O., Franklin Jr, R. G., Wang, E., Stevenson, M. T., Yoshikawa, S., ... & Ambady, N. (2010). Cross-cultural reading the mind in the eyes: An fMRI investigation. *Journal of Cognitive Neuroscience*, 22(1), 97-108.

[2] American Psychiatric Association (2000). *Diagnostic and statistical manual of mental disorders* (4th ed., Text Revision). Washington, DC: Author.

[3] Amodio, D. M., & Bartholow, B. D. (2011). Event-related potential methods in social cognition. In C. Klauer, A. Voss, & C. Stahl (Eds.), *Cognitive methods in social psychology* (pp. 303–339). New York : Guilford Press.

[4] Aron, A., Fisher, H., Mashek, D. J., Strong, G., Li, H., & Brown, L. L. (2005). Reward, motivation, and emotion systems associated with early-stage intense romantic love. *Journal of Neurophysiology*, 94(1), 327–337.

[5] Baron-Cohen, S., & Wheelwright, S. (2004). The empathy quotient: An investigation of adults with Asperger syndrome or high functioning autism, and normal sex differences. *Journal of Autism and Developmental Disorders*, 34(2), 163–175.

[6] Baron-Cohen, S., Wheelwright, S., Hill, J., Raste, Y., & Plumb, I. (2001). The "Reading the Mind in the Eyes" Test Revised Version: A study with normal adults, and adults with Asperger Syndrome or high-functioning Autism. *Journal of Child Psychology and Psychiatry*, 42(2), 241–251.

[7] Baumgartner, T., Fischbacher, U., Feierabend, A., Lutz, K., & Fehr, E. (2009). The neural circuitry of a broken promise. *Neuron*, 64(5), 756–770.

[8] Baumgartner, T., Knoch, D., Hotz, P., Eisenegger, C., & Fehr, E. (2011). Dorsolateral and ventromedial prefrontal cortex orchestrate normative choice. *Nature Neuroscience*, 14(11), 1468–1474.

[9] Behrens, T. E, Hunt, L. T, Woolrich, M. W, Rushworth, M. F (2008). Associative learning of social value. *Nature*, 456(7219), 245–249.

[10] Bhatt, M., & Camerer, C. F. (2005). Self-referential thinking and equilibrium as states of mind in games: fMRI evidence. *Games and Economic Behavior*, 52(2), 424–459.

[11] Bhatt, M. A., Lohrenz, T., Camerer, C. F., & Montague, P. R. (2010). Neural signatures of strategic types in a two-person bargaining game. *Proceedings of the National Academy of Sciences*, 107(46), 19720-19725.

[12] Blanke, O., Mohr, C., Michel, C. M., Pascual-Leone, A., Brugger, P., Seeck, M., et al. (2005). Linking out-of-body experience and self processing to mental own-body imagery at the temporoparietal junction. *The Journal of Neuroscience*, 25(3), 550–557.

[13] Borg, S. J., Hynes, C., Van Horn, J., Grafton, S., & Sinnott-Armstrong, W. (2006). Consequences, action, and intention as factors in moral judgments: An fMRI Investigation. *Journal of Cognitive Neuroscience, 18*(5), 803–817.

[14] Buccino, G., Lui, F., Canessa, N., Pastteri, I., Lagravinese, G., Benuzzi, F., et al. (2004). Neural circuits involved in the recognition of actions performed by nonconspecifics: An fMRI study. *Journal of Cognitive Neuroscience,* 16(1), 114–126.

[15] Buccino, G., Vogt, S., Ritzl, A., Fink, G. R., Zilles, K., Freund, H.-J., et al. (2004). Neural circuits underlying imitation learning of hand actions: An event-related fMRI study. *Neuron*, 42(2), 323–334.

[16] Burke, C. J., Tobler, P. N., Baddeley, M., and Schultz, W. (2010). Neural mechanisms of observational learning. *Proceedings of the National Academy of Sciences*, 107(32), 14431–14436.

[17] Calvert, G. A., Bullmore, E. T., Brammer, M. J., Campbell, R., Williams, S. C. R., McGuire, P. K., et al. (1997). Activation of auditory cortex during silent lipreading. *Science*, 276(5312), 593–596.

[18] Calvo-Merino, B., Glaser, D. E., Grèzes, J., Passingham, R. E., & Haggard, P. (2005). Action observation and acquired motor skills: An fMRI study with expert dancers. *Cerebral Cortex*, 15(8), 1243–1249.

[19] Campbell, R., MacSweeney, M., Surguladze, S., Calvert, G., McGuire, P., Suckling, J., et al. (2001). Cortical substrates for the perception of face actions: An fMRI study of the specificity of activation for seen speech and for meaningless lower-face acts (gurning). *Cognitive Brain Research*, 12(2), 233–243.

[20] Carr, L., Iacoboni, M., Dubeau, M.-C., Mazziotta, J. C., & Lenzi, G. L. (2003). Neural mechanisms of empathy in humans: A relay from neural systems for imitation to limbic areas. *Proceedings of the National Academy of Sciences*, 100(9), 5497–5502.

[21] Cheon, B. K., Im, D.-m., Harada, T., Kim, J.-S., Mathur, V. A., Scimeca, J. M., ..., Chiao, J. Y. (2011). Cultural influences on neural basis of intergroup empathy. *NeuroImage*, 57(2), 642-650.

[22] Chiao, J. Y., Harada, T., Komeda, H., Li, Z., Mano, Y., Saito, D. N., ..., Iidaka, T. (2009). Dynamic cultural influences on neural representations of self. *Journal of Cognitive Neuroscience*, 22 (1), 1–11.

[23] Chiao, J. Y., Iidaka, T., Gordon, H. L., Nogawa, J., Bar, M., Aminoff, E., . . ., Ambady, N. (2008). Cultural specificity in amygdala response to fear faces. *Journal of Cognitive Neuroscience*, 20, 2167–2174.

[24] Cikara, M., & Fiske, S. T. (2011). Bounded empathy: Neural responses to outgroup targets' (mis)fortunes. *Journal of Cognitive Neuroscience*, 23(12), 3791-3803.

[25] Chiu, P. H., Kayali, M. A., Kishida, K. T., Tomlin, D., Klinger, L. G., Klinger, M. R., & Montague, P. R. (2008). Self responses along cingulate cortex reveal quantitative neural phenotype for high-functioning autism. *Neuron*, 57(3), 463-473.

[26] Chong, T. T. J., Cunnington, R., Williams, M. A., Kanwisher, N., & Mattingley, J. B. (2008). fMRI adaptation reveals mirror neurons in human inferior parietal cortex. *Current Biology*, 18(20), 1576–1580.

[27] Christopoulos, G. I., Tobler, P. N., Bossaerts, P., Dolan, R. J., Schultz, W. (2009). Neural correlates of value, risk, and risk aversion contributing to decision making under risk. *Journal of Neuroscience*, 29(40), 12574–12583.

[28] Chua, H. F., Boland, J. E., & Nisbett, R. E. (2005). Cultural variation in eye movements during scene perception. *Proceedings of the National Academy of Science*, 102 (35), 12629–12633.

[29] Coricelli, G., & Nagel, R. (2009). Neural correlates of depth of strategic reasoning in medial prefrontal cortex. *Proceedings of the National Academy of Sciences*, 106(23), 9163–9168.

[30] Cunningham, W. A., Johnson, M. K., Gatenby, J. C., Gore, J. C., & Banaji, M. R. (2003). Neural components of social evaluation. *Journal of Personality and Social Psychology*, 85(4), 639–649.

[31] Cunningham, W. A., Johnson, M. K., Raye, C. L., Gatenby, C. J., Gore, J.C., & Banaji, M.R. (2004). Separable neural components in the processing of Black and White faces. *Psychological Science*, 15(12), 806–813.

[32] Cunningham, W. A., Raye, C. L., & Johnson, M. K. (2004). Implicit and explicit evaluation: fMRI correlates of valence, emotional intensity, and control in the processing of attitudes. *Journal of Cognitive Neuroscience*, 16(10), 1717–1729.

[33] Cunningham, W. A., & Zelazo, P. D. (2007). Attitudes and evaluations: A social cognitive neuroscience perspective. *Trends in Cognitive Sciences*, 11(3), 97–104.

[34] Engell, A. D., Haxby, J. V., & Todorov, A. (2007). Implicit trustworthiness decisions: Automatic coding of face properties in the human amygdala. *Journal of Cognitive Neuroscience*, 19(9), 1508–1519.

[35] Eberhardt, J. L. (2005). Imaging race. *American Psychologist*, 60(2), 181–190.

[36] Falk, E. B., Berkman, E. T., Whalen, D., & Lieberman, M. D. (2011). Neural activity during health messaging predicts reductions in smoking above and beyond self-report. *Health Psychology*, 30(2), 177–185.

[37] Farrer, C., & Frith, C. D. (2002). Experiencing oneself vs another person as being the cause of an action: The neural correlates of the experience of agency. *NeuroImage*, 15(3), 596-603.

[38] Fliessbach, K., Weber, B., Trautner, P., Dohmen, T., Sunde, U., Elger, C. E., & Falk A. (2007). Social comparison affects reward-related brain activity in the human ventral striatum. *Science*. 318(5854), 1305–8.

[39] Freeman, J. B., Rule, N. O., Adams, R. B., & Ambaby, N. (2009). Culture shapes a mesolimbic response to signals of dominance and subordination that associates with behaviour. *NeuroImage*, 47(1), 353–359.

[40] Gallagher, H. L., Happé, F., Brunswick, N., Fletcher, P. C., Frith, U., & Frith, C. D. (2000). Reading the mind in cartoons and stories: An fMRI study of 'theory of mind' in verbal and nonverbal tasks. *Neuropsychologia*, 38(1), 11–21.

[41] German, T. P., Niehaus, J. L., Roarty, M. P., Giesbrecht, B., & Miller, M. B. (2004). Neural correlates of detecting pretense: Automatic engagement of the intentional stance under covert conditions. *Journal of Cognitive Neuroscience*, 16(10), 1805–1817.

[42] Golarai, G., Ghahremani, D. G., Whitfield-Gabrieli, S., Reiss, A., Eberhardt, J. L., Gabrieli, J. D., & Grill-Spector, K. (2007). Differential development of high-level visual cortex correlates with category-specific recognition memory. *Nature Neuroscience*, 10(4), 512–522.

[43] Greenwald, A. G., & Banaji, M. R. (1995). Implicit social cognition: Attitudes, self- esteem, and stereotypes. *Psychological Review*, 102(1), 4–27.

[44] Greenwald, A. G., McGhee, D. E., & Schwartz, J. K. L. (1998). Measuring individual differences in implicit cognition: The implicit association test. *Journal of Personality and Social Psychology*, 74(6), 1464–1480.

[45] Greene, J. D., Sommerville, R. B., , Nystrom, L. E., Darley, J. M., & Cohen, J. D. (2001). An fMRI investigation of emotional engagement in moral judgment. *Science*, 293(5537), 2105-2108.

[46] Haidt, J. (2002). Dialogue between my head and my heart: Affective influences on moral judgment. *Psychological Inquiry*, 13(1), 54–56.

[47] Hampton, A. N., Bossaerts, P., & O'Doherty, J. P. (2008). Neural correlates of mentalizing-related computations during strategic interactions in humans. *Proceedings of the National Academy of Sciences*, 105(18), 6741–6746.

[48] Harenski, C. L., Kim, S., & Hamann, S. (2009). Neuroticism and psychopathy predict brain activation during moral and nonmoral emotion regulation. *Cognitive, Affective, and Behavioral Neuroscience*, 9(1), 1–15.

[49] Harrison, N. A., Singer, T., Rotshtein, P., Dolan, R. J., & Critchley, H. D. (2006). Pupillary contagion: Central mechanisms engaged in sadness processing. *Social Cognitive and Affective Neuroscience*, 1(1), 5–17.

[50] Hart, A.J., Whalen, P.J., Shine, L.M., McInerney, S.C., Fischer, H., & Rauch, S.L. (2000). Differential response in the human amygdala to racial outgroup vs ingroup face stimuli. *Neuroreport*, 11(11), 2351– 2355.

[51] Haruno, M., & Frith, C. (2010). Activity in the amygdala elicited by unfair divisions predicts social value orientation. *Nature Neuroscience*, 13(2), 160–161.

[52] Hedden, T., Park, D.C., Nisbett, R., Ji, L.-J., Jing, Q., & Jiao, S. (2002). Cultural variation in verbal versus spatial neuro- psychological function across the life span. *Neuropsychology*, 16(1), 65–73.

[53] Heekeren, H.R., Wartenburger, I., Schmidt, H., Schwintowski, H.P., & Villringer, A. (2003) An fMRI study of simple ethical decision-making. *Neuroreport*, 14(9), 1215–1219.

[54] Hoffman, E. A., & Haxby, J. V. (2000). Distinct representations of eye gaze and identity in the distributed human neural system for face perception. *Nature Neuroscience*, *3*(1), 80-84.

[55] Hong, Y., Morris, M.W., Chiu, C., & Benet-Martinez, V. (2000). Multicultural minds: A dynamic constructivist approach to culture and cognition. *American Psychology*, 55(7), 709–720.

[56] Hsu, M., Anen, C., & Quartz, S. R. (2008). The right and the good: Distributive justice and neural encoding of equity and efficiency. *Science*, 320(5879), 1092–1095.

[57] Huettel, S. A., Song, A. W., & McCarthy, G. (2009). *Functional Magnetic Resonance Imaging* (2nd ed.). Massachusetts: Sinauer Associates.

[58] Iacoboni, M., Woods, R. P., Brass, M., Bekkering, H., Mazziotta, J. C., & Rizzolatti, G. (1999). Cortical mechanisms of human imitation. *Science, 286*(5449), 2526–2528.

[59] Jackson, P. L., Brunet, E., Meltzoff, A. N., & Decety, J. (2006). Empathy examined through the neural mechanisms involved in imagining how I feel versus how you feel pain. *Neuropsychologia*, 44(5), 752–761.

[60] Jankowiak, W. R., & Fischer, E. F., (1992). A cross-cultural perspective on romantic love. *Ethnology*, 31(2), 149-155.

[61] Kanai, R., Feilden, T., Firth, C., & Rees, G. (2011). Political orientations are correlated with brain structure in young adults. *Current Biology*, 21(8), 1–4.

[62] Kilner, J. M., Neal, A., Weiskopf, N., Friston, K. J., & Frith, C. D. (2009). Evidence of mirror neurons in human inferior frontal gyrus. *The Journal of Neuroscience*, 29(32), 10153–10159.

[63] King-Casas, B., Sharp, C., Lomax-Bream, L., Lohrenz, T., Fonagy, P., & Montague, P. R. (2008). The rupture and repair of cooperation in borderline personality disorder. *Science*, 321(5890), 806–810.

[64] King-Casas, B., Tomlin, D., Anen, C, Camerer, C. F., Quartz, S. R., Montague, P. R. (2005). Getting to know you: Reputation and trust in a two-person economic exchange. *Science*, 308(5718),78-83.

[65] Kitayama, S., Kawamura, T., & Larsen, J. T. (2003). Perceiving an object and its context in different cultures: A cultural look at new look. *Psychological Science*, 14(3), 201–206.

[66] Knutson, K. M., Krueger, F., Koenigs, M., Hawley, A., Escobedo, J. R., Vasudeva, V., Adolphs, R., & Grafman, J. (2010). Behavioral norms for condensed moral vignettes. *Social Cognitive and Affective Neuroscience*, 5(4), 378–384.

[67] Kourtzi, Z., & Kanwisher, N. (2000). Activation in human MT/MST by static images with implied motion. *Journal of Cognitive Neuroscience*, 12(1), 48–55.

[68] Kühn, S., Müller, B. C. N., van Baaren, R. B., Wietzker, A., Dijksterhuis, A., & Brass, M. (2010). Why do I like you when you behave like me? Neural mechanisms mediating positive consequences of observing someone being imitated. *Social Neuroscience*, 5(4), 384–392.

[69] Lawrence, E. J., Shaw, P., Giampietro, V. P., Surguladze, S., Brammer, M. J., & David, A. S. (2006). The role of 'shared representations' in social perception and empathy: An fMRI study. *NeuroImage*, 29(4), 1173–1184.

[70] Leube, D. T., Knoblich, G., Erb, M., Grodd, W., Bartels, M., & Kircher, T. T. J. (2003). The neural correlates of perceiving one's own movements. *NeuroImage*, 20(4), 2084–2090.

[71] Lingnau, A., Gesierich, B., & Caramazza, A. (2009). Asymmetric fMRI adaptation reveals no evidence for mirror neurons in humans. *Proceedings of the National Academy of Sciences*, 106(24), 9925–9930.

[72] Macuga, K. L., & Frey, S. H. (2011). Selective responses in right inferior frontal and supramarginal gyri differentiate between observed movements of oneself vs. another. *Neuropsychologia*, 49(5), 1202–1207.

[73] Mason, M. F., Banfield, J. F., & Macrae, C. N. (2004). Thinking about actions: The neural substrates of person knowledge. *Cerebral Cortex*, 14(2), 209–214.

[74] Mashek, D., Aron, A., & Fisher, H. E. (2000). Identifying, evoking, and measuring intense feelings of romantic love. *Representative Research in Social Psychology*, 24, 48–55.

[75] McKay, L. S., Simmons, D. R., McAleer, P., Marjoram, D., Piggot, J., & Pollick, F. E. (2012). Do distinct atypical cortical networks process biological motion information in adults with Autism Spectrum Disorders? *NeuroImage*, 59(2), 1524-1533.

[76] Mitchell, J. P., Banaji, M. R., & Macrae, C. N. (2005a). General and specific contributions of the medial prefrontal cortex to knowledge about mental states. *NeuroImage,* 28(4), 757–762.

[77] Mitchell, J. P., Banaji, M. R., & Macrae, C. N. (2005b). The link between social cognition and self-referential thought in the medial prefrontal cortex. *Journal of Cognitive Neuroscience,* 17(8), 1306-1315.

[78] Moll, J., de Oliveira-Souza, R., Eslinger P. J., Bramati, I. E., Mourão-Miranda, J., Andreiuolo, P. A., & Pessoa, L. (2002). The neural correlates of moral sensitivity: A functional magnetic resonance imaging investigation of basic and moral emotions. *Journal of Neuroscience,* 22(7), 2730–2736.

[79] Moll, J., de Oliveira-Souza, R., Moll, F.T., Ignacio,F.A., Bramati, I.E., Caparelli-Daquer, E. M., Eslinger, P. J. (2005). The moral affiliations of disgust: A functional MRI study. *Cognitive Behavioural Neurology,* 18(1), 68–78.

[80] Nahab, F. B., Hattori, N., Saad, Z. S., & Hallett, M. (2009). Contagious yawning and the frontal lobe: An fMRI study. *Human Brain Mapping,* 30(5), 1744–1751.

[81] Narumoto, J., Okada, T., Sadato, N., Fukui, K., & Yonekura, Y. (2001). Attention to emotion modulates fMRI activity in human right superior temporal sulcus. *Cognitive Brain Research,* 12(2), 225–231.

[82] Ochsner, K. N., Knierim, K., Ludlow, D. H., Hanelin, J., Ramachandran, T., Glover, G., & Mackey, S. C. (2004). Reflecting upon feelings: An fMRI study of neural systems supporting the attribution of emotion to self and other. *Journal of cognitive neuroscience,* 16(10), 1746-1772.

[83] Oyserman, D., & Lee, S. W. (2008). Priming 'culture': Culture as situated cognition. In Shinobu Kitayama & Dov Cohen (Eds.), *Handbook of Cultural Psychology* (pp. 255–276). New York: Guilford Press.

[84] Parkinson, C., Sinnott-Armstrong, W., Koralus, P., Mendelovici, A., McGeer, V., & Wheatley, T. (2011). Is morality unified? Evidence that distinct neural systems underlie judgments of harm, dishonesty, and disgust. *Journal of Cognitive Neuroscience,* 23(10), 3162–3180.

[85] Pelphrey, K. A., Morris, J. P., Michelich, C. R., Allison, T., & McCarthy, G. (2005). Functional anatomy of biological motion perception in posterior temporal cortex: An fMRI study of eye, mouth and hand movements. *Cerebral Cortex,* 15(12), 1866–1876.

[86] Phelps, E. A., O'Connor, K. J., Cunningham, W. A., Funayama, E. S., Gatenby, J. C., Gore, J. C., & Banaji, M. R. (2000). Performance on indirect measures of race evaluation predicts amygdala activation. *Journal of Cognitive Neuroscience,* 12(5), 729–738.

[87] Platek, S. M., Keenan, J. P., Gallup Jr, G. G., & Mohamed, F. B. (2004). Where am I? The neurological correlates of self and other. *Cognitive Brain Research,* 19(2), 114–122.

[88] Platek, S. M., Loughead, J. W., Gur, R. C., Busch, S., Ruparel, K., Phend, N., et al. (2006). Neural substrates for functionally discriminating self-face from personally familiar faces. *Human Brain Mapping, 27*(2), 91–98.

[89] Premack, D., & Woodruff, G. (1978). Does the chimpanzee have a theory of mind? *Behavioral and Brain Sciences,* 1(04), 515-526.

[90] Poldrack, R. (2006). Can cognitive processes be inferred from neuroimaging data? Trends in Cognitive Sciences. 10(2), 59–63.

[91] Puce, A., Allison, T., Bentin, S., Gore, J. C., & McCarthy, G. (1998). Temporal cortex activation in humans viewing eye and mouth movements. *The Journal of Neuroscience,* 18(6), 2188–2199.

[92] de Quervain, D. J., Fischbacher, U., Treyer, V., Schellhammer, M., Schnyder, U., Buck, A., Fehr, E. (2004). The neural basis of altruistic punishment. *Science,* 305(5688), 1254–1258.

[93] Richeson, J. A., Baird, A. A., Gordon, H. L., Heatherton, T. F, Wyland, C. L., Trawalter, S., & Shelton, J. N. (2003). An fMRI investigation of the impact of interracial contact on executive function. *Nature Neuroscience,* 6(12), 1323–1328.

[94] Rilling, J. K., Sanfey, A. G., Aronson, J. A., Nystrom, L. E., Cohen, J. D. (2004). The neural correlates of theory of mind within interpersonal interaction. *Neuroimage,* 22, 1694–1703.

[95] Rozin, P., Lowery, L., Imada, S., & Haidt, J. (1999). The CAD triad hypothesis: A mapping between three moral emotions (contempt, anger, disgust) and three moral codes (community, autonomy, divinity). *Journal of Personality and Social Psychology,* 76(4), 574–586.

[96] Schulte-Rüther, M., Markowitsch, H. J., Fink, G. R., & Piefke, M. (2007). Mirror neuron and theory of mind mechanisms involved in face-to-face interactions: A functional magnetic resonance imaging approach to empathy. *Journal of Cognitive Neuroscience,* 19(8), 1354–1372.

[97] Sevdalis, V., & Keller, P. E. (2012). Perceiving bodies in motion: expression intensity, empathy, and experience. *Experimental Brain Research,* 222(4), 447-453.

[98] Senior, C., Barnes, J., Giampietroc, V., Simmons, A., Bullmore, E. T., Brammer, M., et al. (2000). The functional neuroanatomy of implicit-motion perception or 'representational momentum'. *Current Biology,* 10(1), 16–22.

[99] Singer, T., Seymour, B., O'Doherty, J., Kaube, H., Dolan, R. J., & Frith, C. D. (2004). Empathy for pain involves the affective but not sensory components of pain. *Science,* 303(5661), 1157–1162.

[100] Spengler, S., von Cramon, D. Y., & Brass, M. (2009). Was it me or was it you? How the sense of agency originates from ideomotor learning revealed by fMRI. *NeuroImage*, 46(1), 290–298.

[101] Strathearn, L., Li, J., Fonagy, P., & Montague, P. R. (2008). What's in a smile? Maternal brain responses to infant facial cues. *Pediatrics*, 122(1), 40–51.

[102] Strathearn, L., Fonagy, P., Amico, J., & Montague, P. R. (2009). Adult Attachment Predicts Maternal Brain and Oxytocin Response to Infant Cues. *Neuropsychopharmacology*, 34(13), 2655–2666.

[103] Sutton, B. P., Goh, J., Hebrank, A., Welsh, R. C., Chee, M. W., & Park, D. C. (2008). Investigation and validation of intersite fMRI studies using the same imaging hardware. *Journal of Magnetic Resonance Imaging*, 28(1), 21-28.

[104] Takahashi, H., Kato, M., Matsuura, M., Mobbs, D., Suhara, T., & Okubo, Y. (2009). When your gain is my pain and your pain is my gain: Neural correlates of envy and schadenfreude. *Science*, 323(5916), 937–939.

[105] Tang, Y., Hojatkashani, C., Dinov, I. D., Sun, B., Fan, L., Lin, X., et al. (2010). The construction of a Chinese MRI brain atlas: A morphometric comparison study between Chinese and Caucasian cohorts. *NeuroImage*, 51(1), 33–41.

[106] Tricomi, E., Rangel, A., Camerer, C. F., & O'Doherty, J. P. (2010). Neural evidence for inequality-averse social preferences. *Nature*, 463(7284), 1089–91.

[107] Uddin, L. Q., Kaplan, J. T., Molnar-Szakacs, I., Zaidel, E., & Iacoboni, M. (2005). Self-face recognition activates a frontoparietal "mirror" network in the right hemisphere: An event-related fMRI study. *NeuroImage*, 25(3), 926–935.

[108] Ueda, Y., & Komiya, A. (2012). Cultural adaptation of visual attention: Calibration of the oculomotor control system in accordance with cultural scenes. *PloS one*, 7(11), e50282.

[109] Vogeley, K., Bussfeld, P., Newen, A., Herrmann, S., Happé, F., Falkai, P., et al. (2001). Mind reading: Neural mechanisms of theory of mind and self-perspective. *NeuroImage*, 14(1), 170-181.

[110] Volz, K.G. & Gigerenzer, G. (2013) The brain is not "as-if" –Taking stock of the neuroscientific approach on decision making. In T.D. Papageorgiou, G. I. Christopoulos & S. M. Smirnakis (Eds.) Advanced Brain Neuroimaging Topics in Health and Disease – Methods and Applications. InTech (Rijeka, Croatia)

[111] Walter, H., Adenzato, M., Ciaramidaro, A., Enrici, I., Pia, L., & Bara, B. G. (2004). Understanding intentions in social interaction: The role of the anterior paracingulate cortex. *Journal of Cognitive Neuroscience*, 16(10), 1854-1863.

[112] Wang, Y., Ramsey, R., & de C. Hamilton, A. F. (2011). The control of mimicry by eye contact is mediated by medial prefrontal cortex. *The Journal of Neuroscience*, 31(33), 12001-12010.

[113] Wicker, B., Keysers, C., Plailly, J., Royet, J.-P., Gallese, V., & Rizzolatti, G. (2003). Both of us disgusted in my insula: The common neural basis of seeing and feeling disgust. *Neuron*, 40(3), 655-664.

[114] Wild, B., Erb, M., Eyb, M., Bartels, M., & Grodd, W. (2003). Why are smiles contagious? An fMRI study of the interaction between perception of facial affect and facial movements. *Psychiatry Research: Neuroimaging*, 123(1), 17-36.

[115] Williams, K. D., Cheung, C. K. T., Choi, W. (2000). Cyberostracism: Effects of being ignored over the internet. *Journal of Personality and Social Psychology*, 79(5), 748–762.

[116] Winston, J. S., Strange, B. A., O'Doherty, J., & Dolan, R. J. (2002). Automatic and intentional brain responses during evaluation of trustworthiness of faces. *Nature Neuroscience*, 5(3), 277–283.

[117] Wolf, I., Dziobek, I., & Heekeren, H. R. (2010). Neural correlates of social cognition in naturalistic settings: A model-free analysis approach. *NeuroImage*, 49(1), 894–904.

[118] Zeki, S. (2007). The neurobiology of love. *Federation of European Biochemical Societies*, 581(14*)*, *2575–2579.*

[119] Zhou, J., Gotch, C., Zhou, Y., & Liu, Z. (2008). Perceiving an object in its context—is the context cultural or perceptual? *Journal of Vision*, 8(12), 1-5.

4

# Social Pain and the Brain: How Insights from Neuroimaging Advance the Study of Social Rejection and Variants of Normal

Richard S. Pond, Jr., Stephanie B. Richman,
David S. Chester and C. Nathan DeWall

## 1. Introduction

Imagine a time when a close loved one has given you the "silent treatment". When describing how this experience made you feel, terms such as "hurt", "pained", and "broken-hearted" may have come to mind. Most everyone at one time or another has experienced the pain of social rejection, whether it was in the form of unrequited love or in the form of punishment, such as when a social click ostracizes an outcast. Over the past decade, social psychologists have conducted a great deal of experimental research to uncover the detrimental effects of social rejection. However, social psychologists are just beginning to understand the neural basis of rejection. In the current chapter, we will review the neuroscientific research on social rejection, and we will discuss the implications from neuroimaging studies that advance theory and research in the area. Specifically, we will highlight how neuroimaging has been used to uncover the neural similarities between physical and social pain.

We will begin this chapter with a brief introduction to social rejection research. Specifically, we will review research that explores the cognitive, emotional, and behavioral consequences of rejection. We will illustrate the effects of rejection within the domains of: antisocial and prosocial behavior, self-regulation, self-defeating behaviors, and intelligent thought. We will end this section with a discussion of the research that suggests an overlap between physical and social pain.

Next we will introduce the neuroscientific approach to the study of social rejection. Specifically, we will review research that has used functional magnetic resonance imaging to help uncover the similarities between social and physical pain. In this section we will focus on activation in the dorsal anterior cingulate cortex and the anterior insula, as they are associated with the affective component of physical and social pain. We will then discuss how acetaminophen, an over-the-counter medication for treating physical pain, reduces activity in these neural regions among rejected people.

Last, we will discuss how neuroimaging has helped social psychologists identify those individuals who are most vulnerable to social rejection. We will review research on the personality characteristics that modulate the neural responses of rejection. Specifically, we will discuss how one's level of attachment anxiety, self-esteem, and emotion differentiation (i.e., aptitude for using discrete emotion categories to capture one's felt experience) either heighten or reduce activity in the neural regions associated with the distress of social rejection.

## 2. Why is there social pain?

The desire for social connection is among the most basic of human motivations. This desire is so strong that is has become known as a need, specifically the "need to belong" (Baumeister & Leary, 1995). All people in all cultures, to at least some degree, have an innate need to form and maintain interpersonal relationships. This need most likely developed over the course of evolutionary history, as social animals like humans have always depended on others for survival. In ancient times, groups provided a variety of advantages to their members (see Axelrod & Hamilton, 1981; Barash, 1977; Buss, 1990, 1991; Hogan et al., 1985; Moreland, 1987). Such advantages include providing mates, sharing resources, and helping to care for offspring. Tasks necessary for survival in ancient times, such as hunting large animals or keeping vigilance against predators, were best accomplished by group cooperation. Even today, people still remain dependent on other people for their survival. Most of us do not grow our own food, sew our own clothes, or build our own houses, just to name a few. Natural selection thus favors those who are motivated to be included, as such people are more likely to survive and reproduce.

In order to ensure that people continued associating with others, they required a system that motivates quick responses to signs of exclusion and punishes those who do not avoid it (MacDonald & Leary, 2005). Such a system would motivate people to identify social acceptance and seek out interpersonal relationships. Over time, humans have developed such a system. The "need to belong" creates in people a fundamental need for positive, enduring relationships with others as well as aversive reactions to a lack of social connection (Baumeister & Leary, 1995). The joy people experience after satisfying their need to belong in a group setting, as well as the consequences they face after their state of belongingness is thwarted, should work as a motivating factor to avoid social exclusion and seek out interpersonal relationships.

## 3. Responses to social pain

If the need to belong is not met or if it is thwarted, people suffer a host of deleterious physical and psychological consequences. Social exclusion thwarts the need to belong, because it is directly contrary to the desired state of social acceptance. Thus, as we present below, exclusion is extremely aversive and people's bodies and minds react accordingly. Exclusion leads people to feel social pain, similar to how being injured leads people to feel physical pain. Additional consequences of social exclusion include impairments in cognitive functioning, increased aggressive behavior, self-defeating behavior, and self-regulatory deficits. Social exclusion can lead to positive behaviors as well, but only if such behaviors have a chance of promoting social acceptance. Each of these consequences to social exclusion will be presented and discussed in the sections below.

### 3.1. Cognitive responses

Social exclusion reduces cognitive performance. Participants who were told they would end up alone later in life (future alone condition), compared to those who were told they would have lots of friends (future belonging condition) or those who were told they would be accident-prone (misfortune control), attempted fewer problems and answered fewer questions correctly on the General Mental Abilities Test (Baumeister et al., 2002: for a description of the GMAT see Janda, 1996 and Janda et al., 1995). Participants in the future alone condition also performed worse on difficult GRE questions about a passage they had read, compared to those in the other two conditions. Finally, future alone participants were no different in their ability to correctly recall nonsense syllables but did show relatively poor performance on analytical GRE questions, compared to participants in the two control conditions (Baumeister et al., 2002). Social exclusion leads to cognitive deficits that specifically impair logic and reasoning ability, although not simple recall. These findings speak to the view that exclusion leads to a deficit in controlled processes and executive functions, potentially because of the need to devote one's self-regulatory resources to stifling emotional distress brought about by social exclusion.

### 3.2. Impact on self-control

As suggested above, social exclusion may impact one's use of self-regulatory resources. Indeed, social exclusion does deplete people's self-regulatory energy. For example, participants who were told they would end up alone later in life, compared to those who were told that they would have lots of friends or those who were told that they would be accident-prone, were less able to make themselves drink a healthy, but bad-tasting beverage (Baumeister et al., 2005). Participants who were excluded by being told no one in a group wanted to work with them ate more cookies in a taste-testing exercise than those who were told everyone in a group wanted to work with them (Baumeister et al., 2005). Excluded participants also persisted less on a frustrating task and performed worse on a dichotic listening task compared to non-excluded participants (Baumeister et al., 2005). Self-regulation is critical in overcoming one's impulses. Decreased ability to eat healthy foods despite their taste, as well as overcoming the desire to eat unhealthy foods and ignoring distractions, are prime examples of self-regulatory failure. Thus, these studies indicate that participants who have just experienced social exclusion are relatively more unwilling or unable to self-regulate effectively.

Perhaps due to these self-regulatory deficits, socially excluded people engage in a variety of self-defeating behaviors. Excluded participants, compared to non-excluded participants, were more likely to choose to participate in a relatively riskier lottery (i.e. one that had an overall lower net gain and in which losing also included listening to aversive noise; Twenge et al., 2002). Excluded participants were also more likely than their non-excluded counterparts to choose a variety of unhealthy over healthy behaviors. These included choosing to eat unhealthier foods, reading entertainment magazines instead of receiving feedback about their health, and opting to receive a resting versus running pulse measure (Twenge et al., 2002). Finally, excluded participants were more likely to procrastinate rather than prepare for an upcoming test, compared to non-excluded participants (Twenge et al., 2002). Following social exclusion, people are more likely to engage in behaviors that are contrary to their own interests.

### 3.3. Behavioral responses: Aggression versus altruism

Not only is social exclusion associated with self-defeating behavior, it is also associated with retaliation. Social exclusion is robustly associated with aggressive behavior (see Leary & Quinlivan, 2006 for a review). Excluded individuals, compared to their non-excluded counterparts, give more damagingly negative job candidate evaluations, make strangers listen to annoying tape recordings, blast strangers with more intense and prolonged noise, and dole out large amounts of hot sauce to people who express a strong dislike for spicy food. Excluded people act more aggressively not only toward their rejecters, but also towards members of a similar social group and even towards people completely unassociated with the rejecters (DeWall et al., 2010). The link between rejection and aggression also extends beyond the laboratory. Feeling rejected is one of the most common precipitating factors associated with domestic violence, in which men murder their wives (Barnard et al., 1982; Crawford & Gartner, 1992). Feeling rejected is also associated with aggression among women towards their husbands (Downey et al., 1998). Finally, there is some evidence that suggests school shootings are associated with social rejection (Leary et al., 2003). Across a variety of different situations both inside and outside a laboratory setting, rejection leads to aggression.

It does not always lead to aggression, however. When the target is the rejecter or when there is no hope for social reconnection, rejected people will act aggressively. In this case, there is no reason for excluded people to overcome their aggressive impulses. However, when it is possible to regain social acceptance, excluded people are motivated to act in a way that will regain their acceptance (see DeWall & Richman, 2011 for a review). Excluded participants, compared to non-excluded participants, awarded more money to a partner based on their partner's average drawing, even though doing so meant they were less likely to win the money back (Maner et al., 2007). This effect only held up if excluded participants expected to meet their partner (thus having the possibility of social reconnection.) If they did not, they had no motivation to behave prosocially and assigned less money to their partner than non-excluded participants did. Participants will behave prosocially in a group setting as well, if doing so can lead to social acceptance. Socially excluded participants, particularly those who were highly sensitive to rejection, ingratiated themselves by contributing more money to a group task than non-excluded participants (Romero-Canyas et al., 2010). Socially excluded people will behave more prosocially if doing so can buy their acceptance.

### 3.4. Emotional responses

Thus far we know how social exclusion affects people both cognitively and behaviorally. Excluded people seem to experience a deficit in controlled processes and executive function as indicated by decreased cognitive performance and self-regulation as well as increased self-defeating behavior and aggression. One hypothesis for this effect is that exclusion causes emotional distress, which requires the use of cognitive resources to reduce its impact. Given what we know about the importance of belongingness (e.g. Baumeister & Leary, 1995), social exclusion should be a distressing and aversive experience. Thus after social exclusion, we would expect participants to report greater negative emotional states than accepted participants. However, empirical research shows that this is not the case. Socially excluded people often report emotional states that do not significantly differ from participants in acceptance or control conditions (Baumeister et al., 2002; Gardner et al., 2000; Twenge et al., 2001; Twenge & Campbell, 2003; Twenge et al., 2002; Zadro et al., 2004). Why are excluded participants numb to negative emotional distress?

One reason socially excluded people report numbness to negative emotional states may be that exclusion leads to a defensive state of cognitive deconstruction (DeWall & Baumeister, 2006). The deconstructed state (Baumeister, 1990) is characterized by emotional numbness, an altered perception of time, thoughts of meaninglessness, lethargy, and avoidance of self-focused attention. Socially excluded people show all of these behaviors (Twenge et al., 2003), suggesting that exclusion may bring about the deconstructed state. This deconstructed state may also explain the deficits in controlled processes as well as the increases in aggressive behavior exhibited by people who have been socially excluded. It may offer excluded people a temporary reprieve from feeling the intense pain or distress that can accompany threats to belongingness. However, after the reprieve, the social pain returns.

## 4. Overlap between social and physical pain

As we have hinted thus far, social and physical pain have much in common. Just as people experiencing social pain suffer deficits in self-regulation and executive functioning, so too do people experiencing physical pain suffer these same consequences. The similarities between the two types of pain extend beyond their consequences. Social and physical pain have numerous other psychological and physiological similarities. For this reason, we propose that severe social pain impacts the body in a similar way as physical injury.

### 4.1. Consequences of physical pain

The consequences of experiencing physical pain are very similar to those of experiencing social pain. People who are in physical pain, similar to people in social pain, experience deficits in cognitive functioning and self-regulation as well as engage in a variety of self-defeating behaviors (for a review, see Solberg Nes et al., 2009). For example, just as people in social pain experience cognitive deficits that impair their logic and reasoning ability, so too do people in physical pain. In particular, chronic pain patients perform relatively worse on tasks that measure working and recognition memory, free recall, verbal fluency, and vocabulary (Landro et al., 1997; Park et al., 2001). Physical pain decreases cognitive functioning on a variety of tasks.

Additionally, similar to participants who are experiencing social pain, participants experiencing physical pain engage in more self-defeating behavior. For example, passive (e.g. relying on doctors, avoiding activities) instead of active (e.g. problem-solving, aiming to control pain) strategies of coping are less likely to help chronic pain patients (Callahan, 2000; Ferrando et al., 2004; Keefe et al., 1989; Snow-Turek et al., 1996; Zautra, 1999). Despite this knowledge, however, chronic pain patients are more likely to attempt to manage their pain through passive strategies (Callahan, 2000; Zautra, 1999). They are also less likely to engage in physical activity (Brown & Nicassio, 1987; Epker & Gatchel, 2000), another behavior that is encouraged and beneficial to the patients' recovery (Abel et al., 2005; Burckardt, 2002; Carlson et al., 2001; Nichols & Glenn, 1992; Smith et al., 2006). Thus, people experiencing chronic physical pain, just like people experiencing social pain, engage in behaviors that are contrary to their own interests.

### 4.2. Psychological similarities

Physical and social pain share several psychological and physiological similarities in addition to their shared consequences. For example, physical pain shares a linguistic similarity with social pain. People describing social pain use metaphors to physical pain such as "broken hearted," "emotionally scarred," or "crushed" (MacDonald & Leary, 2005). In the English language, not only do people describe social pain with reference to physical pain, but there is literally no way to describe it without making that reference (Leary & Springer, 2001). This linguistic link can be found across a wide variety of languages and cultures, including German, Hebrew, Mandarin, and Inuktitut, as well as at least 10 others. (MacDonald & Leary, 2005). Although the linguistic similarity between social and physical pain does not give direct proof of an overlap between their mechanisms, it does show that people think of social and physical pain in extremely similar ways. If social and physical pain share a common psychological or physiological basis, there should be evidence of a crossover between the two types of pain. Specifically, more extreme physical pain should be associated with increased sensitivity to social pain and vice versa. Indeed, the similarity goes beyond mere metaphor.

Personality traits related to a fear of social pain are also associated with pain tolerance, giving further evidence to a relationship between physical and social pain. Introverts, people who are overall less social and more afraid of rejection, have a lower pain tolerance than extraverts, people who are overall more social and less afraid of rejection (Phillips & Gatchel, 2000). This research demonstrates that people who have a lower tolerance for social pain also have a lower tolerance for physical pain. The connection between fear of social pain and pain tolerance is known to work in the opposite direction as well. Increased physical pain, such as chronic pain sufferers experience over time, is associated with behaviors indicative of a fear of social pain.

Chronic pain sufferers become more introverted, socially anxious, and avoidant of social situations the longer their chronic pain continues (Phillips & Gatchel, 2000; Sharp & Harvey, 2001). As people continue to experience physical pain, they become increasingly averse to social pain. These findings show a clear link between physical and social pain. They support the idea that both physical and social pain are managed by the same psychological and physiological systems.

### 4.3. Physiological similarities

Evidence for physiological overlap in physical and social pain stems from the early work of Panksepp and colleagues (Herman & Panksepp, 1978; Panksepp et al., 1978; Panksepp et al, 1978). They noticed the many similarities between the two types of pain and proposed an evolutionary explanation. They hypothesized that the link between social and physical pain exists because evolution piggybacked these neurological systems on top of each other. Animals needed to adapt to increasing social interaction and instead of creating an entirely new system for doing so, evolution used an already existing one. It piggybacked responses to social pain onto the existing systems hard-wired to respond to physical pain. The result of these shared systems is that social events will activate the body's pain response system and possibly have repercussions on how it registers physical pain. This explanation would account for the similarities we have discussed so far, but what evidence do we have for it?

Psychobiological research supports this evolutionary theory and indicates at least two such systems that respond to both physical and social pain. The periaqueductal gray (PAG) brain structures, which receive input from the body's injury detection system (nociceptive system), and anterior cingulated cortex (ACC) are involved in both the detection of physical pain and in animal bonding behavior (Craig & Dostrovsky, 1999). Activation of the PAG elicits separation distress cries from rats (Panksepp, 1998) and lesions to this area lead to reduced separation distress cries (Wiedenmayer et al., 2000). Young rats detect separation from their mother, an occurrence that is socially painful, by means of the same system that detects physical injury. Similarly, lesioning the cingulate eliminates separation distress in hamsters and squirrel monkeys (Maclean & Newman, 1988; Murphy et al., 1981). Administration of oxytocin and opiods such as morphine, used to diminish physical pain, also lead to reduced social pain in the form of reduced separation distress cries in rats (Carden et al., 1996; Carden & Hofer, 1990; Insel & Winslow, 1991). Pharmacological physical pain relief soothes distressed young rats that have been separated from their mothers. These findings indicate that the PAG and ACC are systems that respond to both physical and social pain.

Additional evidence for the overlap between physical and social pain mechanisms stems from research showing that physical pain can be alleviated by social support. Social support, which alleviates social pain, also alleviates physical pain across a variety of situations. Increased social support is associated with reduced chronic pain (Phillips & Gatchel, 2000), labor pain (Klaus et al., 1986; Niven, 1985), cardiac pain (Chalmers et al., 1995; Cogan & Spinnato, 1988), and postoperative pain (Lidderdale & Walsh, 1998). The link between physical pain and social support has also been demonstrated experimentally, which showed that participants had a higher pain threshold, as measured by the cold pressor task (i.e., participants immersed one hand into a container of ice cold water and kept it there until they could no longer tolerate it) when social support was applied before the experience (Brown et al., 2003). Social support can buffer both physical and social pain. This suggests that social and physical pain share many of the same psychological and physiological mechanisms.

### 4.4. Social pain causes physical numbness

Experimental evidence gives further support to the shared mechanisms between the physical and social pain systems. While social support alleviates physical pain, social pain results in physical numbness. That is, socially painful events can have an analgesic effect (i.e., decreased sensitivity to physical pain). As we mentioned earlier, humans experience emotional numbness following social exclusion in the lab (e.g. Baumeister et al., 2002). A similar phenomena is also found among nonhuman animals. Isolation, a phenomenon that is associated with social pain, produces reduced sensitivity to physical pain in rat pups (Kehoe & Blass, 1986a, 1986b; Naranjo & Fuentes, 1985; Spear et al., 1985), mice (Konecka & Sroczynska, 1990), cows (Rushen et al., 1999), and chicks (Sufka & Hughes, 1990; Sufka & Weed, 1994).

Recent research shows that exclusion also produces insensitivity to physical and emotional pain in people. Participants who were told they would end up alone later in life, compared to those who were told they would have lots of friends or those who were told they would be accident-prone, showed significantly higher pain thresholds as evidenced by resisting greater amounts of pressure from a pressure algometer (DeWall & Baumeister, 2006). Exclusion also affected emotional forecasting, simulating emotional responses to possible future events. Excluded participants, compared to those in the two control conditions, predicted relatively neutral emotional reactions to their college football game winning and losing against a rival team (DeWall & Baumeister, 2006). Excluded participants also exhibited significantly less empathy for a person experiencing social pain compared to participants in either control condition. Importantly, increased pain threshold and tolerance scores were a significant predictor of empathy scores. Thus, the increased threshold and tolerance for physical pain following exclusion was related to lack of empathic concern for others. These results were replicated for feeling empathy toward a person in physical pain as well (DeWall & Baumeister, 2006). Next we will introduce the neuroscientific approach to the study of social rejection, reviewing research that has used functional magnetic resonance imaging to help uncover the neural similarities between social and physical pain.

## 5. Neuroscience and social rejection

While the use of a biologically-based approach to understand social-psychological processes can be dated to Ancient Greece and Galen's four humours, neuroscience has only been substantially used to investigate this topic in the past decade or so (Lieberman, 2007). In this time, we have seen a diminished viewpoint among scholars that looking at the brain to understand the complex world of human social dynamics is an irredeemably reductionist endeavor, as well as the emergence of the field of social neuroscience (a.k.a. social cognitive neuroscience) replete with its own dedicated organizations, conferences and journals (see

Harmon-Jones & Winkielman, 2007). As testament to this exponential growth, the number of PsycINFO database hits that return from a search of the term *social neuroscience* have multiplied by an order of more than 16 from 2000 to 2007 (Harris, 2009). Functional magnetic resonance imaging (hereafter fMRI) has been at the forefront of the charge in this neuroscientific revolution of social psychology, providing an unobtrusive avenue through which to elucidate the human mind by measuring the hemodynamic functions of the brain.

As social neuroscience has burgeoned over the past 10-15 years, so has research on social rejection. As we have shown so far in this chapter, conventional methodologies such as overt behavior and self-report have dominated this area of inquiry and have revealed a dizzying amount of information about the powerful and dynamic nature of social rejection. However, as social phenomena are increasingly placed under the lens of investigators using neuroimaging techniques, the literature on social rejection has become infused with a wealth of brain research, though often from researchers without that goal in mind. For instance, Roy Baumeister and Mark Leary's Belongingness Hypothesis (1995), which posits that humans are consummately social beings that require social bonds in the similarly urgent way that they require food and water, was unintentionally substantiated by cognitive neuroscientists who found that the default mode network's regions (i.e., dorsomedial prefrontal cortex, medial prefrontal cortex, ventromedial prefrontal cortex, precuneus, the tempoparietal junction, fusiform gyrus, and temporal poles) are strikingly similar to those involved in social cognition (for a review see Lieberman, 2010). For instance, these areas are crucial for making sense of other people's minds (i.e., mentalizing), for empathizing with others and making moral judgments, as well as for reflecting and forming knowledge about the self (Lieberman, 2010). Thus, when people are not doing other tasks, they engage in thoughts about themselves and their social relationships. Only a remarkably social species would have evolved a brain which, given a lack of external preoccupation, 'prefers' to engage in socially-relevant mental activity. Additional fMRI studies revealed that activation in the ventral striatum, a brain region associated with the feeling of reward, was associated with positive social feedback about oneself (Izuma et al., 2008) and altruistic helping of others (Moll et al., 2006). Demonstrating such a pervasive social-preoccupation and prosocial-orientation of the human brain implicates social rejection as one of the largest threats to our well-being.

Aside from the neuroscience studies that have incidentally advanced the field of social rejection research, relatively few studies have focused explicitly on the topic. Importantly, these studies have garnered a colossal degree of interest (and controversy) from the scientific community and the general populace. For example, the first published fMRI study on social rejection (Eisenberger et al., 2003) has been cited over 400 times in less than eight years. Later in this chapter, we will go into detail about several of these experiments, but beforehand we would like to discuss the features of functional neuroimaging that have made them so impactful.

## 6. Advantages of functional neuroimaging in social rejection research

Given that social rejection research has flourished with the use of conventional measurements such as self-report, overt behavior, and response-time, why should any researcher opt to use neuroimaging techniques in this line of investigation (or any other for that matter)? We argue that functional neuroimaging, fMRI in particular, is a necessary toolbox to fully understand complex social processes, given a laundry list of beneficial attributes that are not available through conventional methodologies. As a most evident benefit, neuroimaging data is not confounded by the psychometric imprecision that is often commensurate with self-report and certain behavioral measures such as response bias and introspective inaccuracy. Additionally, neuroimaging techniques allow researchers to meaningfully distinguish and associate psychological processes on the virtue of whether they are associated with similar or dissimilar neural regions (Lieberman, 2007). Neuroimaging alone can determine when two psychological processes reflect *different* neural mechanisms despite being experientially *similar*, or conversely, when two psychological processes reflect *similar* neural mechanisms despite being perceived as *different*. As an example of the latter capability of fMRI, the medial prefrontal cortex activates similarly to judgments that focus on the self and other individuals who have close relationships with us (Mitchell et al., 2006). By associating or disassociating such mental states, we can further our understanding of the dynamic interactions in the mind and how the brain's structure influences the expression of our thoughts, feelings and behavior. Furthermore, by describing psychological mechanisms in terms of their neural correlates, neuroimaging replaces the often abstract and subjective definitions produced by conventional methods with more objective delineations. Instead of referring to an arbitrarily-defined cognitive sub-mechanism (e.g., the visuospatial sketchpad), we can discuss the neuroanatomical region(s) that process is associated with, its size and position in the brain, the connections that region has to other brain areas and the effects which those connections have (i.e., inhibitory, excitatory). By doing so, psychologists and neuroscientists alike ground models of the mind in concrete parameters that are readily translatable to other fields such as medical and biological sciences. Not only can neuroimaging data help with advances in medical and pharmacological treatments, but can also serve as the basis for understanding behavioral processes, as a result of the novel hypotheses generated via the fMRI technology, which elucidates physiological underpinnings. These powerful advantages of functional neuroimaging are the forces driving the productivity and quality of fMRI research on social rejection.

## 7. Exemplary fMRI studies on social rejection

Now we will focus on four of the aforementioned advantages of adopting neuroimaging methodologies. Each advantage will be accompanied by an fMRI study on social rejection that exemplifies it. It is our hope that in this section we will demonstrate that social rejection research is a line of inquiry that has substantially benefited from the use of fMRI techniques and that these material gains argue for the necessity of functional neuroimaging to understand complex social phenomena. Summary information for each study can be found below in Figure 1 and in Table 1.

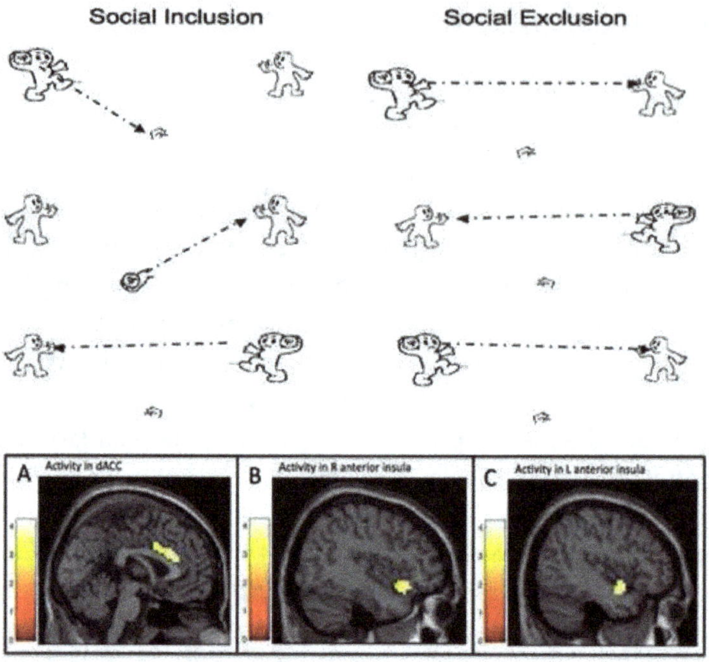


**Figure 1.** The top represents example stimuli from the Cyberball game used in fMRI research on social rejection. Participants typically play the inclusion round during the first scan and the exclusion round during the second scan. The bottom shows areas in the brain that are associated with the affective component of pain (i.e., dACC and anterior insula) which also become activated during exclusion (vs. inclusion) in the Cyberball paradigm.

| Study: | Paradigm: | Analysis of Interest: | Regions of Interest: |
|---|---|---|---|
| Eisenberger et al., 2003 | Cyberball paradigm: 1st scan = included 50% of time 2nd scan = excluded after 7 throws | Whole-brain analysis: Exclusion vs. Inclusion | dACC, RVPFC |
| Eisenberger et al., 2007 | Cyberball paradigm: 1st scan = included 50% of time 2nd scan = excluded after 7 throws | Region of interest regressions with: Daily social support, Cortisol reactivity, Distress | dACC, DSFG |
| DeWall et al., 2010 | Cyberball paradigm: 1st scan = included 33% of time 2nd scan = excluded after 3 throws | Region of interest regression with: Tylenol condition | dACC, anterior insula, amygdala |
| Masten et al., 2011 | Cyberball paradigm: 1st scan = included 33% of time 2nd scan = excluded after 10 throws | Region of interest regression with: Observer ratings of distress, Attributions of discrimination, Self-reported distress | dACC, anterior insula |

**Table 1.** Summary of the studies presented in Section 7. Neural activity of interest is during exclusion vs. inclusion.

### 7.1. Associating seemingly-distinct psychological processes based on shared neural substrates: Eisenberger et al., 2003

Naomi Eisenberger and her colleagues (2003) were not only the first researchers to report fMRI findings on social rejection, but their results confirmed a striking hypothesis that social injury elicits a nearly identical neural response as harm to one's *soma*. To achieve these results, they adapted a computerized, ball-tossing task (Cyberball: Williams et al., 2000) to the fMRI environment that immersed participants in experiences of social acceptance and rejection. Participants were told that they would play a virtual ball-tossing game inside the scanner, via the Internet, with two other participants who were also in scanners. In reality, computer programs represented the other players. During the first round of the game, participants were included (i.e., received a ball toss from one of the virtual players) throughout the round. However, during the second round, the virtual players stopped throwing the participant the ball after he or she had received three throws. Participants were excluded for the remainder of the game and watched as the two virtual players continued without them. After the scanning procedures, participants reported the degree of social distress (a facet of social pain) they experienced due to the rejection manipulation. Traditionally, the neurological mechanisms of pain have been separated into three components: 1. the sensory component, 2. the affective-motivational component, and 3. the evaluative component (Melzack & Casey, 1968). In their study, Eisenberger and colleagues (2003) discovered neural activation that was specific to social rejection in three brain regions previously associated with the affective component of physical pain (e.g., Bush et al., 2000; Carter et al., 2000; Foltz & White, 1968; Lieberman et al., 2007; Price, 2000; Rainville et al., 1997). One of these regions was the dorsal portion of the anterior cingulate cortex (hereafter dACC), a key region for the affective component of pain (see Apkarian et al., 2005 for a review ), which is often conceptualized as an 'alarm system' that monitors the external environment for elements that deviate from the ideal (Bush et al., 2000; Carter et al., 2000). It then responds by eliciting feelings of distress that motivate the individual to repair or assuage the discrepancy (see Eisenberger & Lieberman, 2004). The second region was the anterior portion of the insula, a cortical structure previously associated with both negative affect (e.g., Lane et al., 1997) and visceral pain (e.g., Aziz et al., 2000). Last, this study reported activation in two voxel-clusters of the right-ventral prefrontal cortex (hereafter RVPFC), an area of the neocortex which functions to regulate aversive experiences (e.g., Petrovic & Ingvar, 2002). As predicted, activation in the dACC predicted *greater* levels of social distress, while conversely, the RVPFC predicted *lesser* amounts of social distress. DACC activation also mediated the inhibitory relationship between the RVPFC and social distress, suggesting that the RVPFC reduces subjective distress to social threat by inhibiting the dACC response to it. Taken together, these results are astoundingly analogous to those from physical pain research (e.g., Foltze & White, 1968; Kong et al., 2006; Petrovic et al., 2005; Rainville et al., 1997), establishing the functional similarity between physical and social pain, which has great implications for the understanding and treatment of various psychopathologies, such as post-traumatic stress disorder (PTSD; Felmingham et al., 2007) and anxiety (Simmons et al., 2008). Perhaps most importantly, these findings suggest that maintaining social connections should be conceptualized as a fundamental human need, to the same degree as physical safety, since evolution has given the two equal standing as evidenced by the same neural underpinnings.

The Eisenberger and colleagues (2003) study is exemplary in another related way, in that it largely resolved a decades-long line of research that was previously relegated to harmful experiments on nonhuman animals. Various researchers have suspected the possible social/physical pain overlap that we have discussed here in detail, but since functional neuroimaging techniques were not yet available, their research has taken such forms as measuring the distress vocalizations of socially-isolated bird chicks (Panksepp et al., 1978) and ablating the cingulate cortex of squirrel monkeys (MacLean & Newman, 1988). Thanks to fMRI, it is no longer necessary for a great deal of research questions to be performed on nonhuman animals, who contribute results that are not always readily translatable to humankind and who are often harmed in the process.

### 7.2. Translating psychological processes to their biological mechanisms: Eisenberger et al., 2007

While research on social rejection and isolation had established that a prolonged lack of interpersonal connections is extremely deleterious to physical and mental health (e.g., House et al., 1988; Berkman & Syme, 2007), the biological mechanisms through which this process occurred was largely unknown. Capitalizing on the unique ability of neuroimaging to lay bare the brain's response to social rejection in a format which could then be statistically assessed in relation to other biological processes, Naomi Eisenberger and her colleagues (2007) pitted two popular hypotheses of how social connections improve health outcomes against one another. In these hypotheses, which are not necessarily mutually exclusive, social bonds:

**a.** lessen the extent to which events are perceived as threatening via reduced activation in brain regions associated with HPA activation (namely the dACC, amygdala and insula).

and/or

**b.** increase the coping resources an individual can apply to a threat via greater activation of 'top-down' brain regions associated with self-regulation (namely the ventrolateral- and medial-prefrontal cortices).

Both of these postulated mechanisms would down-regulate the hypothalamic-pituitary-adrenal axis (hereafter HPA axis) response to threats, the activation of which releases the stress hormone, cortisol, into the bloodstream (i.e., cortisol reactivity). Since cortisol suppresses the immune system, both of the aforementioned explanations would ultimately protect individuals by preventing the reduced immune-function that is commensurate with the physiological stress response. To test these competing theories, participants had endogenous cortisol measurements taken before and after a stress-inducing task, with increases in cortisol over the course of the stressful task indicating a larger degree of cortisol reactivity. Self-reported social distress was recorded from each participant immediately after the stress task as well. Over the following 10 days, participants reported the degree of social support they felt at various times throughout that period. At the end of the 10 days, participants had fMRI scans taken of their brain while they performed a variant of the ball-tossing task described in the Eisenberger et al., 2003 study which manipulated experiences of social acceptance and rejection. The authors of the study planned to assess the degree to which neural responses to social rejection were associated with social support, cortisol reactivity during the stress task, and self-reported social distress. The results yielded no support for the hypothesis that social support increases activation in brain regions that would facilitate coping with stressful events, since no neural regions were activated above statistical threshold in the acceptance condition. However, regression analyses on the rejection condition revealed there was substantial evidence for the hypothesis that social support improves physical health by reducing activation in brain regions associated with social distress/pain. Specifically, activation during social rejection in both an *a priori* region-of-interest analysis of the dACC and Brodmann's Area 8 of the dorsal superior frontal gyrus (hereafter DSFG) were both *negatively* correlated with social support and *positively* correlated with both social distress and cortisol reactivity. Rejection-specific activation in both the dACC and DSFG mediated the inhibitory relationship between social support and cortisol reactivity, which implicates these two regions as the mechanism through which social support reduces the physiological stress response. Moreover, rejection-specific activation in the hypothalamus mediated the relationships between the dACC and DSFG and cortisol reactivity. This suggests that the dACC and DSFG influence stress responses by modulating the activity of the HPA axis. Summarizing these findings, this study supports the claim that when people encounter a social threat (e.g., public speaking, social rejection), their everyday levels of social support reduce activation in both the dACC and DSFG. Reduced activation in the dACC and DSFG subsequently reduces HPA axis activation, cortisol release and suppression of the immune system. Aside from the clear implications these findings have for treatments and therapies, this study is a prime example of the process through which functional neuroimaging allows for a more objective delineation of a behavioral response into its physiological components.

### 7.3. Generating novel hypotheses based on physiological principles: DeWall et al., 2010

Recent work from our lab stands as a clear example of the ability of fMRI to produce novel psychological hypotheses based purely on physiological knowledge of neural correlates. Since previous research had established the overlap between brain regions involved in social and physical pain (e.g., Eisenberger et al., 2003), DeWall and colleagues (2010) tested whether a popular physical-pain-reliever, acetaminophen, would have similar analgesic effects for social pain. In the first study, twice-daily ingestion of acetaminophen (compared to placebo) reduced self-reported social pain over a time period of three weeks. To assess whether these self-reports translated to diminished pain responses in the brain, participants who had either taken acetaminophen or placebo twice-daily for three weeks (same as study 1) were placed in an fMRI scanner and then socially-accepted and -rejected by a similar version of the computerized, ball-tossing task used in the two previous studies.

Participants who had taken acetaminophen showed reduced activation (as compared to those who took placebo) during rejection (as compared to acceptance) in both brain regions previously associated with social pain, the dACC and anterior insula. Participants who took acetaminophen also showed lesser activation of the amygdala during social-rejection, a brain region involved in producing 'fight-or-flight' responses. By understanding the physiological similarities between social and physical pain, a novel hypothesis was vetted about a psychological process with powerful implications for our understanding and treatment of social rejection.

### 7.4. Covert measurement of social processes that avoid self-report biases: Masten et al., 2011

Much of the phenomena that interest social psychologists are sensitive to issues of self-presentation and demand characteristics. Thus, psychologists favor measurement tools that avoid or are at least robust to these self-report biases. For example, psychologists interested in studying prejudice may opt for measuring implicit attitudes of their participants, because people may not respond truthfully on self-report questionnaires if holding racist attitudes is looked down upon socially. The fMRI scanner represents a powerful tool that can be used to assess such attitudes in a way that is not subject to self-report biases. A recent rejection study conducted by Masten and colleagues (2011) is an excellent example for how neuroimaging can be utilized to investigate potentially sensitive topics. Specifically, they investigated the neural correlates of negative social treatment associated with racial discrimination.

In their study, African American participants encountered two white (1 male, 1 female) confederates during the informed consent procedure. The participants were told that they would be playing a virtual ball-tossing game (i.e., Cyberball) with the two confederates, while they were each inside fMRI scanners. In reality, participants played the virtual ball-tossing game with a preprogrammed computer. During the initial scan, participants were included by their virtual partners, who threw the ball to the participant one third of the time. However, during the second scan, participants were excluded from their partners after receiving ten throws. After the scanning session, participants completed self-report measures of distress and discriminatory attributions. Observers also rated the participants' level of distress during videotaped interviews, in which the participants discussed their feelings about being excluded during the game.

Using a whole-brain analyses approach, Masten and colleagues (2011) found that exclusion (vs. inclusion) increased activity in the anterior insula, and rACC, and decreased activity in the VLPFC, which was consistent with previous research (Eisenberger et al., 2003, 2007). Yet, in region of interest analyses, self-reported distress was not related to activation in these areas during exclusion, as previous research would suggest. However, observer-rated distress was related to increased activity in the dACC and anterior insula and decreased activity in the VLPFC and ALPFC, which is consistent with previous research. These findings highlight the robustness of fMRI procedures to self-report biases. Last, the authors found that the more participants attributed the exclusion experience to racism, the less activation they experienced in the dACC during exclusion. This last finding suggests that attributing negative social events to discrimination provides a protective function, which allows the individual to better cope with the distress.

## 8. Individual difference factors that moderate neural responses to social rejection

In the previous sections of this chapter, we described how most everyone desires at least some level of social acceptance and that experiences of rejection can have very powerful physical and psychological consequences. We described how the use of fMRI methodologies have helped social psychologists identify the shared neural substrates of physical and social pain, and how this tool has helped psychologists generate and test novel hypotheses about the physiological processes that underlie social pain. In this final section, we will discuss recent research from our lab, which utilized fMRI procedures to identify those individuals who are most vulnerable to social rejection. Specifically, we will concentrate on two individual difference factors that modulate neural responses to rejection, namely one's level of attachment anxiety and one's capacity for identifying and describing emotional experiences. People who are high in attachment anxiety possess an intense desire for intimacy and are highly sensitive to the potential for rejection (Fraley & Shaver, 2000). Thus, they may exhibit heightened neural responses to rejection, compared to individuals who are less anxiously attached. Similarly, people who have a low capacity for identifying and describing their emotional experiences may show heightened neural responses to rejection, because they respond more negatively to stressful situations than people who have a greater capacity for describing their emotions (Barrett et al, 2004; Kashdan et al., 2010; Tugade et al., 2004). Table 2 below presents a brief summary of the two studies that will be described in more detail in sections 8.1 and 8.2

| Study: | Paradigm: | Analysis of Interest: | Regions of Interest: |
|---|---|---|---|
| DeWall et al., 2011a | Cyberball paradigm:<br>1st scan = included 33% of time<br>2nd scan = excluded after 3 throws | Region of interest regressions with:<br>Anxious attachment,<br>Avoidant attachment | dACC,<br>anterior insula |
| DeWall et al., 2011b | Cyberball paradigm:<br>1st scan = included 33% of time<br>2nd scan = excluded after 3 throws | Region of interest regressions with:<br>Emotional differentiation<br>X<br>Self-esteem | dACC,<br>anterior insula |

**Table 2.** Summary of studies presented in Section 8. Neural activity of interest is during exclusion vs. inclusion trials.

### 8.1. Neural responses to rejection depend on attachment style

Prior work has shown that belongingness threats can cause a variety of negative emotional, cognitive, and behavioral outcomes (e.g., Baumeister et al., 2002; DeWall et al., 2009; Twenge et al., 2001, 2003), and that these threats activate some of the same neural substrates as those underlying physical pain (Eisenberger et al., 2003). However, people vary a great deal in how they experience and maintain social relationships. For example, some people may have a high need for social acceptance and are especially attuned to signs of rejection, whereas others may be uncomfortable with close relationships. Such differences in attachment style may have direct implications for neural responses to experiences of rejection.

DeWall and colleagues (2011) tested whether individual differences in anxious and avoidant attachment styles moderated neural responses to social rejection. They predicted that people with high attachment anxiety (depicted as having a great desire for closeness and vigilant to rejection cues; see Fraley & Shaver, 2000) would show heightened neural activity in those regions associated with the processing of social rejection (i.e., dACC and anterior insula). On the other hand, they predicted that those individuals who demonstrated a high level of avoidant attachment (depicted as being uncomfortable with closeness and uses regulatory strategies to minimize attention to attachment-related events and information) would show dampened activity within those same neural regions. In their study, participants completed the Attachment Style Questionnaire (ASQ; Feeney et al., 1994) in the lab, and then returned three weeks later to complete a virtual ball-tossing game in an fMRI scanner. Following Eisenberger and colleagues' (2003, 2007) and DeWall and colleagues' (2010) procedures (i.e., the Cyberball paradigm), participants believed that they were playing the virtual ball-tossing game with two other participants already in fMRI scanners. In reality, computer programs represented the other players. During the first scan, the virtual players regularly tossed the ball to the participants. However, during the second scan, the virtual players excluded those participants who received three throws. After playing the ball-tossing game, participants completed a measure of social distress.

As predicted by DeWall and colleagues (2011), participants with a high level of attachment anxiety exhibited more activity in the dACC and anterior insula while experiencing social exclusion (vs. social inclusion). These results suggest that anxious attachment is associated with greater negative responses to belongingness threats. On the other hand, a high level of avoidant attachment was related to less activation within the dACC and anterior insula during social exclusion (vs. social inclusion). These results suggest that people who reflect the avoidant attachment style detach from attachment-relevant situations, thereby providing a buffer to the negative effects of potential rejection. These findings support and extend prior work on the pain of social rejection. Moreover, they demonstrate how neuroimaging methodologies can be used to allow social psychologists a better understanding of how personality characteristics moderate physiological responses to social situations.

### 8.2. Self-esteem and level of emotional differentiation interact to predict neural responses to rejection

Attachment style represents just one factor that can increase or decrease one's vulnerability to social threats. However, there are surely many other personality characteristics that can intensify or buffer the negative effects of rejection. Self-esteem is one potential factor that has garnered recent attention from social psychologists. People who generally perceive that others reject them tend to have low self-esteem. In contrast, people who generally perceive acceptance from others tend to have high self-esteem (Leary et al., 1995). Using a similar virtual ball-tossing paradigm as the studies above, Onoda and colleagues (2010) have provided some of the first evidence from neuroimaging that people with low self-esteem experience more distress during rejection than people high in self-esteem. They showed that people with low self-esteem exhibit greater activation within the dACC during a simulated rejection experience (vs. inclusion). Similarly, using a social evaluative task, Somerville and colleagues (2010) demonstrated that people with low self-esteem exhibited greater activation in a more ventral area of the anterior cingulate cortex after receiving negative social feedback (versus positive social feedback).

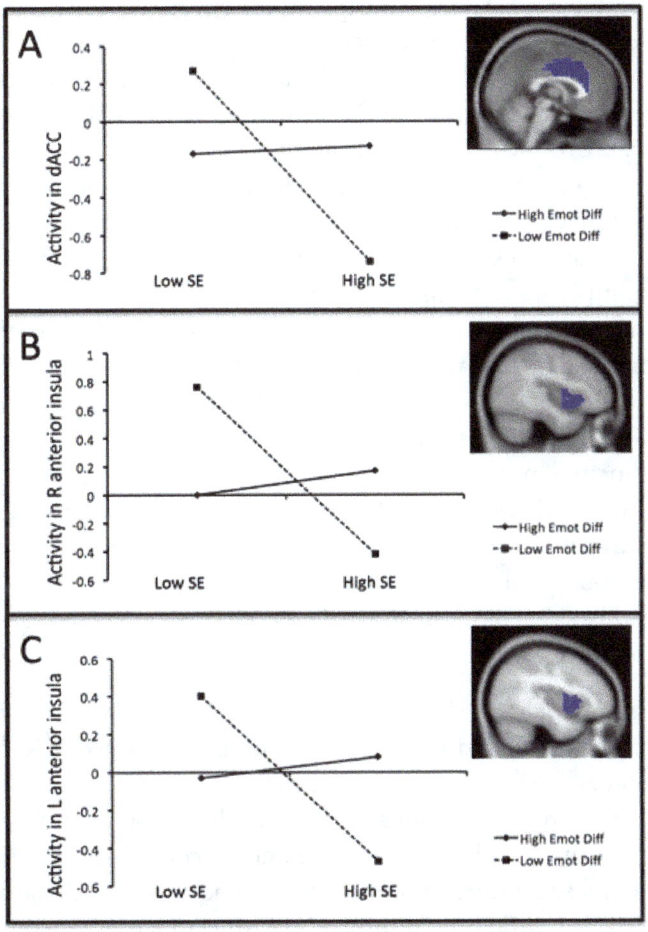


**Figure 2.** Neural activity during exclusion (vs. inclusion) within the dACC (Panel A) and anterior insula (Panels B & C) as a function of self-esteem and emotion differentiation (based on a priori anatomically-defined ROI analyses; significance was defined as $p < .05$). The functionally-defined ROI's are depicted in blue.

Following the work of Onoda and colleagues (2010) and Somerville and colleagues (2010), DeWall and coauthors (2011) explored whether one's capacity for identifying and describing emotional experiences (i.e., emotional differentiation) moderated the effects of self-esteem on neural responses to social rejection. People who are better at differentiating their emotional experiences respond more positively to stress and depend less on maladaptive coping strategies, such as abusing alcohol (Barrett et al, 2004; Kashdan et al., 2010; Tugade et al., 2004). On the other hand, people who are less able to identify and differentiate their emotional experiences react more negatively to stress, possess more negative attitudes, and are more likely to use those maladaptive coping strategies. Thus, DeWall and colleagues (2011) predicted that greater emotional differentiation should be linked to psychological resilience to social rejection experiences. However, among individuals who exhibit a lower capacity for emotional differentiation, those with low self-esteem will be most vulnerable to experiences of rejection, which will be evidenced in heightened responses in the dACC and anterior insula.

In DeWall and colleagues' (2011) study, participants completed daily diary measures of self-esteem and negative emotion for a three-week assessment period. After the diary portion of the study, participants completed the virtual ball-tossing game (i.e., the Cyberball paradigm) with two ostensible partners while in an fMRI scanner (first scan = inclusion round, second scan = exclusion round). Last, participants completed a measure of social distress. All neuroimaging data were preprocessed and analyzed using Statistical Parametric Mapping (SPM8; Wellcome Department of Cognitive Neurology, Institute of Neurology, London, UK). As with the study described in section 8.1, anatomically-defined region of interest (ROI) analyses were implemented based on a priori hypotheses regarding the involvement of the dACC and anterior insula in processing social rejection. Differential activity in each ROI during exclusion vs inclusion was examined, as well as how this activity related to individuals' self-esteem, emotion differentiation, and the interaction between self-esteem and emotion differentiation (significance was defined as $p < .05$). Parameter estimates of activity during exclusion vs inclusion were entered as dependent variables in hierarchical multiple regression analyses, with self-esteem and emotion differentiation scores entered as predictors in the first step and their interaction entered as a predictor in the second step. Finally, supplemental whole-brain analyses were implemented, thresholded at $p < .005$ and 20 voxels for a priori defined regions of interest, while all other regions were examined at a threshold corrected for false discovery rate.

As predicted, regression analyses showed that among low emotional differentiators, lower self-esteem was strongly associated with greater activation in the dACC and the anterior insula during exclusion (vs. inclusion). However, high emotional differentiation bore no relation to activity in these neural regions during exclusion (vs. inclusion), regardless of selfesteem level (see Figure 2). These findings extend prior neuroimaging research linking low self-esteem to increased vulnerability to social rejection, by demonstrating that one's level of emotional differentiation may reinforce or buffer this relationship. Additionally, this research is an example of how neuroimaging can be utilized to explore the physiology of psychological resilience and expand upon prior conclusions drawn from behavioral and/or self-report methodologies.

## 9. Criticisms of the Cyberball paradigm

For the most part, the fMRI literature on social rejection is nested within the Cyberball paradigm (Williams et al., 2000), in which participants believe that they are playing a ball-tossing computer game over the Internet with two other participants who are, ostensibly, also in MRI scanners. However, the nature of the rejection experience during Cyberball is not without its limitations. For example, in order for the rejection manipulation to maintain believability and ecological validity, all participants are included by their virtual partners during the first fMRI scan and excluded by those same partners during the second scan. The blocks must be presented in this order to ensure that all participants have the same expectations from one scan to the next. That is, if the blocks were presented randomly, then those participants who encountered exclusion during the first scan would naturally expect exclusion on the second scan. Inclusion during the second scan might appear unrealistic.

Although the presentation of inclusion blocks and exclusion blocks are not usually randomized in the Cyberball paradigm, follow-up fMRI research has replicated the patterns of brain activation commonly reported with Cyberball, using other manipulations of rejection. For example, participants show increased activity within the dorsal ACC while viewing rejection-themed images as opposed to acceptance-themed images or abstract paintings of positive and negative valence (Kross et al., 2007). Similarly, people show increased dACC activity while viewing pictures with disapproving facial expressions (Burklund et al., 2007). Moreover, Sebastian and colleagues (2010) found that activation within the amygdala and subgenual ACC increased when participants viewed social threat words (e.g., pathetic), as opposed to neutral words, during a rejection-themed emotional Stroop task. They also found an Age x Valence interaction, such that adults who viewed rejection-themed words, in contrast to acceptance or neutral control words, exhibited decreased activity within the right VLPFC. However, this activity was not present in adolescents who viewed the rejection-themed words. This finding suggests that maturation of the right VLPFC, an area associated with affect regulation, continues during adolescence. Last, a recent study conducted by Bolling and colleagues (2011) actually modified the Cyberball paradigm, such that participants played several blocks of the game, which alternated between inclusion and exclusion. They found that participants' self-reported distress after Cyberball was comparable to previous research and did not decline or become less upsetting over time. Additionally, the authors replicated previous research by showing, in whole-brain and region of interest analyses, that brain activity within the ventral anterior cingulate cortex (vACC), the posterior cingulate cortex (PCC), and the right anterior insula increased during exclusion (vs. inclusion). Each of these studies give support for the validity of the Cyberball paradigm for fMRI research.

Another criticism of the Cyberball paradigm for fMRI research is that the manipulation may not be strong enough to mimic the sensation of physical pain, nor is it especially prolonged. Thus, experiences of intense social pain that are drawn out over time may prove to be more beneficial in examining the neural similarities between physical and social pain. For example, a recent study by Kross and colleagues (2011) shows that the overlap between social and physical pain may be more extensive than previously understood. They argued that neural activation during social pain should not just mirror the affective component of physical pain (e.g., activation within the dACC and anterior insula), but if the socially painful experience is extreme enough then it should also mirror the sensory component of physical pain (e.g., activation within the secondary somato-sensory cortex and the dorsal posterior insula). In their study, they recruited participants who have recently experienced an unwanted romantic break-up. Those participants then performed two counterbalanced tasks during an fMRI scanning session: 1. a Social Rejection task, and 2. a Physical Pain task. During the rejection-trials of the social rejection task, participants viewed a headshot of their ex-partner and thought about their specific break-up. During friend-trials of the social rejection task, participants viewed a headshot of a close friend of the same sex as the ex-partner and thought of a positive experience with that friend. During the physical pain task, participants experienced painfully hot thermal stimulation to an area on their left arm during hot trials and non-noxious thermal stimulation to the same area during warm trials. In a whole-brain conjunction analyses and region of interest analyses, the authors found that the brain activation during social rejection overlapped with the brain activation during physical pain in the areas associated with the affective component of pain (i.e., dACC and anterior insula), replicating previous research (e.g., Eisenberger et al., 2003). Moreover, the brain activation during social rejection also overlapped with the brain activation during physical pain in areas associated with the sensory component of pain (i.e., the thalamus and the secondary somatosensory cortex). Thus, one of the implications of this research is that to fully understand the overlap between physical and social pain, researchers must employ stronger manipulations of rejection than what the Cyberball paradigm might provide.

## 10. Future directions

There are many possible directions for future neuroscientific research concerning social pain. One avenue that will provide fruitful exploration concerns how the brain regulates the immune system in response to physical and social threats. The current literature supports the idea that the neural mechanisms for social and physical pain overlap, but how far does this overlap extend and what implications does this overlap have for people in terms of health and disease? A recent study from Slavich and colleagues (2010) provides initial evidence that individual differences in neural responses to social threat may make one more or less susceptible to disease. In their study, participants performed the Trier Social Stress Test (TSST; Kirschbaum et al., 1993), in which they prepared and delivered an unrehearsed speech and performed mental arithmetic in front of a panel of socially rejecting raters. Participants then provided a saliva sample, which was assayed for two markers of inflammatory response: 1. a soluble receptor for tumor necrosis factor-$\alpha$ (sTNF$\alpha$RII) and 2. interleukin-6 (IL-6). At a second laboratory session, a subsample of these participants played the Cyberball game, in which they experienced exclusion, during an fMRI scanning session. The authors found that the TSST increased levels of sTNF$\alpha$RII and IL-6, compared to baseline levels. Once more, in region of interest analyses, increased activity within the dACC and anterior insula during exclusion (vs. inclusion) was associated with increased levels of sTNF$\alpha$RII after the TSST, but not IL-6. These findings give initial evidence that the neural mechanisms underlying social pain are associated with susceptibility to inflammatory responses in socially stressful situations, which has implications for the link between stress and disease.

Another future direction for fruitful research centers around the emerging area of genomic imaging, in which investigators are able to model the neural responses towards a stimulus among individuals genetically predisposed for various characteristics or not. For example, Way and colleagues (2009) conducted initial research that applied this method to the study of social rejection. They were interested in whether variation in the μ-opioid receptor gene (a site where morphine acts) was associated with individual differences in sensitivity to social rejection. In their study, participants completed a rejection sensitivity questionnaire and provided a saliva sample that was assayed for the A118G polymorphism (a measure of the μ-opioid receptor gene). A subsample of participants then completed the Cyberball game, in which they experienced exclusion, during a second laboratory session. The investigators expected that participants with the G allele on the A118G polymorphism would be more sensitive to rejection, because the G allele is related to the reduced potency of opiates. As expected, participants who were G allele carriers reported more sensitivity to rejection. Additionally, in region of interest analyses, activity in the dACC and anterior insula during exclusion (vs. inclusion) was greater for G allele carriers than A allele homozygotes. Moreover, activity in the dACC during exclusion (vs. inclusion) significantly mediated the association between individual variation in the A118G polymorphism and individual differences in rejection sensitivity. These findings provide initial evidence for the genetic overlap between physical and social pain, however much more work still needs to be done in this area.

## 11. Conclusion

Humans are social creatures, and the need to belong is a powerful motivator for sustenance of social integration. Over the past decade, social psychologists have worked hard to understand the consequences of rejection at the cognitive, emotional, and behavioral levels. However, we are just beginning to understand the neural basis underlying social rejection. Recently, social psychologists have been able to apply functional magnetic resonance imaging to this research area. Doing so, we have gained a better understanding of the neural similarities between physical and social pain. Specifically, psychologists have identified the dorsal anterior cingulate cortex and the anterior insula (areas associated with the affective component of physical pain) as particularly important in the processing of social rejection. More recently, researchers have employed fMRI procedures to extend upon this work. Through neuroimaging, psychologists have shown that an over-the-counter medication, acetaminophen, reduces feelings of rejection by dampening activity in the dACC and anterior insula during rejection experiences. Neuroimaging has also been useful in helping researchers identify those individuals who are most vulnerable to social rejection, exclusion, and ostracism.

As technology becomes more advanced and user-friendly, the researcher's toolkit will expand to incorporate new scientific approaches. Functional brain imaging can be applied in a variety of ways to the study of human behavior. This chapter is just one example of an area in which neuroimaging procedures can be easily adapted. Although we don't fully understand the neural basis of social pain, psychologists have been able to gain ground in this area because of the availability of fMRI technology.

The brain is an immensely complex organ. In order to gain a better understanding of the behaviors that it produces, we need to make full use of the research tools at our disposal.

Functional brain imaging can offer valuable insights to the social sciences. These insights lead to better questions, the generation of novel hypotheses, and more elegant methods for testing those hypotheses.

## Author details

Richard S. Pond, Jr., Stephanie B. Richman, David S. Chester and C. Nathan DeWall

University of Kentucky, United States of America

## References

[1] Abell, J.E., Hootman, J.M., Zack, M.M., Moriarty, D., Helmick, C.G. (2005). Physical activityand health related quality of life among people with arthritis. *Journal of Epidemiology and Community Health,* Vol. 59, No.5, (May 2005), pp. 380–385, ISSN 1470-2738.

[2] Apkarian, A.V., Bushnell, M.C., Treede, R., & Zubieta, J. (2005). Human brain mechanisms of pain perception and regulation in health and disease. *European Journal of Pain,* Vol.9, No.4, (August 2005), pp. 463–484, ISSN 1090-3801.

[3] Axelrod, R., & Hamilton, W.D. (1981). The evolution of cooperation. *Science.* Vol. 211,No.4489, (March 1981), pp. 1390-1396, ISSN 0036-8075.

[4] Aziz, Q., Schnitzler, A., & Enck, P. (2000). Functional neuroimaging of visceral sensations. *Journal of Clinical Neurophysiology,* Vol.17, No.6, (November 2000), pp. 604-612, ISSN 0736-0258.

[5] Barash. D.P. (1977). *Sociobiology and behavior,* Elsevier, ISBN 0444990364, New York.

[6] Barnard, G.W., Vera, H., Vera, M.I., & Newman, G. (1982). Til death do us part: A study of spouse murder. *Bulletin of the American Academy of Psychiatry and the Law,* Vol. 10, No.4, (December 1982), pp. 271-280, ISSN 7165803.

[7] Barrett, L.F., Tugade, M.M., & Engle, R.W. (2004). Individual differences in working memory capacity and dual-process theories of the mind. *Psychological Bulletin,* Vol. 130, No.4, (July 2004), pp.553-573, ISSN 00332909.

[8] Baumeister, R.F. (1990). Suicide as escape from the self. Psychological Review, Vol. 97, No.1,(January 1990), pp. 90-113, ISSN 1939-1471.

[9] Baumeister, R.F., & Leary, M.R. (1995). The need to belong: Desire for interpersonal attachments as a fundamental human motivation. *Psychological Bulletin,* Vol.117, No. 3, (May 1995), pp. 497-529, ISSN 0033-2909.

[10] Baumeister, R.F., Twenge, J.M., & Nuss, C.K. (2002). Effects of social exclusion on cognitive processes: Anticipated aloneness reduces intelligent thought. *Journal of Personality and Social Psychology,* Vol.83, No.4, (October 2002), pp. 817-827, ISSN 1939-1315.

[11] Baumeister, R.F., DeWall, C.N., Ciarocco, N.J., & Twenge, J.M. (2005). Social exclusion impairs self-regulation. *Journal of Personality and Social Psychology,* Vol.88, No.4 (April 2005), pp. 589-604, ISSN 1939-1315.

[12] Berkman, L.F., & Syme, S.L. (1979). Social networks, host resistance, and mortality: A nine-year follow-up study of Alameda county residents. *American Journal of Epidemiology,* Vol.109, No.2, (February 1979), pp. 186-204, ISSN 0002-9262.

[13] Bolling, D.Z., Pitskel, N.B., Deen, B., Crowley, M.J., McPartland, J.C., Mayes, L.C., & Pelphrey, K.A. (2011). Dissociable brain mechanisms for processing social exclusion and rule violation. *Neuroimage,* Vol.54, No.3, (February 2011), pp. 2462-2471, ISSN 1095-9572.

[14] Brown, G., & Nicassio, P. (1987). Development of a questionnaire for the assessment of active and passive coping strategies in chronic pain patients. *Pain.* Vol.31, No.1, (October 1987), pp. 53–64, ISSN 0304-3959.

[15] Brown, J.L., Sheffield, D., Leary, M.R., & Robinson, M.E. (2003). Social support and experimental pain. *Psychosomatic Medicine,* Vol.65, No.2, (March-April 2003), pp.276–283, ISSN 1534-7796.

[16] Buckley, K., Winkel, R., & Leary, M.R. (2004). Reactions to acceptance and rejection: Effects of level and sequence of relational evaluation. *Journal of Experimental Social Psychology,* Vol.40, No.1, (January 2004), pp.14-28, ISSN 0022-1031.

[17] Burckardt, C.S. (2002). Nonpharmacologic management strategies in fibromyalgia. *Rheumatic Disease Clinics of North America,* Vol.28, No.2, (May 2002), pp. 291–304, ISSN 0889-857X.

[18] Burklund, L.J., Eisenberger, N.I., & Lieberman, M.D. (2007). The face of rejection: Rejection sensitivity moderates dorsal anterior cingulated activity to disapproving facial expressions. *Social Neuroscience,* Vol.2, No.3–4, (July 2007), pp. 238–253, ISSN 1747-0919.

[19] Bush, G., Luu, P., & Posner, M.I. (2000). Cognitive and emotional influences in anterior cingulated cortex. *Trends in Cognitive Sciences,* Vol.4, No.6, (June 2000), pp. 215–222, ISSN 1879-307X.

[20] Buss, D.M. (1990). The evolution of anxiety and social exclusion. *Journal of Social and Clinical Psychology,* Vol.9, No.2, (June 1990), pp. 196-210, ISSN 0736-7236.

[21] Buss, D.M. (1991). Evolutionary personality psychology. *Annual Review of Psychology,* Vol. 42, pp. 459-491, ISSN 0-8243-0242-7.

[22] Callahan, C.D. (2000). Stress, coping, and personality hardiness in patients with temporomandibular disorders. *Rehabilitative Psychology,* Vol.45, No.1, (February 2000), pp. 38–48, ISSN 1939-1544.

[23] Carden, S.E., & Hofer, M.A. (1990). Socially mediated reduction of isolation distress in rat pups is blocked by naltrexone but not by Ro 15–1788. *Behavioral Neuroscience,* Vol. 104, No.3, (June 1990), pp. 457–463, ISSN 1939-0084.

[24] Carden, S.E., Hernandez, N., & Hofer, M.A. (1996). The isolation and companion comfort responses of 7- and 3-day-old rat pups are modulated by drugs active at the opioid receptor. *Behavioral Neuroscience,* Vol.110, No.2, (April 1996), pp. 324–330, ISSN 1939-0084.

[25] Carlson, C.R., Bertrand, P.M., Ehrlich, A.D., Maxwell, A.W., & Burton, R.G. (2001). Physical self-regulation training for the management of temporomandibular disorders. *Journal of Orofacial Pain,* Vol.15, No.1, (Winter 2001), pp. 47–55, ISSN 11889647.

[26] Carter, C.S., MacDonald, III, A.M., Botvinick, M.M., Ross, L.L., Stenger, V.A., Noll, D., & Cohen, J. (2000). Parsing executive processes: Strategic vs. evaluative functions of the anterior cingulate cortex. *Proceedings of the National Academy of Sciences,* Vol.97, No.4, (February 2000), pp. 1944 – 1948, ISSN 0027-8424.

[27] Chalmers, B., Wolman, W.L., Nikodem, V.C., Gulmezoglu, A.M., & Hofmeyer, G.J. (1995). Companionship in labour: Do the personality characteristics of labour supporters influence their effectiveness? *Curationis,* Vol.18, No.4, (December 1995), pp. 77–80, ISSN 8697543.

[28] Cogan, R., & Spinnato, J.A. (1988). Social support during premature labor: Effects on labor and the newborn. *Journal of Psychosomatic Obstetrics and Gynecology,* Vol.8, No.3, (June 1988), pp. 209–216, 1743-8942.

[29] Craig, A.D., & Dostrovsky, J.O. (1999). Medulla to thalamus. In: *Textbook of pain,* P. Wall & R. Melzack (Eds.), pp. 183–214, Churchill Livingstone, ISBN 0443062528, New York.

[30] Crawford, M., & Gartner, R. (1992). *Women killing: Intimate femicide in Ontario, 1974-1990.* Women We Honour Action Committee, Toronto.

[31] DeWall, C.N., & Baumeister, R.F. (2006). Alone but feeling no pain: Effects of social exclusion on physical pain tolerance and pain threshold, affective forecasting, and interpersonal empathy. *Journal of Personality and Social Psychology,* Vol.91, No.1, (July 2006), pp. 1-15, ISSN 1939-1315.

[32] DeWall, C.N., MacDonald, G., Webster, G.D., Masten, C.L., Baumeister, R.F., Powell, C., Combs, D., Schurtz, D.R., Stillman, T.F., Tice, D.M., & Eisenberger, N.I. (2010). Acetaminophen reduces social pain: Behavioral and neural evidence. *Psychological Science,* Vol.21, No.7, (June 2010), pp. 931-937, ISSN 1467-9280.

[33] DeWall, C.N., Masten, C.L., Kashdan, T.B., Pond, Jr., R.S., Powell, C., Combs, D., & Schurtz, D.R. (2011). *Who is Most Vulnerable to Social Rejection? The Toxic Combination*

*of Low Self-Esteem and Lack of Emotional Differentiation on Neural Responses to Rejection.* Unpublished manuscript, University of Kentucky.

[34] DeWall, C.N., Masten, C.L., Powell, C., Combs, D., Schurtz, D.R., & Eisenberger, N.I. (2011). Does the pain of rejection depend on attachment style? An fMRI study. *Social Cognitive & Affective Neuroscience,* Advance Access, (April 2011), ISSN 1749-5016.

[35] DeWall, C.N. & Richman, S.B. (2011). Social exclusion and the desire to reconnect. *Social and Personality Psychology Compass,* Vol.5, No.11, (November 2011), pp. 919-932, ISSN1751-9004.

[36] DeWall, C.N., Twenge, J.M., Gitter, S.A., & Baumeister, R.F. (2009). It's the thought that counts: The role of hostile cognition in shaping aggressive responses to social exclusion. *Journal of Personality and Social Psychology,* Vol.96, No.1, (January 2009), pp. 45-59, ISSN 1939-1315.

[37] DeWall, C.N., Twenge, J.M., Bushman, B.J., Im, C., & Williams, K.D. (2010). Acceptance by one differs from acceptance by none: Applying social impact theory to the rejection-aggression link. *Social Psychological and Personality Science,* Vol.1, No.2, (April 2010), pp. 168-174, ISSN 1948-5506.

[38] Downey, G., Freitas, A.L., Michaelis, B., & Khouri, H. (1998). The self-fulfilling prophecy in close relationships: Rejection sensitivity and rejection by romantic partners. *Journal of Personality and Social Psychology,* Vol.75, No.2, (August 1998), pp. 545-560, 1939-1315.

[39] Eisenberger, N.I., & Lieberman, M.D. (2004). Why rejection hurts: A common neural alarm system for physical and social pain. *Trends in Cognitive Sciences,* Vol.8, No.7, (July 2004), pp.294-300, ISSN 1364-6613.

[40] Eisenberger, N.I., Lieberman, M.D., & Williams, K.D. (2003). Does rejection hurt? An fMRI study of social exclusion. *Science,* Vol.302, No.5643, (October 2003), pp. 290-292, ISSN 1095-9203.

[41] Eisenberger, N.I., Taylor, S.E., Gable, S.L., Hilmert, C.J., & Lieberman, M.D. (2007). Neural pathways link social support to attenuated neuroendocrine stress responses. *Neuroimage,* Vol.35, No.4, (May 2007), pp. 1601-1612, ISSN 1053-8119.

[42] Epker, J., & Gatchel, R.J. (2000). Coping profile differences in the biopsychosocial functioning of patients with temporomandibular disorder. *Psychosomatic Medicine,* Vol.62, No.1, (January 2000), pp. 69–75, ISSN 1534-7796.

[43] Feeney, J.A., Noller, P., & Hanrahan, M. (1994). Assessing adult attachment. In: *Attachment in adults: Clinical and developmental perspectives,* M.B. Sperling, and W.H. Berman (Eds.), pp. (128–152). Guilford Press, ISBN 0898625475, New York.

[44] Felmingham, K., Kemp, A., Williams, L., Das, P., Hughes, G., Peduto, A., and Bryant, R. (2007). Changes in anterior cingulate and amygdala after cognitive behavior thera-

py of posttraumatic stress disorder. *Psychological Science,* Vol.18, No.2, (February 2007), pp. 127–129, ISSN 1467-9280.

[45] Ferrando, M., Andreu, Y., Galdon, M.J., Dura, E., Poveda, R., & Bagan, J.V. (2004) Psychological variables and temporomandibular disorders: Distress, coping, and personality. *Oral Surgery, Oral Medicine, Oral Pathology, Oral Radiology, and Endodontics,* Vol.98, No.2, (August 2004), pp. 153–160, ISSN 1531-6541.

[46] Foltz, E.L., & White, L.E. (1968). The role of rostral cingulotomy in "pain" relief. *International Journal of Neurology,* Vol.6, pp. 353–373, ISSN 0020-7446.

[47] Fraley, R.C., & Shaver, P.R. (2000). Adult romantic attachment: theoretical developments, emerging controversies, and unanswered questions. *Review of General Psychology,* Vol.4, No.2, (June 2000), pp.132–154, ISSN 1089-2680.

[48] Gaertner, L., JIuzzini, J., & O'Mara, E.M. (2008). When rejection by one fosters aggression against many: Multiple-victim aggression as a consequence of social rejection and perceived groupness. *Journal of Experimental Social Psychology,* Vol.44, No.4 (July, 2008), pp. 958-970, ISSN 0022-1031.

[49] Gardner, W.L., Pickett, C.L., & Brewer. M.B. (2000). Social exclusion and selective memory: How the need to belong influences memory for social events. *Personality and Social Psychology Bulletin,* Vol.26, No.4, (April 2000), pp. 486–496, ISSN 1552-7433.

[50] Harmon-Jones, E., & Winkielman, P. (Eds.). (2007). *Social Neuroscience: Integrating Biological and Psychological Explanations of Social Behavior,* Guilford Publications, ISBN 978-159-3854-04-1, New York, NY.

[51] Harris, M.J. (2009). *Bullying, Rejection, and Peer Victimization: A Social Cognitive Neuroscience Perspective.* Springer Publishing Company, ISBN 978-082-6103-78-9, New York, NY.

[52] Herman, B.H., & Panksepp, J. (1978). Effects of morphine and naloxone on separation distress and approach attachment: Evidence for opiate mediation of social affect. *Pharmacology, Biochemistry, & Behavior,* Vol.9, No.2, (August 1978), pp. 213–220, 0091-3057.

[53] Hogan, R., Jones, W.H., & Cheek, J.M. (1985). Socioanalytic theory: An alternative to armadillo psychology. In: *The self and social life,* B.R. Schlenker (Ed.), pp. (175-198). McGraw-Hill, ISBN 0070553076, New York.

[54] House, J.S., Landis, K.R., & Umberson, D. (1988). Social relationships and health. *Science,* Vol.241, No.4865, (July 1988), pp. 540-545, ISSN 0036-8075.

[55] Insel, T.R., & Winslow, J.T. (1991). Central administration of oxytocin modulates the infant rat's response to social isolation. *European Journal of Pharmacology,* Vol.203, No. 1, (October 1991), pp. 149–152, ISSN 1665788.

[56] Izuma, K., Saito, D.N., & Sadato, N. (2008). Processing of social and monetary rewards in the human striatum. *Neuron,* Vol.58, No.2, (April 2008), pp. 284-294, ISSN 0896-6273.

[57] Janda, L.H., Fulk, J., Janda, M., & Wallace, J. (1995). *The development of a test of General Mental Abilities.* Unpublished manuscript, Old Dominion University.

[58] Janda, L. (1996). *The psychologists' book of self-tests.* Berkley, ISBN 0399522115, New York.

[59] Kashdan, T.B., Ferssizidis, P., Collins, R.L., & Muraven, M. (2010). Emotion differentiation as resilience against excessive alcohol use: An ecological momentary assessment in underage social drinkers. *Psychological Science,* Vol.21, No.9, (September 2010), pp.1341-1347, ISSN 1467-9280.

[60] Keefe, F.J., Brown, G.K., Wallston, K.A., Caldwell, D.S. (1989). Coping with rheumatoid arthritis pain: Catastrophizing as a maladaptive strategy. *Pain,* Vol.37, No.1, (April 1989), pp. 51–56, ISSN 0304-3959.

[61] Kehoe, P., & Blass, E. M. (1986). Opioid-mediation of separation distress in 10-day-old rats: Reversal of stress with maternal stimuli. *Developmental Psychobiology,* Vol.19, No.4, (July 1986), pp. 385–398, ISSN 1098-2302.

[62] Kirschbaum, C., Pirke, K.M., & Hellhammer, D.H. (1993). The 'Trier Social Stress Test'—a tool for investigating psychobiological stress responses in a laboratory setting. *Neuropsychobiology,* Vol.28, No.1–2, (June 1993), pp. 76–81, ISSN 0302-282X.

[63] Klaus, M., Kennel, J., Robertson, S., & Rosa, R. (1986). Effects of social support during parturition on maternal and infant mortality. *British Medical Journal,* Vol.293, No. 6547, (September 1986), pp. 585–597, ISSN 0267-0623.

[64] Konecka, A.M., & Sroczynska, I. (1990). Stressors and pain sensitivity in CFW mice: Role of opioid peptides. *Archives Internationales de Physiologie et de Biochimie,* Vol.98, No.5, pp. 245–252, ISSN 0003-9799.

[65] Kong, J., Gollub, R. L., Rosman, I. S., Webb, J. M., Vangel, M. G., Kirsch, I., and Kaptchuk, T.J. (2006). Brain activity associated with expectancy-enhanced placebo analgesia as measured by functional magnetic resonance imaging. *The Journal of Neuroscience,* Vol.26, No.2, (January 2006), pp. 381–388, ISSN 0270-6474.

[66] Kross, E., Berman, M.G., Mischel, W., Smith, E.E., & Wager, T.D. (2011). Social rejection shares somatosensory representations with physical pain. *Proceedings of the* National Academy of Sciences, Vol.108, No.15, (April 2011), pp. 6270-6275, ISSN 1091-6490.

[67] Kross, E., Egner, T., Ochsner, K., Hirsch, J., & Downey, G. (2007). Neural dynamics of rejection sensitivity. *Journal of Cognitive Neuroscience,* Vol.19, No.6, (June 2007), pp. 945–956, ISSN 1530-8898.

[68] Landro, N.I., Stiles, T.C., & Sletvold, H. (1997). Memory functioning in patients with primary fibromyalgia and major depression and healthy controls. *Journal of Psychosomatic Research,* Vol.42, No.3, (March 1997), pp. 297-306, ISSN 0022-3999.

[69] Lane, R.D., Reiman, E.M., Ahern, G.L., Schwartz, G.E., & Davidson, R.J. (1997). Neuroanatomical correlates of happiness, sadness, and disgust. *American Journal of Psychiatry,* Vol.154, No.7, (July 1997), pp. 926-933, ISSN 0002-953X.

[70] Leary, M.R. & Springer, C.A. (2001). Hurt feelings: The neglected emotion. In: *Aversive behaviors and interpersonal transgression,* R. Kowalski (Ed.), pp. (151-175). American Psychological Association, ISBN 1-55798-716-5, Washington DC.

[71] Leary, M.R., Kowalski, R.M., Smith, L., & Phillips, S. (2003). Teasing, rejection, and violence: Case studies of the school shootings. *Aggressive Behavior,* Vol.29, No.3, (June 2003), pp. 202-214, ISSN 1098-2337.

[72] Leary, M.R., Tambor, E.S., Terdal, S.J., & Downs, D.L. (1995). Self-esteem as an interpersonal monitor: The sociometer hypothesis. *Journal of Personality and Social Psychology,* Vol.68, No.3, (March 1995), pp.518-530, ISSN 0022-3514.

[73] Leary, M.R., Twenge, J.M., & Quinlivan, E. (2006). Interpersonal Rejection as a Determinant of Anger. *Personality and Social Psychology Review,* Vol.10, No.2, (May, 2006), pp. 111-132, ISSN 1532-7957.

[74] Lidderdale, J.M., & Walsh, J.J. (1998). The effects of social support on cardiovascular reactivity and perinatal outcome. *Psychology and Health,* Vol.13, No.6, (May 1998), pp. 1061–1070, ISSN 1476-8321.

[75] Lieberman, M.D. (2007). Social cognitive neuroscience, In: *Encyclopedia of Social Psychology Vol. 2,* Baumeister, R.F., & Vohs, K.D. (Eds.), pp. 885-887, Sage Press, ISBN 978-141-2916-70-7, Thousand Oaks, CA.

[76] Lieberman, M.D. (2010). Social cognitive neuroscience, In: *Handbook of Social Psychology 5th ed.,* Fiske, S.T., Gilbert, D.T., & Lindzey, G. (Eds.), pp. 143-193, McGraw-Hill, ISBN 047-013-7479, New York, NY.

[77] Lieberman, M.D., Eisenberger, N.I., Crockett, M.J., Tom, S.M., Pfeifer, J.H., & Way, B.M. (2007). Putting feelings into words: Affect labeling disrupts amygdala activity in response to affective stimuli. *Psychological Science,* Vol.18, No.5, (May 2007), pp. 421–428, ISSN 0956-7976.

[78] MacDonald, G., & Leary, M.R. (2005). Why does social exclusion hurt? The relationship between social and physical pain. *Psychological Bulletin,* Vol.131, No.2, (March 2005), pp. 202–223, ISSN 1939-1455.

[79] MacLean, P.D., & Newman, J.D. (1988). Role of midline frontolimbic cortex in production of the isolation call of squirrel monkeys. *Brain Research,* Vol.450, No.1-2, (May 1988), pp. 111-123, ISSN 0006-8993.

[80] Maner, J.K., DeWall, C.N., Baumeister, R.F., & Schaller, M. (2007). Does social exclusion motivate withdrawal or reconnection? Resolving the "porcupine problem." *Journal of Personality and Social Psychology,* Vol.92, No.1, (January 2007), pp. 42-55, ISSN 1939-1315.

[81] Masten, C.L., Telzer, E.H., & Eisenberger, N.I. (2011). An fMRI investigation of attributing negative social treatment to racial discrimination. *Journal of Cognitive Neuroscience,* Vol.23, No.5, (May 2011), pp. 1042-1051, ISSN 1530-8898.

[82] Melzack, R. & Casey, K. (1968). Sensory, motivational and central control determinants of pain: A new conceptual model. In: *The Skin Senses,* D. Kenshado (Ed.), (pp. 423-439). C. C. Thomas, ISBN BWB5857742, Springfield, IL.

[83] Mitchell, J.P., Cloutier, J., Banaji, M.R., & Macrae, C.N. (2006). Medial prefrontal dissociations during processing of trait diagnostic and nondiagnostic person information. *Social Cognitive and Affective Neuroscience,* Vol.1, No.1, (May 2006), pp. 49-55, ISSN 0006-8993.

[84] Moll, J., de Oliveira-Souza, R., Eslinger, P.J., Bramati, I.E., Mourão-Miranda, J., Andreiuolo, P.A., & Pessoa, L. (2002). The neural correlates of moral sensitivity: A functional magnetic resonance imaging investigation of basic and moral emotions. *The Journal of Neuroscience,* Vol.22, No.7, (April 2002), pp. 2730 -2736, ISSN 1529-2401.

[85] Moreland, R.L. (1987). The formation of small groups. In: *Group processes: Review of personality and social psychology Vol 8,* C. Hendrick (Ed.), pp. (80-110). Sage, ISBN 0803930720, Newbury Park, CA.

[86] Murphy, M.R., MacLean, P.D., & Hamilton, S.C. (1981). Species-typical behavior of hamsters deprived from birth of the neocortex. *Science,* Vol.213, No.4506, (July 1981), pp.459–461, ISSN 0036-8075.

[87] Naranjo, J.R., & Fuentes, J.A. (1985). Association between hypoalgesia and hypertension in rats after short-term isolation. *Neuropharmacology,* Vol.24, No.2, (February 1985), pp. 167–171, ISSN 0028-3908.

[88] Nichols, D.S., Glenn, T.M. (1994). Effect of aerobic exercise on pain perception, affect, and level of disability in individuals with fibromyalgia. *Physical Therapy,* Vol.74, No. 4, (April 1994), pp. 327–332, ISSN 8140145.

[89] Niven, C. (1985). How helpful is the presence of the husband at childbirth? *Journal of Reproductive and Infant Psychology,* Vol.3, No.2, pp. 45–53, ISSN 1469-672X.

[90] Onoda, K., Okamoto, Y., Nakashim, K., Nittono, H., Yoshimura, S., Yamawaki, S., Yamaguchi, S., & Ura M. (2010). Does low self-esteem enhance social pain? The relationship between trait self-esteem and anterior cingulate cortex activation induced by ostracism. *Social Cognitive and Affective Neuroscience,* Vol.5, No.4, (December 2010), pp.385-391, ISSN 1749-5016.

[91] Panksepp, J. (1998). *Affective neuroscience: The foundations of human and animal emotions.* Oxford University Press, ISBN 0-19-509673-8, London.

[92] Panksepp, J., Herman, B.H., Conner, R., Bishop, P., & Scott, J.P. (1978). The biology of social attachments: Opiates alleviate separation distress. *Biological Psychiatry,* Vol.13, No.5, (October 1978), pp. 607–618, ISSN 0006-3223.

[93] Panksepp, J., Vilberg, T., Bean, N.J., Coy, D.H., & Kastin, A.J. (1978). Reduction of distress vocalization in chicks by opiate-like peptides. *Brain Research Bulletin,* Vol.3, No.6,(November 1978), pp. 663-667, ISSN 0361-9230.

[94] Park, D.C., Glass, J.M., Minear, M., & Crofford, L.J. (2001). Cognitive function in fibromyalgia patients. *Arthritis and Rheumatism,* Vol.44, No.9, (September 2001), pp. 2125-2133, ISSN 0004-3591.

[95] Petrovic, P., Dietrich, T., Fransson, P., Andersson, J., Carlsson, K., & Igvar, M. (2005). Placebo in emotion processing—induced expectations of anxiety relief activate a generalized modulatory network. *Neuron,* Vol.46, No.6, (June 2005), pp. 957–969, ISSN 0896-6273.

[96] Petrovic, P., & Ingvar, M. (2002). Imaging cognitive modulation of pain processing. *Pain,* Vol.95, No.1-2, (January 2002), pp. 1-5, ISSN 0304-3959.

[97] Phillips, J.M., & Gatchel, R.J. (2000). Extraversion–introversion and chronic pain: Locus of control in the patient with chronic pain. In: *Personality characteristics of patients with pain,* R. Gatchel & J. Weisberg (Eds.), pp. (181–202). American Psychological Association, ISBN 1-55798-646-0, Washington, DC.

[98] Price, D.D. (2000). Psychological and neural mechanisms of the affective dimension of pain. *Science,* Vol.288, No.5472, (June 2000), pp. 1769–1772, ISSN 0036-8075.

[99] Rainville, P., Duncan, G.H., Price, D.D., Carrier, B., & Bushnell, M.C. (1997). Pain affect encoded in human anterior cingulated but not somatosensory cortex. *Science,* Vol.277, No.5328, (August 1997), pp. 968–971, ISSN 0036-8075.

[100] Rushen, J., Boissy, A., Terlouw, E.M., & de Passille, A.M. (1999). Opioid peptides and behavioral and physiological responses of dairy cows to social isolation in unfamiliar surroundings. *Journal of Animal Science,* Vol.77, No.11, (November 1999), pp. 2918-2924, ISSN 1525-3163.

[101] Sebastian, C.L., Roiser, J.P., Tan, G.C., Viding, E., Wood, N.W., & Blakemore, S.J. (2010). Effects of age and MAOA genotype on the neural processing of social rejection. *Genes, Brain & Behavior,* Vol.9, No.6, (June 2010), pp. 628-637, ISSN 1601-183X.

[102] Sharp, T.J., & Harvey, A.G. (2001). Chronic pain and post-traumatic stress disorder: Mutual maintenance? *Clinical Psychology Review,* Vol.21, No.6, (August 2001), pp. 857– 877, ISSN 0272-7358.

[103] Simmons, A., Matthews, S.C., Feinstein, J.S., Hitchcock, C., Paulus, M.P., & Stein, M.B. (2008). Anxiety vulnerability is associated with altered anterior cingulate re-

sponse to an affective appraisal task. *NeuroReport,* Vol.19, No.10, (July 2008), pp. 1033–1037, ISSN 0959-4965.

[104] Slavich, G.M., Way, B.M., Eisenberger, N.I., & Taylor, S.E. Neural sensitivity to social rejection is associated with inflammatory responses to social stress. *Proceedings of the National Academy of Sciences,* Vol.107, No.33, (August 2010), pp. 14817-14822, ISSN 0027-8424.

[105] Smith, A.K., White, P.D., Aslakson, E., Vollmer-Conna, U., & Rajeevan, M.S. (2006). Polymorphisms in genes regulating the HPA axis associated with empirically delineated classes of unexplained chronic fatigue. *Pharmacogenomics,* Vol.7, No.3, (April 2006), pp 387–394, ISSN 16610949.

[106] Snow-Turek, A.L., Norris, M.P., Tan, G. (1996) Active and passive coping strategies in chronic pain patients. *Pain,* Vol.64, No.3, (March 1996). pp. 455–462, ISSN 0304-3959.

[107] Solberg Nes, L., Roach, A.R., & Sergerstrom, S.C. (2009). Executive functions, self-regulation, and chronic pain: a review. *Annals of Behavioral Medicine,* Vol.37, No.2, (April 2009), pp. 173-183, ISSN 0883-6612, 1532-4796.

[108] Somerville, L.H., Kelley, W.M., & Heatherton, T.F. (2010). Self-esteem modulates medial prefrontal cortical responses to evaluative social feedback. *Cerebral Cortex,* Vol. 20, No.12, (December 2010), pp.3005-3013, ISSN 1047-3211.

[109] Spear, L.P., Enters, E.K., Aswad, M.A., & Louzan, M. (1985). Drug and environmentally induced manipulations of the opiate and serotonergic systems alter nociception in neonatal rat pups. *Behavioral and Neural Biology,* Vol.44, No.1, (July 1985), pp. 1–22, ISSN 0163-1047.

[110] Sufka, K.J., & Hughes, R.A. (1990). Dose and temporal parameters of morphine-induced hyperalgesia in domestic fowl. *Physiology & Behavior,* Vol.47, No.2, (February 1990), pp. 385–387, ISSN 0031-9384.

[111] Sufka, K.J., & Weed, N.C. (1994). Construct validation of behavioral indices of isolation stress and inflammatory nociception in young domestic fowl. *Physiology & Behavior,* Vol.55, No4., (April 1994), pp. 741–746, ISSN 0031-9384.

[112] Tugade, M.M., Fredrickson, B.L., & Barrett, L.F. (2004). Psychological resilience and emotional granularity: Examining the benefits of positive emotions on coping and health. *Journal of Personality,* Vol.72, No.6, (December 2004), pp.1161-1190, ISSN 1467-6494.

[113] Twenge, J.M., Baumeister, R.F., Tice, D.M., & Stucke, T.S. (2001). If you can't join them, beat them: Effects of social exclusion on aggressive behavior. *Personality and Social Psychology,* Vol.81, No.6, (December, 2001), pp.1058-1069, ISSN 1939-1315.

[114] Twenge, J.W., Cantanese, K.R., & Baumeister, R.F. (2002). Social exclusion causes self-defeating behavior. *Journal of Personality and Social Psychology,* Vol.83, No.3, (September, 2002), pp. 606-615, ISSN 1939-1315.

[115] Twenge, J.M., Catanese, K.R., & Baumeister, R.F. (2003). Social exclusion and the deconstructed state: Time perception, meaninglessness, lethargy, lack of emotion, and self-awareness. *Journal of Personality and Social Psychology,* Vol.85, No.3, (September 2003), pp. 409–423, ISSN 1939-1315.

[116] Way, B.M., Taylor, S.E., & Eisenberger, N.I. (2009). Variation in the mu-opioid receptor gene (OPRM1) is associated with dispositional and neural sensitivity to social rejection.*Proceedings of the National Academy of Sciences,* Vol.106, No.35, (September 2011), pp. 15079-15084, 0027-8424.

[117] Wiedenmayer, C.P., Goodwin, G.A., & Barr, G.A. (2000). The effect of periaqueductal gray lesions on responses to age-specific threats in infant rats. *Developmental Brain Research,* Vol.120, No.2, (April 2000), pp. 191–198, ISSN 0165-3806.

[118] Williams, K.D., Cheung, C.K.T., & Choi, W. (2000). CyberOstracism: Effects of being ignored over the Internet. *Journal of Personality and Social Psychology,* Vol.79, No.5, (November 2000), pp.748–762, ISSN 00223514.

[119] Zadro, L., Williams, K.D., & Richardson, R. (2004). How low can you go? Ostracism by a computer is sufficient to lower self-reported levels of belonging, control, self-esteem, and meaningful existence. *Journal of Experimental Social Psychology,* Vol.40, No. 4, (July 2004), pp. 560-567, ISSN 0022-1031.

[120] Zautra, A.J., Hamilton, N.A., & Burke, H.M. (1999). Comparison of stress responses in Women with two types of chronic pain: Fibromyalgia and osteoarthritis. *Cognitive Therapy and Research,* Vol.23, No.2, (April 1999), pp. 209–230, ISSN 1573-2819.

# 5

# The Brain is not "as-if" — Taking Stock of the Neuroscientific Approach on Decision Making

Kirsten G. Volz and Gerd Gigerenzer

## 1. Introduction

How do we make decisions? This question has long engaged researchers from various disciplines, including philosophy, psychology, economics, and cognitive neuroscience. Recently, a new discipline – neuroeconomics – emerged, devoted to addressing exactly this question by means of interdisciplinary endeavors. Broadly stated, neuroeconomics sets out "to promote interdisciplinary collaborations on the topics lying at the intersection of the brain and decision sciences in the hope of advancing both theory and research in decision making" (Society for Neuroeconomics, www.neuroeconomics.org), so that it can be used "for discriminating among standard economic models" (Maskin, 2008, p. 1788) and thus inform economic theory.

Neuroeconomics evolved as a field in the late 1990s, an offspring of behavioral economics and cognitive neuroscience. Behavioral economics is itself a relatively new field, just two decades old, and is commonly traced back to Herbert Simon's concept of bounded rationality (Simon, 1989). All three fields share the same goal of making theories of decision making more realistic by using insights from psychology or cognitive neuroscience. But what may be unrealistic about classical theories of decision making? It appears that there is little evidence that humans make decisions by calculating the expected utility (EU) or any of its variants outside the world of choices between gambles, if at all (e.g., Kahneman & Tversky, 2000; Lopes, 1981; Rubinstein, 1988; Russo & Dosher, 1983). Daniel Friedman and Shyam Sunder (2011) reviewed the literature on risky choice from 1950 up to 2010:

Most theories of risky choice postulate that a decision maker maximizes the expectation of a Bernoulli (or utility or similar) function. We tour 60 years of empirical search and conclude that no such functions have yet been found that are useful for out-of-sample predictions. Nor do we find practical applications of Bernoulli functions in major risk-based industries such as finance, insurance and gambling. (p. 1)

The important methodological concept is "out-of-sample prediction." There is plenty of evidence that EU theory and its variants, such as prospect theory, can *fit* their parameters to data after the fact, but the real test is in *prediction*. "Out of sample" means that a utility function is fitted to a randomly chosen part of the data – say one half – and the fitted function is then tested on the other part (known as *cross-validation*). If the fitted utility function captures the actual process of decision making, then that function should predict the same person's or group's choices. Friedman and Sunder (2011) claim having found no evidence of this in the 60 years of research they reviewed, neither for individual utility functions nor for group utility functions, where groups are defined by demography, gender, and the like.

Neoclassical economists have, in fact, never proposed that people actually weight utilities with probabilities and carry out computations to maximize expected utility. On the contrary, they insist that their theory says nothing about processes either at the level of cognitive psychology and/or its neural implementation. Following Milton Friedman's (1953) "as-if" methodology of "positive economics," neoclassical economists, like the behaviorist B. F. Skinner, saw value only in predicting behavior, not in modeling cognitive processes. EU theory, prospect theory, equity aversion theory, and other utility theories are "as-if" models that are deliberately *not* meant to model the cognitive processes or give information on the neural implementation. The theoretical direction that much of cognitive neuroscience on decision making has taken, however, is to apply the as-if framework as a theory for how the brain works. For example, Glimcher and his colleagues suggested that "the neoclassical/revealed preference framework might prove a useful theoretical tool for neuroscience" (Glimcher et al., 2009, p. 7). Subsequently, the concepts of 'expected value' and 'expected utility' found their ways into neuroeconomics, and there is broad consensus that neuroeconomics is about studying "the computations that the brain carries out in order to make value-based decisions, as well as the neural implementation of those computations" (Rangel et al., 2008, p. 545).

In this chapter, we will provide a positive alternative to the main path pursued by the cognitive neuroscience of decision making. One of the authors (GG) has spent decades on opening the "black box" and investigating the cognitive processes of decision making in humans (Gigerenzer, 2008; Gigerenzer et al., 1999, 2011), including expert groups of doctors, judges, and managers (Gigerenzer & Gray, 2011). Consistent with D. Friedman and Sunder (2011), Gigerenzer and colleagues found little evidence that utility functions predict (as opposed to fit) laypersons' and experts' behavior. Moreover, none of the professional groups investigated uses EU maximization in practice, while there is evidence that they rely strongly on heuristics (Gigerenzer et al., 2011). Given these findings and the overall aim of unraveling human decision making processes, we argue that the neuroscience of decision making would benefit from the following principles so as to approach a psychologically valid account of human decision making (in the brain):

1. *Study the neural correlates of process theories, not of as-if theories*. As explained above, the aim of as-if models, such as EU theory and its modifications is to explain behavior on an aggregate level by explicitly ignoring the underlying cognitive processes. Examples are

the explanation of cabdrivers' labor supply decisions (Crawford & Meng, 2010), farmers' decision behavior given new Common Agricultural Policy (Serrao & Coelho, 2004), or individuals' risky choice behavior (Kahneman & Tversky, 1979). Cognitive neuroscience, however, is explicitly dedicated to the process level, i.e., cognitive neuroscientists want to understand "*how* [emphasis added] the brain enables mind" (Gazzaniga, 2000, p. xii). That is, the object of interest is "the cognitive rules that people follow and the knowledge representations that those rules operate on" (Gazzaniga, 2000, p. 6). Accordingly, the two disciplines work at different levels of description, paying – by definition – no or only little attention to how descriptions at one specific level are related to descriptions at other levels (e.g., Craver, 2007; Marr, 1982). Thus, testing for the neural correlates of EU theory or its variants appears to us as if researchers would interpret an as-if model as a cognitive process model. One solution to this inconsistency would be to test for the neural correlates of process models of decision making, such as heuristics and their adaptive use (Gigerenzer et al., 2011; Payne et al., 1992, 1993; Volz et al. 2006, 2010). For instance, research on investigating how the brain encodes magnitude and probability (e.g., Tobler et al., 2005; Preuschoff et al., 2006, 2008) or how risk is coded (Christopoulos et al., 2009) does not need the EU framework of weighting and integration (of all utilities and probabilities). Magnitude and probability are also components of heuristic models, such as the priority heuristic (Brandstätter et al. 2006; see below). Researchers testing for the neural correlates of an as-if model – such as EU and its variants – however, need to explain why they reinterpret these models in a way they were explicitly not meant to be interpreted.

2. *Study decision making in uncertain ("large") worlds, not only certain ("small") worlds.* The large majority of neuroscientific studies on decision making examines behavior predominantly in situations where everything is known for certain, including all alternatives, consequences, and their probabilities (a so-called small world). A prototypical example is the gambling paradigm. Variants are probabilistic learning-or probabilistic tracking paradigms, in which events are exclusively governed by a specific probability function and individuals are encouraged to estimate the probability of reward. Tasks of the latter sort might be more or less difficult (e.g., depending on whether encountering a volatile or a stable environment, cp. Beherns et al., 2007), but individuals know on which variable(s) to concentrate, i.e., they know about the structure of the task.

To study decision making in gambling and similar small worlds can be an interesting subject. Yet as a study of cognitive processes, it is unclear what this approach can tell us about decision making under uncertainty, that is, situations where not all alternatives, consequences, and probabilities are known for sure. Recent research indicates that neither the normative nor the descriptive results can be automatically generalized. First, what is rational in small worlds is *not* generally rational in uncertain worlds (Gigerenzer et al., 2011). On the contrary, models that are optimal in a small world are typically only second-best when uncertainty is introduced, as in out-of-sample prediction or out-of-population prediction (Czerlinski et al., 1999; Gigerenzer & Brighton, 2009). One reason is that optimization models tend to overfit. Second, small worlds and large worlds may require entirely different skills and strategies. For example, whereas it might suffice to calculate the expected value in a lottery, this skill will not be sufficient for deciding whether or not to be vaccinated against swine flu, which share to buy, or whom to marry. Decision making under risk (small worlds) and under uncertainty (large worlds) do require different skills: statistical thinking and heuristic thinking. It is not possible to extrapolate from small to large worlds except for the rare case in which the former approximates the latter. Savage, known as the father of Bayesian decision theory, has drawn a clear line between the study of small and large worlds:

Jones is faced with the decision whether to buy a certain sedan for a thousand dollars, a certain convertible also for a thousand dollars, or to buy neither and continue carless. The simplest analysis, and the one generally assumed, is that Jones is deciding between three definite and sure enjoyments, that of the sedan, the convertible, or the thousand dollars. Chance and uncertainty are considered to have nothing to do with the situation. This simple analysis may well be appropriate in some contexts; however, it is not difficult to recognize that Jones must in fact take account of many uncertain future possibilities in actually making his choice. The relative fragility of the convertible will be compensated only if Jones's hope to arrange a long vacation in a warm and scenic part of the country actually materializes; Jones would not buy a car at all if he thought it is likely that he would immediately be faced by a financial emergency arising out of the sickness of himself or of some member of his family; he would be glad to put the money on a car, or almost any durable goods, if he feared extensive inflation." (Savage, 1954, p. 83).

Note that studying decision making under uncertainty (as opposed to risk) does not require bringing the complexity of the world into the scanner. It only requires studying tasks where not all alternatives, consequences, and probabilities are known for sure. Well-known examples of large world paradigms are the city task by Goldstein and Gigerenzer (2002), in which individuals are presented with pairs of cities (e.g., Portland – Virginia Beach) and have to infer which city in each pair had the larger population, the fever task by Persson & Rieskamp (2009), and Bröder et al.'s (2010) tasks in which individuals have to judge which of two patients (each with a specific combination of symptoms) had reached the more advanced and dangerous stage.

*Implement predictive and competitive tests as methodological standards.* The practice of using good fits to support theories has been very popular, in psychology as well as in behavioral economics in the past. However, a good fit by itself is not an adequate test of a theory (Roberts & Pashler, 2000; Roberts & Sternberg, 1993; Wexler, 1978). Fitting means that the data is already known, and dependent on the number and kind of adjustable parameters, one can always achieve a good fit. Accordingly, the practice is now changing and researchers now determine how the theory constrains possible outcomes (i.e., how well it predicts), how actual outcomes agree with those constraints, and whether plausible alternative outcomes would have been inconsistent with the theory (Ahn et al., 2008; Roberts & Pashler, 2000; Bröder et al., 2010; Persson & Rieskamp, 2009). Besides fitting, a second limitation of many tests is that only one theory is being tested, and one does not know whether other theories would predict behavior better. Examples for competitive tests are found in Brandstätter et al., (2006) on models predicting choice between lotteries (small worlds), and in Dhami (2003) on British magistrates' bail decisions (uncertain worlds). Following up on this progression, we would like to push forward the implementation of predictive and competitive tests also in the cognitive neuroscience of decision making, which only now started to be pursued (e.g., Christopoulos et al., 2009; Venkatraman et al., 2009). Obviously, we specifically would like to suggest incorporating heuristic models in competitive testing on the neural level since this hasn't been pursued intensively yet. Exceptions are from our own research: In an fMRI study on the neural correlates of the Recognition Heuristic (RH)[1], we predicted the neuronal activation patterns that different theories for RH-based decisional processes made. Results revealed that processes underlying RH-based decisions go beyond simply choosing the recognized alternative and are rather distinguished by judgments about the ecological rationality of the RH (Volz et al., 2006).

The three issues are linked. We begin our discussion of them by introducing the basic concepts of modern decision theory and methodology.

## 2. As-If models and process models

It is often worthwhile to ask where ideas come from. That helps to understand why we ask the questions we ask. Expected value theory has its origin in the social gambling behavior of aristocrats. Its year of birth is commonly dated 1654, when the Chevalier de Méré asked the mathematicians Pierre Fermat and Blaise Pascal for advice in gambling. Their exchange of letters is seen as the beginning of probability and decision theory (for the psychological interpretation of the classical theory, and decline, see Daston, 1988; Gigerenzer et al., 1989). The resulting theory of rational choice is known today as expected value (EV) theory:

$$\mathrm{EV}(x) = \Sigma p_i x_i \tag{1}$$

where $p_i$ is the probability and $x_i$ the (monetary) value of each outcome ($i$=1, …, $n$) of a given alternative $x$. For example, being offered the choice between two alternatives, Gamble A: 490.000€ with $p$=1.0 and Gamble B: 1 million with $p$=.5 and 0€ with $p$=.5, which would you choose? According to EV theory, you should choose the risky Gamble B because it maximizes EV. However, the choices of reasonable people did not always conform to theory. This discrepancy received the greatest attention in the St. Petersburg problem, which led Daniel Bernoulli (1738/1954) to modify EV theory into what is now called expected utility (EU) theory:

$$\mathrm{EU}(x) = \Sigma p_i u_i \tag{2}$$

As one can see, the basic idea is the same: Instead of choosing the alternative that maximizes EV, one now chooses the alternative that maximizes EU. Bernoulli assumed that $u$=log($x$), modeling diminishing returns, but other functions have been proposed, including nonmono-

1 The RH can be stated as follows: "If one of two objects is recognized and the other is not, then infer that the recognized object has the higher value with respect to the criterion." (Goldstein &Gigerenzer, 2002, p. 76).

tonic functions (e.g., Friedman & Savage, 1948). In the second half of the 20th century, systematic deviations from EU theory were shown in experimental studies, including the Allais paradox and the fourfold pattern (Kahneman & Tversky, 2000; Lopes, 1994). Simon (1989) and Selten (2001) proposed a radical break from EU theory, based on empirical psychological principles, such as the study of adaptive heuristics (Gigerenzer et al., 1999; Leland, 1994; Payne, Bettman, & Johnson, 1993; Tversky, 1972). However, most of the economic community retained the EU framework but modified it by adding more adjustable parameters, as in prospect theory (Kahneman & Tversky, 1979):

$$V(x) = \sum_{i=0}^{n} \pi_i^{+} v(x_i) + \sum_{i=-m}^{0} \pi_i^{-} v(x) \tag{3}$$

where $\pi$ are the decision weights for positive and negative domains (gains and losses). The added flexibility – five adjustable parameters – fitted the data better than EU theory, as long as the additional parameter values were suitably chosen. Given that the form of the relation between $u$ and $x$ is left unspecified, one has to estimate it for each person or group. Yet, as mentioned above, the fitted utility functions of EU and its modifications have not been shown to be useful in out-of-sample prediction of behavior (Friedman & Sunder, 2011). The problem that Bernoulli functions lack predictive power is rarely mentioned in the neuroscience literature.

Prospect theory and similar attempts to make models of decision making more realistic led to "the paradoxical result that the models became even less psychologically plausible" (Gigerenzer & Selten, 2001, p. 5). For example, try to compute the subjective values of risky prospects following prospect theory:

An individual chooses among two or more lotteries according to the following procedure. First, transform the probabilities of all outcomes associated with a particular lottery using a nonlinear probability-transformation function. Then transform the outcomes associated with that lottery (i.e., all elements of its support). Third, multiply the transformed probabilities and corresponding transformed lottery outcomes, and sum these products to arrive at the subjective value associated with this particular lottery. Repeat these steps for all remaining lotteries in the choice set. Finally, choose the lottery with the largest subjective value, computed according to the method above. (Berg & Gigerenzer, 2010, pp. 4-5)

Yet, as explained above, prospect theory should not be mistaken as a cognitive process model. On the contrary, economists since Samuelson (1937) and Friedman (1953) have thought of EU and its variants as *as-if-models*, not as theories that describe the cognitive or neural processes, and neoclassical economists treat the mind as a black box. Economic theory is about the prediction of behavior, not of process. This is the main reason why many economists see little value in neuroeconomics (for economic research) (e.g., Gul & Pesendorfer, 2008; Harrison, 2008; Marchionni & Vromen, 2010; Rubinstein, 2008).

Hitherto, most of the neuroscience of decision making set out to investigate the neural correlates of as-if models, assuming that the mind engages in some form of utility calculations. A great number of neuroeconomic studies aimed at identifying "the brain activations coding the key decision parameters of expected value (magnitude and probability)." (Tobler et al., 2007, p. 1621). Fox and Poldrack (2009, p. 165) claim that there "has been substantial progress in understanding the neural correlates of prospect theory." Others present the assumptions of EU theory as true with regard to the cognitive processes weighting and integrating, but did neither proof whether individuals indeed engaged in these cognitive processes nor elaborated on the issue of as-if models vs. process models. "Decision makers integrate the various dimensions of an option into a single measure of its idiosyncratic subjective value and then choose the option that is most valuable. Comparisons between different kinds of options rely on this abstract measure of subjective value, a kind of "common currency" for choice" (Kable & Glimcher, 2009, p. 734).

The assumption that choice is always based on a weighted integration of all relevant aspects is the most widely held belief across disciplines when it comes to decision making processes; irrespective of whether decisions entail choosing between risky prospects, such as in gambling situations, or between uncertain options, such as a suitable capital investment, a proper university degree, or a life partner: "When deciding between different options, individuals are guided by the expected (mean) value of the different outcomes and by the associated degrees of uncertainty." (Tobler et al., 2007, p. 1621).

These claims are somewhat astounding, at least to us. The experimental literature indicates that full integration (compensation) of the various attributes is the exception rather than the rule (e.g., Gigerenzer & Gaissmaier, 2011; Hauser, 2011; Marewski et al., 2010). Often, humans rely on heuristics that are noncompensatory, such as one good reason or lexicographic decisions. A classic review of 45 studies in which the process of decision making was analyzed by means of eye movement, mouse lab, and other process tracking studies concluded (Ford et al., 1989):

The results firmly demonstrate that non-compensatory strategies were the dominant mode used by decision makers. Compensatory strategies were typically used only when the number of alternatives and dimensions were small or after a number of alternatives have been eliminated from consideration. (p. 75)

Influential neuroeconomic papers, including those cited above, yet, seem to focus on the EU framework and hence seem to accept its basic assumptions as a realistic description of cognitive and neural processes. These assumptions about the nature of decision making thus include (Katsikopoulos & Gigerenzer, 2008):

1. *Independent evaluations:* Every option has a value that is measured by a single number (options are not evaluated relative to other options).
2. *Exhaustive search:* The value of an option is calculated by using all available information (for gambles, the probabilities and values for all possible outcomes).

3. *Trade-offs:* To calculate an option's value, low values on one attribute (e.g., a value) can be compensated by high values on another attribute (e.g., a probability).
4. *Optimization.* The final choice is based on the maximization of utility or some other function of value.

These four assumptions are maintained through almost all modifications of EU theory; what is modified in reaction to inconsistent data are the functions of the probabilities and values, as illustrated in Equations 2 and 3. Most important, the optimization assumption requires studying a small world in which all alternatives, consequences, and probabilities are known, as in a lottery. We will turn to the consequences of this assumption below.

What would a process model look like? A process model would not take the four assumptions as axiomatic, but consider the empirical evidence. In brief, evidence shows that the first three assumptions sometimes hold, typically in small worlds, but are most of the time not descriptively correct (e.g., Bröder & Gaissmaier, 2007; Hauser, 2011). Specifically, there is little evidence that individuals use the same strategy for each decision; instead it implements an "adaptive toolbox" with multiple strategies, called heuristics (Bröder, Persson? Gigerenzer & Selten 2001; Honda et al., 2011; Payne et al., 1993). One interesting result is that whereas modifications of EU such as the Allais paradox grow increasingly complex in order to represent deviating behavior in the EU framework, simple heuristics that are based on evidence on cognitive processes can dispense with this added complexity. One illustration of a process model is the priority heuristic, which applies to lotteries (Brandstätter et al., 2006). Like many heuristics, it has three building blocks: a search rule, a stopping rule, and a decision rule.[2] The priority heuristic consists of the following steps:

*Search rule*: Go through reasons in the following order: Minimum gain, probability of minimum gain, maximum gain.

*Stopping rule*: Stop examination if the minimum gains differ by 1/10 (or more) of the maximum gain; otherwise, stop examination if probabilities differ by 1/10 (or more) of the probability scale.

*Decision rule*: Choose the gamble with the more attractive gain (probability).

The term "attractive" refers to the gamble with the higher (minimum or maximum) gain and the lower probability of the minimum gain. The priority heuristic models difficult choices (same or similar expected values of the alternatives) and nontrivial choices (no alternatives dominates the other, weakly or strongly). The search, stopping, and decision rules were derived from psychological studies (Brandstätter et al., 2006, 2008).

Consider one of the problems, known as the Allais paradox, which shows an inconsistency between the actual observed choices and the predictions of EU theory, or more specifically the transgression of the common consequence effect (Allais 1953, p. 527):

2 Note that EU theory has no search and stopping rules, because it assumes full information or exhaustive search.

| | | | |
|---|---|---|---|
| $A$: | 100 | million | for sure |
| $B$: | 500 | million | $p = .10$ |
| | 100 | million | $p = .89$ |
| | 0 | | $p = .01$ |

| | | | |
|---|---|---|---|
| $C$: | 100 | million | $p = .11$ |
| | 0 | | $p = .89$ |
| $D$: | 500 | million | $p = .10$ |
| | 0 | | $p = .90$ |

Most people prefer *A* over *B*, but *D* over *C*, violating EU theory (because *C* and *D* are obtained from *A* and *B* by eliminating a.89 probability to win 100 million from both gambles). EU does not predict whether *A* or *B* will be chosen; it simply makes predictions of the type "if *A* is chosen over *B*, then it follows that *C* is chosen over *D*." The priority heuristic, in contrast, makes stronger predictions: It predicts whether *A* or *B* will be chosen, and whether *C* or *D* will be chosen. Consider the choice between *A* and *B*. The maximum payoff is 500 million, and therefore the aspiration level is 50 million; 100 million and 0 represent the minimum gains of the choice problem. Because the difference (100 million) exceeds the aspiration level of 50 million, the minimum gain of 100 million is considered good enough and people are predicted to select gamble *A*. That is, the heuristic predicts the majority choice correctly.

In the second choice problem, the minimum gains (0 and 0) do not differ. Hence, the probabilities of the minimum gains are attended to, $p$=.89 and.90, a difference that does not meet the aspiration level. Thus, the higher maximum gain (500 million versus 100 million) decides the choice, and the prediction is that people will select gamble *D*. Again, this prediction is consistent with the choice of the majority. Together, the pair of predictions amount to the Allais paradox.

This simple three-step process generates not only the Allais paradox, but several other so-called anomalies as well. It simultaneously implies common consequence effects, common ratio effects, reflection effects, and the fourfold pattern of risk attitude (Katsikopoulos & Gigerenzer, 2008). Note that the priority heuristic logically *implies* these behaviors, whereas prospect theory is only *consistent* with these.

The priority heuristic is an example of a process model that assumes dependent rather than independent evaluation: The two alternatives are compared, one by one, on the attributes, rather than each alternative having a utility independent of the other. Second, it assumes limited rather than exhaustive search, that is, it does not always use all of the information but employs a stopping rule. Third, it makes no trade-offs between the attributes: For instance, the first attribute alone can determine the decision. Finally, it is not based on the computation of a maximum or minimum of a function including weighting and summing, but is a model of bounded rationality in the sense of Simon.

In sum, EU theory and its modifications have been proposed as as-if models in neoclassical economics precisely because there is little evidence that they describe the psychological or neuronal processes underlying a decision. Behavioral economics largely retained the as-if framework, adding realism in the form of one or a few adjustable parameters and continuing to produce as-if models (Berg & Gigerenzer, 2010). Given this fact and the case that cognitive neuroscience investigations are by definition foremost interested in process models, we wonder why most of neuroeconomic research attempted to locate the computations involved in as-if theories in the brain and did not turn to distinct process models of decision making. Thus, an alternative is to study the neural correspondents of heuristic processes, such as search rules, stopping rules, and decision rules (e.g., Volz et al., 2006, 2010).

## 3. The brain is adapted to the uncertainty of large worlds, not to the certainty of lotteries and small worlds

EU and its modifications all involve optimization. Optimization means finding the maximum or minimum of a function and proving that it is the best choice. Optimization requires a world in which all alternatives, consequences, and probability distributions are known for certain (otherwise one cannot know what the optimal alternative is). The father of modern Bayesian decision theory, L. J. Savage (1954), distinguished between small worlds in which these conditions are met and where Bayesian theory is optimal, and large worlds in which these conditions are not met and where it would be "ridiculous" to use Bayesian decision theory (Binmore, 2008). The prototype for a small-world problem is the lottery. Many of the standard neuroscientific tasks on choice and decision making have been modeled after the lottery: two-armed bandit tasks, intertemporal choice tasks, and the ultimatum game, among others. For example, in the financial decision-making task by De Martino and colleagues (2006), participants had the choice between a sure option, i.e., how much money can be won on a specific trial ($v$=£20 with $p$=1.0) and a gamble option, i.e., the exact specification of the probabilities of winning or losing a specific amount of money ($v$=£50 with $p$=.37 and $v$=£0 with $p$=.63). Likewise, outcomes are certain in intertemporal choice paradigms, where, for instance, participants have to choose between smaller monetary rewards delivered immediately (€13.83 today) and larger monetary rewards delivered only later (€17.29 in 4 weeks) (e.g., Albrecht et al., 2011; McClure et al., 2004).

Without any disparagement intended, we note that these conditions rarely apply to real-world decisions. In the real world, part of the relevant information is missing or has to be estimated from small samples and the future is naturally unpredictable, so that optimization is out of reach. Such decisions include which capital investment to favor, which used car to buy, or whether to take a specific cancer check-up. Moreover, even if all alternatives, consequences, and probabilities are known, computing the best alternative in such situations can be computationally intractable. For example, computing Bayes' rule is NP-hard, that is, it becomes computationally intractable for brain and computers alike when large numbers of attributes are involved. Even in the simplest case with binary predictors only and a binary criterion, the number of leaves (exits) of the full decision tree increases exponentially ($2^n$) with the number $n$ of predictors. In contrast, in a fast-and-frugal tree, which is a heuristic model of Bayesian-type decision making, the number of leaves increases with $n$+1 only (Martignon et al., 2011).

### 3.1. Cognitive processes in large worlds differ from those in small worlds

The crucial question is, what can we learn about the brain if we focus experimental tasks on small worlds? Can we generalize the findings from small world studies to large worlds? Consider first the sub-question: Can we generalize the norms? To begin with, note that the very reason to construct small worlds is that EU theory or some other optimization model can be used to determine the best alternative. But the best strategy in a small world is not necessarily the best one in a large world. By way of illustration, two examples may suffice. Consider financial investment once again. A normative theory of how to allocate a sum of money to *N* assets is Markowitz's Nobel prize-winning mean-variance model. Like all optimizing theories, it assumes perfect knowledge about the relevant parameters. Is the theory optimal in the real world of financial investment, where parameter values are not known for certain but need to be estimated? The answer is no. De Miguel and colleagues (2009) showed that the simple 1/*N* heuristic (allocate your money equally to *N* assets) performs better in out-of-sample prediction. Note that the heuristic achieves better performance because it ignores part of the information, which makes it robust, while the mean-variance portfolio tries to integrate all information to estimate the weights and suffers from overfitting.

Second, consider sequential decision making where cues need to be ordered in a way that improves inductive inferences. The optimal ordering can be determined easily in a small world, and it leads to more accurate inferences than when cues are ordered simply, as with the take-the-best heuristic. Yet, in out-of-sample prediction, the optimal ordering is no longer best, and the simple ordering leads to more accurate inferences (Gigerenzer & Brighton, 2009; Martignon & Hoffrage, 1999). These results illustrate *less-is-more effects*, that is, situations where less computation and information enables more accurate inferences. They also explain why a certain degree of memory and capacity limitations can be beneficial (e.g., Goldstein & Gigerenzer, 2002; Hertwig & Todd, 2003). The study of ecological rationality answers the question of the worlds in which a given heuristic is successful, relative to other strategies. For instance, to allocate one's money to *N*=50 assets, an estimated 500 years of stock data would be needed for the mean-variance portfolio to finally exceed the performance of the 1/*N* heuristic (DeMiguel et al, 2009).

In sum, good decision making in large worlds requires different cognitive processes than those studied in small worlds. Studying a world of certainty may very likely miss the cognitive processes in the brain that deal with uncertainty (such as limited search and aspiration levels), thus extrapolation is simply not feasible. Furthermore, one cannot extend claims about a person's cognitive processes based on a rational or irrational behavior in a small world to corresponding claims for the same person in a large world.

### 3.2. Bounded rationality is the study of cognition in "Large worlds"

In behavioral economics, the term "bounded rationality" is correctly attributed to H. A. Simon but incorrectly identified with a program that is not his: the study of deviations from optimality. For instance, Daniel Kahneman (2003, p. 1449) noted: "Our research attempted to obtain a map of bounded rationality, by exploring the systematic biases that separate the beliefs that people have and the choices they make from the optimal beliefs and choices assumed in rational-agent models." In this research, it is assumed that the conditions for rational models (i.e., for a small world) hold and can thus define optimal reasoning. Simon (1989), however, asked a fundamentally different question, leading to a different research program.

Simon's question: "How do human beings reason when the conditions for rationality postulated by the model of neoclassical economics are not met?" (p. 377)

The study of behavior in lotteries – and other small worlds where the conditions of rationality are met – does not address Simon's question. In large worlds, people cannot optimize, but need to satisfice by relying on heuristics from the brain's adaptive toolbox. The term 'satisficing', originally introduced by Simon, is the Northumbrian term for 'satisfying' and is used to refer to decision strategies that ignore part of the available information and involve little computation. For example, when having to decide quickly whether an incoming patient should be treated as low-risk or high-risk in an emergency room, medical decisions implement fast and frugal heuristics (cp. Gigerenzer et al., 1999). We believe that as long as research continues to focus on small worlds, we will learn little about the brain's decision processes that people use *outside the laboratory*, i.e., in uncertain decision situations, which structurally differ from small world problems.

Why are lotteries studied so extensively in decision research and neuroeconomics and used to define rational choice? This appears particularly surprising given that we do not come across gambling situations very frequently in the real world, nor that most of our daily decision situations structurally resemble gambling situations. There are probably three reasons for this tradition. The first is the historical origin of aristocrats asking mathematicians for advice on gambling problems – not on whom to marry, what job offer to accept, or how to invest money wisely. The second reason is the fondness for optimization models. And the third is the misinterpretation of Simon's concept of bounded rationality as constrained optimization, or the deviation of human judgment from optimization.

In sum, much of cognitive neuroscience studies decision making in small worlds, where optimization is defined. This focus imposes limits on the understanding of brain processes, both normatively and descriptively. Normative behavior in a small world is not necessarily so in large worlds, where robustness counts. Furthermore, cognitive processes underlying bounded rationality, such as heuristic search, stopping rules, and aspiration levels, have little chance of being "detected" when one is looking for the neural correlates of EU theory and other as-if theories.

## 4. Methodology

### 4.1. Prediction versus fitting

In their methodological critique of behavioral economics, Binmore and Shaked (2010) recall the importance of distinguishing between data fitting and prediction:

The scientific gold standard is prediction. It is perfectly acceptable to propose a theory that fits existing experimental data and then to use the data to calibrate the parameters of the model.

But, before using the theory in applied work, the vital next step is to state the proposed domain of application of the theory and to make specific predictions that can be tested with the data that was used neither in formulating the theory nor in calibrating its parameters. (p. 89)

Whereas the dependent variable in behavioral decision research is the actual choice behavior of individuals, groups, or the entire economy, the primary dependent variable in almost all neuroeconomic studies to date is the BOLD signal change. Accordingly, the gold standard in neuroscience is the prediction of the BOLD response as a function of the manipulation of the independent variable(s). Neuroeconomic studies thus aim at predicting the BOLD signal changes as a function of choice behavior, or, in the words of Glimcher and colleagues (2009, p. 7): "Neuroscientists [...] were interested in describing the algorithmic mechanisms of choice. Their goal was to describe the neurobiological hardware that supported choice behavior in situations ranging from perceptual decision making to the expression of more complicated preferences." Yet the authors also noted that "what they [the neuroscientists] lacked was an overarching theoretical framework for placing their neural measurements into context." This lacuna was filled by Glimcher and colleagues' (2009) suggestion "that the neoclassical/revealed preference framework might prove a useful theoretical tool for neuroscience. What followed was the rapid introduction to the neuroscientific literature of such concepts as expected value and expected utility" (p. 7).

This statement reveals three issues that we propose to characterize the state of the art in current neuroeconomic research:

1. Cognitive neuroscientific and neuroeconomic research on decision making primarily pursues the neoclassical as-if approach while so far neglecting process theories, such as the program on fast-and-frugal heuristics (cp. Gigerenzer, Hertwig, & Pachur, 2011; for exceptions, see Volz et al., 2006, 2010).

2. The predominant focus on concepts such as expected value and expected utility has led to the generally accepted assumption in the cognitive neuroscience literature on decision making that the choice process comprises a first evaluation stage in which values for each option are determined and a subsequent decision phase in which the individual chooses on the basis of this common currency. Accordingly, these two stages have been investigated separately, and a considerable number of studies have focused on the neurobiological implementation of the anticipation/valuation phase, which is – by definition – characterized by a lack of choice behavior. As noted above, there is no compelling empirical evidence supporting the assumption that decision makers go through the stages of the expected value or utility model (e.g., Ford et al., 1989; Friedman & Sunder, 2011; Venkatraman et al., 2009). Even in gambling situation, individuals seem to process information in a way that is incompatible with the EU framework, as revealed by imaging studies (Venkatraman et al., 2009), verbal protocol studies (Cokely & Kelley, 2009), eye tracking studies (Russo & Dosher, 1983), and information board studies (Mann & Ball, 1994; Payne & Braunstein, 1978).

3. The presentation of data on the neurobiology of value-based decision making, which are considered to "yield new insights into behavior" (Kable & Glimcher, 2009, p. 734), may

> make researchers forget that neuroimaging does *not* allow "to look into the head" objectively or "watch the brain while deciding". Rather, by setting up an experiment, researchers are driven by their theoretical assumptions, which subsequently lead to very specific experimental manipulations, such as manipulating the probability and the value of choice options, as well as to very specific analyses, such as conducting an analysis "to identify candidate regions whose activity correlated with a linear model of EV." (Knutson et al., 2005; p. 4807). Thus, fMRI data themselves do not tell us what is going on in the brain. The data are always interpreted in light of a theory; more important, the very choice of a theory determines a study's problems and experimental set-up. For instance, optimization theory, such as EU and Bayes, confines studies to small worlds, where *the* best outcome is computationally tractable.

Returning to the issue of the degree to which neuroeconomic studies use prediction, we would like to recapitulate that the scientific method is hypothesis-driven. In other words, (neuroeconomic) researchers *first* hypothesize about the alleged brain areas being crucially involved in the respective cognitive process(es) and *then* conduct significance testing. Hypothesis-driven research needs to be distinguished from so-called "see-and-tell" studies or "fishing expeditions." The latter are appropriate for finding hypotheses, but should not be presented as testing hypotheses by performing significant tests after the fact. The practice of (mis)presenting a hypothesis-finding study as a hypothesis-testing study is possibly due to disregard for the value of hypotheses finding, high degrees of freedom in data collection and post hoc analysis, and the practice of null-hypothesis significance testing (NHST) (Loftus, 1996; Simmons et al., 2011; Vul et al., 2009). This is not to say that we take issue with research that describes the data of an experiment, which may lead to specific testable predications; we solely disapprove of presenting significant results after the fact, that is, selling ad hoc interpretations as genuine experimental hypotheses testing.

The very majority of neuroeconomic studies use prediction. That is, as a function of the experimental design, more or less elaborated anatomical hypotheses are made. For example, in the realm of value-based decision making, it has been predicted and shown that the ventral striatum encodes the subjective value of both primary (e.g., pleasant sweet taste [O'Doherty et al., 2002], naturalistic food aromas [Bragulat et al., 2010], or erotic stimuli [Sescousse et al., 2010]) and secondary rewards (e.g., money [Delgado et al., 2000; Elliott et al., 2000; Knutson et al., 2000]); that the ventral striatum reflects the anticipation and expectation of (monetary) rewards (Breiter et al., 2001; Knutson et al., 2000, 2003, 2005; Preuschoff et al., 2006;); and that the ventral striatum is directly related to an individual's actual behavioral preferences (Kable & Glimcher, 2007; O'Doherty et al., 2006;). A similar story seems to hold for the medial prefrontal cortex (mPFC) (e.g., Elliott et al., 2003; Lebreton et al., 2009; Plassmann et al., 2007; Tom et al., 2007; for a review see Rushworth et al., 2011). That is, the mPFC seems to reflect the "some aspect of both expected reward value prior to the making of a choice and the received reward value after a choice is made" (Rushworth et al., 2011, p. 1056). Contemporary research suggests that the mPFC valuation signal is an automatic one reflecting the value of an option even in the absence of any choice (Lebreton et al., 2009; Smith et al., 2010). Further endeavors to differentiate the roles of the mPFC and the ventral striatum suggested that the latter specifically represents anticipated gain magnitude, whereas the mPFC also represents anticipated gain probability; it was also suggested that the mPFC integrates the two components of expected value (Knutson et al., 2005; Knutson & Wimmer, 2007; but see also Behrens et al., 2007; Rushworth & Behrens, 2008, for the suggestion that anterior cingulate cortex activity encodes the integrated value of actions).

In the realm of intertemporal choice, it has been predicted and shown that decisions involving immediately available rewards draw specifically on limbic structures, whereas intertemporal choices per se, irrespective of delay, draw on the lateral prefrontal cortex and associated structures (Albrecht et al., 2010; McClure et al., 2004; Mitchell et al., 2011). Moreover, by taking into account the actual choice behavior of subjects, it has been predicted and shown that activity in the ventral striatum, the mPFC, and within the posterior cingulate cortex "tracks the revealed subjective value of delayed monetary rewards" (Kable & Glimcher, 2007, p. 1625). In the realm of social decision making, activation within neural structures that are involved in emotional processing, such as the insula and amygdala, have been predicted and shown to be activated for a number of so-called decision anomalies such as rejecting unfair offers in the UG (Sanfey et al., 2003; Tabibnia et al., 2008), reciprocating trust (van den Bos et al., 2009), displaying inequity aversion (Haruno & Frith, 2010), or third-party punishment decisions (Buckholtz et al., 2008); for an overview, see Rilling & Sanfey, 2011). Amygdala or insula activation has generally been considered to provide important affective biases to social decisions.

All these predictions were made in small world settings, where all alternatives, consequences, and probability distributions were known or could be learned from experience. That is, participants had to value specific items such as food, money, or specific abstract symbols representing money, or had to choose between (two) risky outcomes. As outlined before, these results are very interesting by itself and can help in determining the cognitive processes involved in different decision making tasks. For example, individuals using the priority heuristic (PH) when making decisions between risky gambles, by definition, first go through the reasons in the order of minimum gain, probability of minimum gain, maximum gain and they stop their examination if the minimum gain differs by 1/10 (or more) of the maximum gain; otherwise they stop the examination if probabilities differ by 1/10 (or more) of the probability scale. Given the formal description of the PH, individuals applying the PH simply compare the numbers of the two gambles and thus the corresponding anatomical hypothesis would predict activation within a parietal network, which has been shown to support number comparison processes (Deheaene & Cohen, 1995; Pinel et al., 2001). Yet, if activation within striatal, dorsal anterior cingulate cortex, or inferior frontal cortex would elicit, i.e., within the network suggested to reflect processes involved in EU calculations, this finding would raise issues.

### 4.2. Competitive tests of models versus testing only one

Given the abundance of evidence on the neurobiology of choice behavior, "for a neuroeconomist, then, these studies constitute overwhelming evidence that a value system exists and can be functionally localized" (Glimcher, 2009, p. 514). This may certainly apply to small world settings. Yet, achieving a good fit of the expected value model/neoclassical framework to the neuroscientific observations does not necessarily mean that a good model or *the* best model is found. This is because "all models are wrong, but some of them predict better than others and may lead to novel questions." (Gigerenzer & Gaissmaier, 2011). Thus, although EV models and their variants may capture the algorithmic mechanisms of choice behavior for small-world problems, a convincing argument would require tests of several models to determine how well the model of choice performs against competing ones. This procedure differs from the widespread practice of null hypothesis testing. Since neuroeconomics seeks an algorithmic description of the mechanisms for choice behavior and the cognitive strategies underlying economic and everyday decisions, implementing comparative tests of formal models seems indispensable. Only by pursuing this strategy, we consider, can one accomplish the ambitious aim of describing the mechanisms of how decisions are made (in the brain).

To our knowledge, hitherto there are only a handful of imaging studies that use competitive testing on the neural level, for example in risky decision making (Basten et al., 2010; Christopolous et al., 2010; Hsu et al., 2009; Venkatraman et al., 2009) and we are not aware of imaging studies that tested whether competing models such as heuristic models (e.g., priority heuristic for risky gambles) fit to the neural data. We would be eager to learn whether the activation in a specific area may also or better be explained by a competing (heuristic) model of choice.

One reason for this may be that in the implemented small-world problems, the very experimental set-up primes one specific strategy, namely EV calculations. Experimenters may have thereby induced the decision strategy in which they were interested. For example, in gambling paradigms the only information that is presented concerns probabilities and incentives (e.g., Behrens et al., 2007; Cooper & Knutson, 2008; De Martino et al., 2006; Elliott et al., 2000; Hsu et al., 2009; Knutson et al., 2005; Shiv et al., 2005; Preuschoff et al., 2006, 2008; Tom et al., 2007; Yacubian et al., 2006). Nevertheless, different decision strategies are also conceivable in gambling paradigms, such as probability matching, the priority heuristic, guessing, win-stay/lose-shift and others whose correlates could be investigated and compared (for probability matching in monkeys, see Morris et al., 2006; Niv et al., 2006). Indeed, Venkatraman and colleagues (2009) when investigating risky choice behavior on the neural level, found neural predictors of strategic variability in decision making: "Choices that maximized gains or minimized losses were predicted by fMRI activation in ventromedial prefrontal cortex or anterior insula, respectively. However, choices that followed a simplifying strategy (i.e., attending to overall probability of winning) were associated with activation in parietal and lateral prefrontal cortices." (p. 593). Most interestingly, activation within the mPFC predicted individual variability in strategic preferences through differential functional connectivity with parietal and insular cortex. In our view, studies like Venkatraman's et al. are very promising and should be extended to large world decision situations.

With these exceptions, the focus hitherto has been on the investigation of the anticipation/expectation phase, in which participants are presented with a specific gamble, bet, or other well-defined option and are encouraged to choose advantageously. For example, in the probabilistic monetary incentive delay task by Knutson and colleagues, participants in the anticipation phase were presented with an icon indicating exactly the incentive that could be obtained on that specific trial and its probability. After having seen the trial specification, participants awaited the feedback, which was probabilistically determined, sometimes even independent of participants' choice. The fMRI analyses in studies using such small world settings are generally stimulus-dependent, that is, regressors are generated on the basis of measures built into the task, such as magnitude of gain/loss, probability of gain/loss, valence or salience of events, trial-specific EVs, or the like. Accordingly, analyses reveal activation in areas responsible for processing specific task characteristics.

Recently, further progress has been made in showing – for risky decisions– that in combining information from the three areas that are particularly responsive to changes in magnitude (striatum), objective risk coding (doral anterior cingulate cortex (dACC)), and risk aversion (inferior frontal gyrus (IFG)), "these BOLD responses were informative enough to allow an ideal observer to detect the overt choice: a risky choice was more probably when striatal and cingulate activity was higher, whereas increased BOLD signals from IFG correlated with increased probability of a safe choice." (Christopoulos et al., 2009, p. 12581). In other words, the BOLD responses from these areas combined essentially decoded the behavioral choice.

Such findings are very interesting by itself and especially give information on how the brain (in small world settings) encodes and processes specific task characteristics and combines them to produce overt choice behavior; yet, it remains an open and interesting issue whether these processes will manifest themselves in large world decision situations alike. In other words, the description of the neurobiology of value-based decisions in the small world does not necessarily imply these processes and activations in large-world decisions, yet this remains to be seen. To clarify this problem, we recommend imaging studies on large-world decisions that determine and compare the neural correlates of different decision strategies, including those modeled by the neoclassical approach and the heuristic approach.

Another recent development, which we think should be pursued and extended, is model-based fMRI, "which involves the application of computational models in the design and analysis of neuroimaging experiments" (O'Doherty et al., 2007, p. 35). The standard operating procedure is to "first fit the computational model to subjects' actual behavior to find specific values for the free parameters in the model []. Once the best-fitting model parameters have been found, then the different model components can be regressed against the fMRI data [] to identify areas where the model-predicted time series show significant correlations with the actual changes in blood oxygenation level-dependent (BOLD) signal over time." (O'Doherty et al., 2007, p. 37). This model-based approach has been used to investigate questions of how the brain integrates cost and benefits during decision making (Basten et al., 2010), how it trades off between amount and delay during intertemporal decisions (Kable & Glimcher, 2007), how different experiences (volatility) are weighted in guiding future actions (Behrens et al., 2007), and whether the brain encodes a nonlinear probability function when evaluating risky choices as predicted by prospect theory (Hsu et al., 2009; Boorman & Sallet, 2009). Accordingly, in the various studies, the authors fitted several functions to the subjects' actual choices (e.g., various nonlinear probability-weighting functions or discount functions) and used the best fitting ones for the fMRI analyses. Results were interpreted to show that "the brain, thus, weighs costs against benefits by combining neural benefit and cost signals into a single, difference-based neural representation of net value" (Basten et al., 2010, p. 21767); that "the neural tradeoffs between amount and delay that are captured by the neurometric discount functions match the behavioral tradeoffs between these variables that are captured by the psychometric discount functions" (Kable & Glimcher, 2007, p. 1631); that "humans repeatedly combine prior and subsequent information as data accumulate over time," as reflected by ACC activity; and "that activity in the striatum during valuation of monetary gambles are nonlinear in probabilities in the pattern predicted by prospect theory, suggesting that probability distortion is reflected at the level of the reward encoding process." (Hsu et al., 2009, p. 2231). Despite these impressive results, it should be kept in mind that only different forms of neoclassical models were applied and compared, that is, competitive tests were carried out only within the same model class of as-if models. Moreover, these models were fit to the behavioral data (for problems with data fitting, see above), and the results cannot conclusively demonstrate that the respective activated regions implement the process specified within the model. Yet, in our view, it is a step in the right direction and should definitely be pursued and extended.

## 5. Taking stock: As-If models, small worlds and comparative tests

### 5.1. As-If models and neuroeconomics

In reviewing the neuroeconomic literature it appears that the overarching theoretical framework is the neoclassical as-if theory. The consensus that "the brain must perform multiple value computations to make sound choices" (Hare et al., 2008, p. 5623) just as in the as-if theory seems too strong and questionable given that hitherto only few studies investigated competing process models.

### 5.2. Small worlds and neuroeconomics

The majority of cognitive neuroscience studies on decision making use variants of small-world problems, prototypical gambling tasks, in which all alternatives, consequences and their probabilities are known. In nongambling decision situations, such as intertemporal choice paradigms, decisions are not even risky, but have certain outcomes. Examples are: "Do you prefer $24 now or $33 in 4 weeks?" or "How much are you willing to pay for a candy bar?" (cp. Hare et al., 2008; Kable & Glimcher, 2007; Lebreton et al., 2009; McClure et al., 2004; Plassmann et al., 2007). Moreover, in several other decision making and conditioning tasks, participants had extensive experience with the stimuli and the associated rewards, so that choice might simply have entailed assessing the likelihoods of rewards, as for example in probability-tracking tasks and their variants (cp., Behrens et al., 2007; Huettel et al., 2005). Subsuming conditioning under decision making is a questionable practice that leads to every response, conscious or unconscious, being called decision making, so that the term becomes meaningless. Accordingly, decisions such as whether to select surgery or radiation therapy for a tumor, to invest retirement savings in the stock market or treasury bills, to pursue a university degree, or to accept a new job – all of which were mentioned as prototypical for decision making (examples taken from Rustichini, 2009; Tom et al., 2007; Trepel et al., 2005) – have almost nothing in common with the experimental investigations of decision making processes in neuroeconomic studies (so far).

At this point, we return to Savage's distinction between small worlds and large worlds. Savage, the father of modern Bayesian decision theory, considered Bayesian rationality as normative for small worlds, holding the opinion that a decision maker should engage in subjective EU maximization when making decisions under risk in such a world. But Savage also wrote that it would be "ridiculous" to use Bayesian rationality outside small worlds. Instead, he emphasized that rational models cannot be automatically assumed to provide the correct answer in real-life decision situations. Large worlds need a different kind of rationality, and the study of heuristic decision making is one way to model rationality under uncertainty.

With that said, we agree with Glimcher (2009) that it might be the case that "dopamine neurons lead to the direct computation of SV [subjective value] under some conditions" (p. 514), whereby "some conditions" should be translated to "small-world problems". Although we believe that none of the proposed subjective EU maximization strategies is computationally feasible in large worlds, those who make the claim that dopamine neurons compute EU in small worlds need to show this by performing competitive tests with models that do not involve optimization.

A promising course of research, we think, is based on modeling cognitive decision making processes by means of alternative models, including models of heuristics, and testing and comparing their respective neural correlates.

Given that we share neuroscientists' overall aim of understanding how decisions are made, our main concern, however, is to promote the use of uncertain large-world paradigms in the neuroeconomic literature. For one, it is indispensable to incorporate heuristics into the theoretical portfolio, since previous research on large-world problems has shown that laypeople and experts (e.g., doctors, judges, managers) use heuristics in an ecologically rational way, that is, when the heuristics are adapted to the structure of the environment (Dhami, 2003; Gigerenzer & Gaissmaier, 2011; Gigerenzer et al., 2011; Wübben & Wangenheim, 2008). This research indicated that individuals, especially under time pressure and information overload, switch to simple noncompensatory strategies that use few cues rather than engaging in exhaustive compensatory strategies such as EU maximization.

### 5.3. Predictive and competitive tests and neuroeconomics

The inventory for this issue is elaborated in section 4. In short, neuroeconomics does a good job of predicting BOLD signal changes as a function of the manipulation of the independent variable(s), but we hold that neuroeconomic studies have a large developmental potential for competitive tests, especially with regard to heuristic models. As outlined above, our second concern is to promote predictive and competitive tests as methodological standards in neuroeconomics (where it is feasible). For example, cognitive neuroscience investigations shall compare different decision strategies that individuals actually used (cp. Venkatraman et al., 2009). Examples of general methodological approaches to determine which decision rules people (very likely) follow are the use of outcome-based strategy classification such as the maximum-likelihood strategy classification (Bröder & Schiffer, 2003; Bröder, 2010) or ACT-R (Anderson, 2007), cognitive process analysis (if it is useful) (Witteman & van Geenen, 2010), or a multiple measure strategy classification combining outcomes and decision times (Bergert & Nosofsky, 2006; Bröder & Gaissmaier, 2007; Glöckner, 2010; Rieskamp & Otto, 2006).

## 6. Conclusion

Neuroeconomics or the study of the neurobiology of decision making set out with ambitious aims, namely, "revealing the neurobiological mechanisms by which decisions are made" (Glimcher & Rustichini, 2004, p. 447) and "providing a biologically sound theory of how humans make decisions that can be applied in both the natural and the social sciences." (Rangel et al., 2008, p. 545). Back in 2005, Camerer, Loewenstein, and Prelec outlined two types of contributions that they suggested neuroscience could make to economics, or more broadly to decision sciences, namely, an incremental and a radical approach. The incremental approach was formulated as "neuroscience adds variables to conventional accounts of decision making or suggests specific functional forms to replace "as if" assumptions that have never been well supported empirically." (Camerer et al., 2005, p. 10).

We highly appreciate this statement, yet, as the previous literature review showed, in most neuroeconomic studies, the as-if models were not replaced (e.g., by models of heuristic decision making) but instead retained as descriptions of how the brain works.

The radical approach, on the other hand, is about neuroscience informing economic theory. According to Camerer and colleagues (2005), neuroscience "points to an entirely new set of constructs to underlie economic decision making. The standard economic theory of constrained utility maximization is most naturally interpreted either as the result of learning based on consumption experiences (which is of little help when prices, income, and opportunity sets change), or careful deliberation – a balancing of the costs and benefits of different options [...]." (p.10). In this passage, the authors appear to be in line with us. First, they acknowledge that for most of our real-life decisions we cannot rely on an extensive learning history and thus cannot define priors (as necessary for Bayesian calculations), and second, they admit that the decision process as prescribed in (neo-)classical decision theory for actual flesh-and-blood human beings is simply intractable: "The variables that enter into the formulation of the decision problem are precisely the variables that should affect the decision if the person had unlimited time and computing ability." (p. 10). In this way, Camerer and colleagues seem to concur with Savage that small-world and large-world decision situations differ fundamentally and that the investigation of small-world experiments alone may produce unrealistic data having no relevance for understanding how the brain deals with the real world. Yet, as we have shown in this contribution, the study of optimization in small worlds is still the norm of present-day neuroeconomics.

We find the advent of neuroeconomics promising and hope that it will continue on its original course so that we can arrive at psychologically valid accounts of human decision making. This, in our view, is only possible if the neuroscience of decision making forsakes as-if theories, investigates decision making under uncertainty (large worlds) rather than only under risk (small worlds), and implements competitive testing that includes heuristic models.

## Author details

Kirsten G. Volz[1] and Gerd Gigerenzer[2]

1 Werner Reichardt Centre for Integrative Neuroscience, Tuebingen, Germany

2 Max Planck Institute for Human Development, Berlin, Germany

## References

[1] Ahn, W.-Y., Busemeyer, J.R., Wagenmakers, E.-J., & Stout, J.C. (2008). Comparison of decision learning models using the generalization criterion method. *Cognitive Science,* Vol. 32, pp. 1376-1402

[2] Albrecht et al. (2011). What is for me is not for you: Brain correlates of intertemporal choice for self and other. *Social Cognitive and Affective Neuroscience,* Vol. 6, pp. 218-225

[3] Allais, M. (1953). Le comportement de l'homme rationnel devant le risque: Critique des postulates et axioms de l'école américaine. *Econometrica,* Vol. 21, pp. 503-546

[4] Anderson, J.R. (2007). Using brain imaging to guide the development of a cognitive architecture, In: *Integrated models of cognitive systems,* W.D. Gray, (Ed.), pp. 49-62, Oxford University Press, New York

[5] Basten, U., Biele, G., Heekeren, H.R. & Fiebach, C.J. (2010). How the brain integrates costs and benefits during decision making, *Proceedings of the National Academy of Sciences,* Vol. 107, pp. 21767-21772

[6] Behrens, T.E.J., Wollrich, M.W., Walton, M.E. & Rushworth, M.F.S. (2007). Learning the value of information in an uncertain world. *Nature Reviews Neuroscience,* Vol. 10, pp. 1214-1221

[7] Berg, N. & Gigerenzer, G. (2010). As-if behavioral economics: Neoclassical economics in disguise? *History of Economic Ideas,* Vol. 18, pp. 133-166

[8] Bergert, F.B. & Nosofsky, R.M. (2007). A response-time approach to comparing generalized rational and take-the-best models of decision making. *Journal of Experimental Psychology: Learning, Memory, and Cognition,* Vol. 331, pp. 107-129

[9] Bernoulli, D. (1738/1954). Specimen theoriae novae de mensura sortis. *Comentarii academiae scientarum imperialis Petropolitanae,* Vol. 5, pp. 175-192. (Engl. Transl. by L.

Sommer, Exposition of a new theory on the measurement of risk. *Econometrica,* Vol. 22, pp. 23-26

[10] Binmore, K. & Shaked, A. (2010). Experimental economics: Where next? *Journal of Economic Behavior & Organization,* Vol. 73, pp. 87-100

[11] Binmore, K. (2008). Behavioral economics and its applications. *The Economic Journal,* Vol. 118, pp. F248-F251

[12] Boorman, E. D. & Sallet, J. (2009). Mean-variance or prospect theory? The nature of value representations in the human brain. *The Journal of Neuroscience,* Vol. 29, pp. 7945-7947

[13] Bragulat, V., Dzemidzic, M., Bruno, C., Cox, C.A., Talavage, T., Considine, R.V. & Kareken, D.A. (2010). Food-related odor probes of brain reward circuits during hunger: A pilot fMRI study. *Obesity,* Vol. 18, pp. 1566-1571

[14] Brandstätter, E., Kühberger, A. & Schneider, F. (2002). A cognitive-emotional account of the shape of the probability weighting function. *Journal of Behavioral Decision Making,* Vol. 15, pp. 79-100

[15] Brandstätter, E., Gigerenzer, G. & Hertwig, R. (2006). The priority heuristic: Making choices without trade-offs. *Psycholocial Review,* Vol. 113, pp. 409-432

[16] Brandstätter, E., Gigerenzer, G. & Hertwig, R. (2008). Risky choice with heuristics: Reply to Birnbaum (2008), Johnson, Schulte-Mecklenbeck, and Willemsen (2008) and Rieger and Wang (2008). *Psychological Review,* Vol. 115, pp. 281-290

[17] Breiter, H.C., Aharon, I., Kahnemann, D., Dale, A. & Shizgal, P. (2001). Functional imaging of neural responses to expectancy and experience of monetary gains and losses. *Neuron,* Vol. 30, pp. 619-639

[18] Bröder, A. & Gaissmaier, W. (2007). Sequential processing of cues in memory-based multi-based multi-attribute decisions. *Psychonomic Bulletin and Review,* Vol. 45, pp. 895-900

[19] Bröder, A., Newell, B.R., & Platzer, C. (2010). Cue integration vs. Exemplar-based reasoning in multi-attribute decisions from memory: A matter of cue representation. *Judgment and Decision Making,* Vol. 5, pp. 326-338

[20] Bröder, A. & Schiffer, S. (2003). Bayesian strategy assessment in multi-attribute decision making. *Journal of Behavioral Decision Making,* Vol. 16, pp. 193-213

[21] Bröder, A. (2010). Outcome-based strategy classification, In: *Foundations for Tracing Intuition: Challenges and Methods,* A. Glöckner & C. Witteman, (eds.), pp. 61–82, Psychology Press, 978-1-84872-019-0, New York

[22] Buckholtz, J.W., Asplund, C.L., Dux, P.E., Zald, D.H., Gore, J.C., Jones, O.D. & Marois, R. (2008). The neural correlates of third-party punishment. *Neuron,* Vol. 60, pp. 930-940

[23] Camerer, C., Loewenstein, G., & Prelec, D. (2005). Neuroeconomics: How neuroscience can inform economics. *Journal of Economic Literature*, Vol. XLIII, pp. 9-64

[24] Christopoulos, G.I., Tobler, P.N., Bossaerts, P., Dolan, R.J., & Schultz, W. (2009). Neural correlates of value, risk, and risk aversion contributing to decision making under risk. *Journal of Neuroscience*, Vol. 29, pp. 12574-12583

[25] Cokely, E.T. & Kelley, C.M. (2009). Cognitive abilities and superior decision making under risk: A protocol analysis and process model evaluation. *Judgment and Decision Making*, Vol. 4, pp. 20-33

[26] Cooper , J.C. & Knutson, B. (2008). Valence and salience contribute to nucleus accumbens activation. *NeuroImage*, Vol. 39, pp. 538-547

[27] Craver, C.F. (2007). Explaining the brain: Mechanisms and the mosaic unity of neuroscience. Oxford: Oxford University Press.

[28] Crawford, V.P. & Meng, J. (2010). New York City cabdrivers' labor supply revisited: reference-dependent preferences with rational-expectations targets for hours and income. Available at SSRN: http://ssrn.com/abstract=1851878

[29] Czerlinski, J., Gigerenzer, G., & Goldstein, D.G. (1999). How good are simple heuristics? In: *Simple heuristics that make us smart*, G. Gigerenzer, P.M. Todd, and the ABC research group (eds.), pp. 97-118, New York: Oxford University Press

[30] Daston, L.J. (1988). *Classical Probability in the Enlightenment*, Princeton Univ. Press, Princeton, NJ

[31] Dhami, M.K. (2003). Psychological models of professional decision making. *Psychological Science*, Vol. 14, pp. 175-180

[32] De Martino, B., Kumaran, D., Seymour, B. & Dolan, R.J. (2006). Frames, biases, and rational decision-making in the human brain. *Science*, Vol. 313, pp. 684-687

[33] Dehaene, S. & Cohen, L. (1995). Towards an anatomical and functional model of number processing. *Mathematical Cognition*, Vol. 1, pp. 83-120

[34] Delgado. M.R., Nystrom, L.E., Fissell, C., Noll, D.C. & Fiez, J.A. (2000). Tracking the hemodynamic responses to reward and punishment in the striatum. *Journal of Neurophysiology*, Vol. 84, pp. 3072-3077

[35] DeMiguel, V., Garlappi, L., Nogales, F.J. & Uppal, R. (2009). A generalized approach to portfolio optimization: Improving performance by constraining portfolio norms. *Management Science*, Vol. 55, pp. 798-812

[36] Dhami, M. (2003). Psychological models of professional decision making. *Psychological Science*, Vol. 14, pp. 175-180

[37] Elliot, R., Friston, K.J. & Dolan, R.J. (2000). Dissociable neural responses in human reward systems. *The Journal of Neuroscience*, Vol. 20, pp. 6159-6165

[38] Elliot, R., Newman, J.L., Longe, O.A. & Deakin, J.F.W. (2003). Differential response patterns in the striatum and orbitofrontal cortex to financial reward in humans: A parametric functional magnetic resonance imaging study. *The Journal of Neuroscience,* Vol. 23, pp. 303-307

[39] Ford, J.K., Schmitt, N., Schlechtman, S.L., Hults, B.H. & Doherty, M.L. (1989). Process tracing methods: contributions, problems and neglected research questions. *Organizational Behavior and Human Decision Processes,* Vol. 43, pp. 55-117

[40] Fox, C.R. & Poldrack, R.A. (2009). Prospect theory and the brain, In: *Neuroeconomics: Decision Making and the Brain,* P.W. Glimcher, C. Camerer, E. Fehr, & R.A. Poldrack, (eds.), pp. 145-173, New York, NY: Academic Press, 978-0-12-374176-9

[41] Friedman, D. & Sunder, S. (2011). Risky curves: From unobservable utility to observable opportunity sets, *Cowles Foundation Discussion Paper No. 1819,* Cowles Foundation for Research in Economics, Yale University, New Haven CT

[42] Friedman, M. & Savage, L.J. (1948). The utility analysis of choices involving risk. *Journal of Political Economy,* Vol. 56, pp. 279-304

[43] Friedman, M. (1953). *Essays in Positive Economics,* Chicago Press, Chicago

[44] Friedmann, D. & Sunder, S. (2011). Risky curves: From unobservable utility to observable opportunity sets. *Cowles Foundation Discussion Paper No. 1819,* Cowles Foundation for Research in Economics, Yale University, New Haven CT

[45] Gazzaniga, M.S. (2000). Cognitive Neuroscience: A reader. Malden, MA: Blackwell Publishers

[46] Gigerenzer, G. (2008). Why heuristics work. *Perspectives on Psychological Science,* Vol. 3, pp. 20-29

[47] Gigerenzer, G. & Brighton, H. (2009). Homo heuristics: Why biased minds make better inferences. *Topics in Cognitive Science,* Vol. 1, pp. 107-143

[48] Gigerenzer, G. & Gaissmaier, W. (2011). Heuristic decision making. *Annual Review Psychology,* Vol. 62, pp. 451-482

[49] Gigerenzer, G. & Gray J.A.M. (2011). Launching the century of the patient, In: *Better Doctors, Better Patients, Better Decisions: Envisioning Health Care 2020,* G. Gigerenzer & J.A.M. Gray, (eds.), pp. 3-29, MIT Press, 978-0-262-01603-2, Cambridge MA

[50] Gigerenzer, G. & Selten, R. (2001). Rethinking rationality. In: *Bounded rationality: The adaptive toolbox.* , G. Gigerenzer & R. Selten, (eds.), pp. 1-12, MIT Press, Cambridge MA

[51] Gigerenzer, G., Hertwig, R. & Pachur, T. (eds.) (2011). *Heuristics: The Foundations of Adaptive Behavior,* Oxford University Press, New York

[52] Gigerenzer, G., Swijtink, Z., Porter, T., Daston, L., Beatty, J. & Krüger, L. (1989). *The Empire of Chance. How Probability Changed Science and Everyday Life,* Cambridge University Press, Cambridge

[53] Gigerenzer, G., Todd, P.M. & the ABC Research Group (1999). *Simple Heuristics that Make Us Smart,* Oxford University Press, New York

[54] Glimcher, P.W. (2009). Choice: Towards a standard back-pocket model. In: *Neuroeconomics: Decision Making and the Brain,* P.W. Glimcher, C. Camerer, E. Fehr, & R.A. Poldrack, (eds.), pp. 503-521, New York, NY: Academic Press, 978-0-12-374176-9

[55] Glimcher, P.W. & Rustichini, A. (2004). Neuroeconomics: The consilience of brain and decision. *Science,* Vol. 306, pp. 447-452

[56] Glimcher, P.W., Camerer, C., Fehr, E., & Poldrack, R.A. (2009). Introduction: A brief history of neuroeconomics, In: *Neuroeconomics: Decision Making and the Brain,* P.W. Glimcher, C. Camerer, E. Fehr, & R.A. Poldrack, (eds.), pp. 1-12, New York, NY: Academic Press, 978-0-12-374176-9

[57] Glöckner, A. (2010). Multiple measure strategy classification: Outcomes, decision times and confidence ratings, In: *Foundations for Tracing Intuition: Challenges and Methods,* A. Glöckner & C. Witteman, (eds.), pp. 83-105, Psychology Press, 978-1-84872-019-0, New York

[58] Goldstein, D.G. & Gigerenzer, G. (2002). Models of ecological rationality: The recognition heuristic. *Psychological Review,* Vol. 109, pp. 75-90

[59] Gul, F. & Pesendorfer, W. (2008). The case for mindless economics, In: *The Foundations of Positive and Normative Economics: A Handbook,* A. Caplin & A. Schotter, (eds.), pp. 3-39, Oxford, Oxford University Press

[60] Hare, T.A., O'Doherty, J., Camerer, C.F., Schultz, W. & Rangel, A. (2008). Dissociating the role of the orbitofrontal cortex and the striatum in the computation of goal values and prediction errors. *The Journal of Neuroscience,* Vol. 28, pp. 5623-5630

[61] Harrison, G.W. (2008). Neuroeconomics: A critical reconsideration. *Economics and Philosophy,* Vol. 24, pp. 303-344

[62] Haruno, M. & Frith, C.D. (2010). Activity in the amygdala elicited by unfair divisions predicts social value orientation. *Nature Neuroscience,* Vol. 13, pp. 160-161

[63] Hauser, J. (2011). A marketing science perspective on recognition-based heuristics (and the fast-and-frugal paradigm). *Judgment and Decision Making,* Vol. 6, pp. 396-408

[64] Hertwig, R. & Todd, P.M. (2003). More is not always better: The benefits of cognitive limits, In: *Thinking: Psychological Perspectives on Reasoning, Judgment and Decision making,* D. Hardman & L. Macchi, pp. 213-233, John Wiley & Sons Ltd, 0-471-49457-7, Chichester, United Kingdom

[65] Honda, H., Abe, K., Matsuka, T., & Yamagishi, K. (2011). The role of familiarity in binary choice inferences. *Memory and Cognition*, Vol. 39, pp. 851-863

[66] Hsu, M., Krajbich, I., Zhao, C. & Camerer, C.F. (2009). Neural response to reward anticipation under risk is nonlinear in probabilities. *The Journal of Neuroscience*, Vol. 29, pp. 2231-2237

[67] Huettel, S.A., Song, A.W. & McCarthy, G. (2005). Decisions under uncertainty: Probabilistic context influences activation of prefrontal and parietal cortices. *The Journal of Neuroscience*, Vol. 25, pp. 3304-3311

[68] Kable, J.W. & Glimcher, P.W. (2007). The neural correlates of subjective value during intertemporal choice. *Nature Reviews Neuroscience*, Vol. 10, pp. 1625-1633

[69] Kable, J.W. & Glimcher, P.W. (2009). The neurobiology of decision: Consensus and controversy. *Neuron*, Vol.63, pp. 733-745

[70] Kahneman, D. & Tversky, A. (1979). Prospect theory: An analysis of decision under risk. *Econometrica*, Vol. 47, pp. 163-291

[71] Kahneman, D. & Tversky, A. (eds.) (2000). *Choices, Values and Frames*, Cambridge University Press, Cambridge

[72] Kahneman, D. (2003). Maps of bounded rationality: Psychology for behavioral economics. *The American Economic Review*, Vol. 93, pp. 1449-1475

[73] Katsikopoulos, K.V. & Gigerenzer, G. (2008). One reason decision-making: Modeling violations of expected utility theory. *Journal of Risk and Uncertainity*, Vol. 37, pp. 35-56

[74] Knutson, B. & Wimmer, G.E. (2007). Splitting the difference: How does the brain code reward episodes? *Annals of the New York Academy of Sciences*, Vol. 1104, pp. 54-69

[75] Knutson, B., Fong, G.W., Bennett, S.M., Adams, C.M. & Hommer, D. (2003). A region of mesial prefrontal cortex tracks monetarily rewarding outcomes: Characterization with rapid event-related FMRI. *NeuroImage*, Vol. 18, pp. 263-272

[76] Knutson, B., Taylor, J., Kaufman, M., Peterson, R. & Glover, G. (2005). Distributed neural representation of expected value. *The Journal of Neuroscience*, Vol. 25, pp. 4806-4812

[77] Knutson, B., Westdorp, A., Kaiser, E. & Hommer, D. (2000). fMRI visualization of brain activity during a monetary incentive delay task. *NeuroImage*, Vol. 12, pp. 20-27

[78] Lebreton, M., Jorge, S., Michel, V., Thirion, B. & Pessiglione, M. (2009). An automatic valuation system in the human brain. Evidence from functional neuroimaging. *Neuron*, Vol. 64, pp. 431-439

[79] Leland, H.E. (1994). Corporate dept value, bond convenants, and optimal capital structure. *The Journal of Finance*, Vol. 49, pp. 1213-1252

[80] Lopes, L.L. (1981). Decision making in the short run. *Journal of Experimental Psychology: Human Learning and Memory,* Vol. 7, pp. 377-385

[81] Lopes, L.L. (1994). Psychology and economics. Perspectives on risk, cooperation, and the marketplace. *Annual Review of Psychology,* Vol. 45, pp. 197-227

[82] Loftus, G.R. (1996). Psychology will be a much better science when we change the way we analyze data. *Current Directions in Psychological Science,* Vol. 5, pp. 161-171

[83] Mann, L. & Ball, C. (1994). The relationship between search strategy and risky choice. *Australian Journal of Psychology,* Vol. 46, pp. 131-136

[84] Marchionni, C. & Vromen, J. (2010). Neuroeconomics: hype or hope? *Journal of Economic Methodology,* Vol. 17, pp. 103-106

[85] Marewski, J.N., Gaissmaier, W. & Gigerenzer, G. (2010). Good judgments do not require complex cognition. *Cognitive Processing,* Vol. 11, pp. 103-121

[86] Martignon, L. & Hoffrage, U. (1999). Why does one-reason decision making work? A case study in ecological rationality, In: *Simple heuristics that make us smart,* G. Gigerenzer, P.M. Todd & the ABC Research Group, pp. 119– 140, Oxford University Press, New York

[87] Martignon, L., Vitouch, O., Takezawa, M. & Forster, M. R. (2011). Naive and yet enlightened: From natural frequencies to fast and frugal decision trees, In: *Heuristics: The Foundations of Adaptive Behavior,* G. Gigerenzer, R. Hertwig & T. Pachur (eds.), pp. 136-150, Oxford University Press, Oxford

[88] Marr, D. (1982). Vision. San Francisco: W.H. Freeman

[89] Maskin, E. (2008). Can neural data improve economics? *Science,* Vol. 321, pp. 1788-1789

[90] McClure, S.M., Laibson, D.I., Loewenstein, G. & Cohen, J.D. (2004). Separate neural systems value immediate and delayed monetary rewards. *Science,* Vol. 306, pp. 503-507

[91] Mitchell, J.P., Schirmer, J., Ames, D.L. & Gilbert, D.T. (2011). Medial prefrontal cortex predicts intertemporal choice. *Journal of Cognitive Neuroscience,* Vol. 23, pp. 857-866

[92] Morris, G., Nevet, A., Arkadir, D., Vaadia, E. & Bergman, H. (2006) Midbrain dopamine neurons encode decisions for future action. *Nature Neuroscience,* Vol. 9, pp. 1057-1063

[93] Niv, Y., Daw, N.D. & Dayan, P. (2006). Choice values. *Nature Neuroscience,* Vol. 9, pp. 987-988

[94] O'Doherty, J.P., Hampton, A. & Kim, H. (2007). Model-based fMRI and its application to reward learning and decision making. *Annals of the New York Academy of Sciences,* Vol., 1104, pp. 35-53

[95] O'Doherty, J.P., Buchanan, T.W., Seymour, B. & Dolan, R.J. (2006). Predictive neural coding of reward preference involves dissociable responses in human ventral midbrain and ventral striatum. *Neuron,* Vol. 49, pp. 157-166

[96] O'Doherty, J.P., Deichmann, R., Critchley, H.D. & Dolan, R.J. (2002). Neural responses during anticipation of a primary taste reward. *Neuron,* Vol. 33, pp. 815-826

[97] Payne, J.W., Bettman, J.R., Coupey, E.,& Johnson, E.J. (1992). A constructive process view of decision making – Multiple strategies in judgment and choice. *Acta Psychologica,* Vol. 80, pp. 107-141

[98] Payne, J.W., Bettman, J.R. & Johnson, E.J. (1993). *The Adaptive Decision Maker,* Cambridge University Press, Cambridge

[99] Payne, J.W. & Braunstein, M.L. (1978). Risky choice: An examination of information acquisition behavior. *Memory and Cognition,* Vol. 6, pp. 554-561

[100] Persson, M., & Rieskamp, J. (2009). Inferences from memory: Strategy- and exemplar-based judgment models compared. *Acta Psychologica,* Vol. 130, pp. 25-37

[101] Pinel, P., Dehaene, S., Riviere, D., & LeBihan, D. (2001). Modulation of parietal activation by semantic distance in a number comparison task. *Neuroimage,* Vol. 14, pp. 1013-1026

[102] Plassmann, H., O'Doherty, J. & Rangel, A. (2007). Orbitofrontal cortex encodes willingness to pay in everyday economic transactions. *The Journal of Neuroscience,* Vol. 27, pp. 9984-9988

[103] Preuschoff, K., Bossaerts, P. & Quartz, S.R. (2006). Neural differentiation of expected reward and risk in human subcortical structures. *Neuron,* Vol. 51, pp. 381-390

[104] Preuschoff, K., Quartz, S.R. & Bossaerts, P. (2008). Human insula activation reflects risk prediction errors as well as risk. *The Journal of Neuroscience,* Vol. 28, pp. 2745-2752

[105] Rangel, A., Camerer, C. & Montague, P.R. (2008). A framework for studying the neurobiology of value-based decision making. *Nature Reviews Neuroscience,* Vol. 9, pp. 545-556

[106] Rieskamp, J. & Otto, P.E. (2006). SSL: A theory of how people learn to select strategies. *Journal of Experimental Psychology: General,* Vol. 135, pp. 207-236

[107] Rilling, J.K. & Sanfey, A.G. (2011). The neuroscience of social decision-making. *Annual Review of Psychology,* Vol. 62, pp. 23-48

[108] Roberts, S. & Pashler, H. (2000). How persuasive is a good fit? A comment on theory testing. *Psychological Review,* Vol. 107, pp. 358-367

[109] Roberts, S. & Sternberg, S. (1993).The meaning of additive reaction-time effects: Tests of three alternatives. In: Attention and Performance XIV: Synergies in experimental

psychology, artificial intelligence, and cognitive neuroscience – A Silver Jubilee, D.E. Meyer & S. Kornblum (eds.), pp. 611-653, Cambridge, MA: MIT Press

[110] Rubinstein, A. (1988). Similarity and decision-making under risk (is there a utility theory resolution tot he Allais Paradox?). *Journal of Economic Theory,* Vol. 46, pp. 145-153

[111] Rubinstein, A. (2008). Comments on neuroeconomics. *Economics and Philosophy,* Vol. 24, pp. 485-494

[112] Rushworth, M.F.S. & Behrens, T.E.J. (2008). Choice, uncertainty and value in prefrontal and cingulate cortex. *Nature Neuroscience,* Vol. 11, pp. 389-397

[113] Rushworth, M.F.S., Noonan, M.P., Boorman, E.D., Walton, M.E. & Behrens, T.E. (2011). Frontal cortex and reward-guided learning and decision-making. *Neuron,* Vol. 70, pp. 1054-1069

[114] Russo, J.E., & Dosher, B.A. (1983). Strategies for multiattribute binary choice. Journal of Experimental Psychology: *Learning, Memory, and Cognition,* Vol. 9, pp. 676-696

[115] Rustichini, A. (2009). Neuroeconomics: What have we found, and what should we search for. *Current Opinion in Neurobiology,* Vol. 19, pp. 672-677

[116] Samuelson, P.A. (1937). A note on the measurement of utility. *The Review of Economic Studies,* Vol. 4, pp. 155-161

[117] Sanfey, A.G., Rilling, J.K., Aronson, J.A., Nystrom, L.E. & Cohen, J.D. (2003). The neural basis of economic decision-making in the ultimatum game. *Science,* Vol. 300, pp. 1755-1758

[118] Savage, L.J. (1954). *Foundations of Statistics.* Wiley, New York

[119] Selten, R. (2001) What is bounded rationality? In: *Bounded Rationality: The Adaptive Toolbox,* G. Gigerenzer & R. Selten (eds.), pp. 13-36, MIT Press, Cambridge MA

[120] Serrao, A. & Coelho, L. (2004). Cumulative Prospect Theory : A study oft he farmers' decision behavior in the Alentejo dryland region of Protugal. Presentation at the American Agricultural Economics Association Annual Meeting, Denver, Colorado, August 1-4, 2004.

[121] Sescousse, G., Redouté, J. & Dreher, J.-C. (2010). The architecture of reward value coding in the human orbitofrontal cortex. *The Journal of Neuroscience,* Vol. 30, pp. 13095-13104

[122] Shiv, B., Loewenstein, G., Bechara, A., Damasion, H., & Damasio, A.R. (2005). Investment behavior and the negative side of emotion. *Psychological Science,* Vol. 16, pp. 435-439

[123] Simon, H.A. (1989). The scientist as a problem solver. In: *Complex Information Processing: The Impact of Herbert A. Simon*, D. Klar & K. Kotovsky (eds.), pp. 373-398, Erlbaum, Hillsdale NJ

[124] Simmons, J.P., Nelson, L.D. & Simonsohn, U. (2011). False-positive psychology: Undisclosed flexibility in data collection and analysis allows presenting anything as significant. *Psychological Science*, in press

[125] Smith, D.V., Hayden, B.Y., Truong, T.K., Song, A.W., Platt, M.L., & Huettel, S.A. (2010). Distinct value signals in anterior and posterior ventromedial prefrontal cortex. *Journal of Neuroscience*, Vol. 30, 2490-2495

[126] Tabibnia, G., Satpute, A.B. & Lieberman, M.D. (2008). The sunny side of fairness: Preference for fairness activates reward circuitry (and disregarding unfairness activates self-control circuitry). *Psychological Science*, Vol. 19, pp. 339-347

[127] Tobler, P.N., Fiorillo, C.D., & Schultz, W. (2005). Adaptive coding of reward value by dopamine neurons. *Science*, Vol. 307, pp. 1642-1645

[128] Tobler, P.N., O`Doherty, J.P., Dolan, R.J. & Schultz, W. (2007). Reward value coding distinct from risk attitude-related uncertainty coding in human reward systems. *Journal of Neurophysiology*, Vol. 97, pp. 1621-1632

[129] Tom, S.M., Fox, C.R., Trepel, C., & Podrack, R.A. (2007). The neural basis of loss aversion in decision-making under risk. *Science*, Vol. 315, pp. 515-518

[130] Trepel, C., Fox, C.R. & Poldrack, R.A. (2005). Prospect theory on the brain? Toward a cognitive neuroscience of decision under risk. *Cognitive Brain Research*, Vol. 23, pp. 34-50

[131] Tversky, A. (1972). Elimination by aspects: A theory of choice. *Psychological Review*, Vol. 79, pp. 281-299

[132] Van den Bos, W., van Dijk, E., Westenberg, M., Rombouts, S.A., & Crone, E.A. (2009). What motivates repayment? Neural correlates of reciprocity in the Trust Game. *Social Cognitive and Affective Neuroscience*, Vol. 4, pp. 294-304

[133] Venkatraman, V., Payne, J.W., Bettman, J.R., Luce, M.F., & Huettel, S.A. (2009). Separate neural mechanisms underlie choice and strategic preferences in risky decision making. *Neuron*, Vol. 62, pp. 593-602

[134] Vul, E., Harris, C., Winkielman, P. & Pashler, H. (2009). Puzzling high correlations in fMRI studies of emotion, personality, and social cognition. *Perspectives on Psychological Science*, Vol. 4, pp. 274-2980

[135] Volz, K.G., Schooler, L.J. & von Cramon, D.Y. (2010). It just felt right: The neural correlates of the fluency heuristic. *Consciousness and Cognition*, Vol. 19, pp. 829-837

[136] Volz K.G., Schooler, L.J., Schubotz, R.I., Raab, M., Gigerenzer, G. & von Cramon, D.Y. (2006). Why you think Milan is larger than Modena: Neural correlates of the recognition heuristic. *Journal of Cognitive Neuroscience,* Vol. 18, pp. 1924-1936

[137] Wexler, K. (1978). A review of John R. Andereson's Language, Memory, and Thought. *Cognition,* Vol. 6, pp. 327-351

[138] Witteman, C. & van Geenen, E. (2010). Cognitive process analysis, In: *Foundations for Tracing Intuition: Challenges and Methods,* A. Glöckner & C. Witteman, (eds.), pp. 45-60, Psychology Press, 978-1-84872-019-0, New York

[139] Wübben, M. & von Wangenheim, F. (2008). Instant customer base analysis: Managerial heuristics often "get it right". *Journal of Marketing,* Vol. 72, pp. 82-93

[140] Yacubian, J., Gläscher, J., Schroeder, K., Sommer,T., Braus, D.F. & Büchel, C. (2006). Dissociable systems for gain- and loss-related value predictions and errors of prediction in the human brain. The Journal of Neuroscience, Vol. 26, pp. 9530-9537

# 6

# Active and Passive fMRI for Presurgical Mapping of Motor and Language Cortex

Victoria A.L. Mosher, Einat Liebenthal and
Bradley G. Goodyear

## 1. Introduction

### 1.1. Overview of fMRI and its use in presurgical mapping

Functional magnetic resonance imaging (fMRI) using the blood-oxygenation level dependent (BOLD) contrast measures local changes in the concentration of paramagnetic deoxyhemoglobin associated with an increase in blood flow to active regions of the brain (Bandettini, Wong, Hinks, Tikofsky, & Hyde, 1992; Kwong, et al., 1992; Ogawa, Lee, Kay, & Tank, 1990). Together with structural MRI, BOLD fMRI is increasingly being used for presurgical functional mapping of epilepsy and brain tumor patients (Binder, et al., 1996; Haberg, Kvistad, Unsgard, & Haraldseth, 2004; Hall & Truwit, 2008; Krings, et al., 2001; Lee, et al., 1999; Van Westen, Skagerberg, Olsrud, Fransson, & Larsson, 2005; Liebenthal, 2011). Presurgical fMRI provides patient-specific functional information that may facilitate maximal tumor or epileptic tissue surgical resection, with minimal damage to surrounding gray and white matter structures that support vital sensory and cognitive functions. Presurgical mapping of brain regions and their spatial relationship to the lesion can in some cases help predict possible deficits in sensory, motor or cognitive functions due to surgery or due to continued lesion growth (Haberg, Kvistad, Unsgard, & Haraldseth, 2004). In this way, presurgical mapping can guide the decision for course of intervention (extent of resection, alternative treatment, etc.) and the decision to conduct additional intra-operative functional mapping (e.g., intra-cortical stimulation-ICS). Finally, presurgical mapping is also valuable for planning the pathway of surgical approach.

The main advantages of fMRI in particular for clinical applications are its high spatial resolution, non-invasive nature, relative safety, and the good access to MRI scanners in most medical centers. Compared to functional mapping using ICS, or the intracarotid sodium amobarbital procedure (Wada test) to assess hemispheric language and memory dominance, fMRI is far less unpleasant to the patient and it is also less expensive (Medina et al., 2004). Unlike ICS, fMRI is performed prior to the surgery, without the time constraints and limitations on patient cognitive ability imposed by the surgery. The Wada test, named after Canadian neurologist and epileptologist Juhn Atsushi Wada, was developed 50 years ago to assess the hemispheric dominance of language and thereby the risk of language decline in patients undergoing brain surgery (Wada & Rasmussen, 1960). The procedure involves some risk to the patient, however, and it is unpleasant, consisting of intracarotid injection of a barbiturate to one brain hemisphere, during which time the other hemisphere is examined for language and memory functions.

One concern sometimes raised with respect to fMRI presurgical mapping is that it identifies neuronal networks involved in a specific function, including regions that may actually be expendable (Desmond & Annabel Chen, 2002). The problem is that, surgical resection of expendable areas of a functional network identified with fMRI should not cause a post-surgical functional decline, and it would therefore be safe and desirable for achieving the surgery goals to resect them. In contrast, ICS is thought to indicate strictly regions that are essential for a function, and should therefore be preserved during surgery in order to prevent functional damage. However it is important to understand that, as with fMRI, a similar concern actually applies to ICS in that regions that are remote from the stimulated region but connected to it may also be affected by the stimulation and 'erroneously' considered essential.

Another difficulty relates to the high inter-and intra-subject variability in the extent of activation foci observed with fMRI even with constant scanning parameters and consistent task performance (Liu, Zhang, Brown, Yue, 2004). This problem usually arises because the extent of active areas is determined by a statistical significance threshold that depends on the quality and quantity of the acquired signal, irrespective of the physiological boundaries of functional fields. In an effort to address this issue, recent work examined the spatial and temporal reproducibility of the relative amplitude of the fMRI signal and found it to be more stable than the absolute amplitude (Voyvodic, 2006). It was further determined empirically that thresholding individual activation maps at 40% of the most active voxels resulted in highly reproducible activity in the sensorimotor hand region during a finger tapping task, both within and across subjects (Voyvodic, Petrella, Friedman, 2009). Thus, relative amplitude maps can be used to improve the reliability and anatomical specificity of functional MR mapping.

Despite the differences between the techniques, there is generally very good concordance between fMRI and ICS mapping of somatosensory and motor functions (Bartos, et al., 2009; Hirsch, et al., 2000; Holodny, et al., 2000; Jack, et al., 1994; Krishnan, et al., 2004; Lehericy, Duffau, et al., 2000; Pujol, et al., 1996; Yetkin, et al., 1997). Nevertheless, in language mapping, reported levels of task sensitivity and specificity are variable and strongly dependent on the particular task that is used (Bookheimer, 2007). High sensitivity (i.e., fMRI activates all or most sites identified by ICS) but low specificity (i.e., fMRI activates additional sites not identified by ICS) has been reported for auditory tasks and in particular word generation to auditory cues (FitzGerald, et al., 1997). Higher sensitivity can generally be achieved with the conjunction of several fMRI language tasks, but specificity remains low (Pouratian, Bookheimer, Rex, Martin, & Toga, 2002; Rutten, Ramsey, van Rijen, Noordmans, & van Veelen, 2002).

Perhaps the most serious concern with regard to fMRI presurgical mapping (and functional mapping in general) is that the predictive value of this technique for patient outcome has not yet systematically been established in different patient types and using specific activation paradigms. Several studies in small cohorts of brain tumor patients suggest that fMRI mapping can be predictive of surgical outcome. A distance of 10 mm or more between tumor and functional cortex has been suggested to carry reduced risk for postsurgical neurological deficits (Haberg, et al., 2004; Krishnan, et al., 2004). In epilepsy, fMRI of language has been demonstrated to be strongly correlated with Wada language asymmetry (Binder, et al., 1996; Lehericy, Cohen, et al., 2000; Liegeois, et al., 2002) and to predict language (Sabsevitz, et al., 2003) and verbal memory (Binder et al., 2008) outcome after left anterior temporal lobe resection. Despite these recent advances, more work is required to establish guidelines for the use of fMRI in presurgical mapping.

### 1.2. Selection of fMRI paradigms

Factors related to the choice of fMRI activation paradigm (active or passive experimental task, control task, level of task performance, and the number of trials per task condition) have a critical impact on the resulting functional maps and their interpretation, particularly for mapping cognitive functions such as language and memory (Binder, Swanson, Hammeke, & Sabsevitz, 2008; Bookheimer, 2007). In terms of motor paradigms, simple hand/finger movements are usually sufficient to get a reliable map of motor cortex activity. These types of paradigms will be presented later in the chapter when we compare task-based fMRI with passive resting-state paradigms.

In terms of language tasks, active tasks requiring an overt response are generally considered more reliable because they allow monitoring of the patient's performance, and are thought to engage targeted brain regions more strongly (Lee, Jack, & Riederer, 1998). An active control task rather than passive rest (i.e., no task) is recommended as a baseline for contrasting with an active language task, because activation in the control condition can account for general executive, attentional and motor processes that are nonspecific to the tested cognitive function (Binder, Swanson, et al., 2008; Demonet, et al., 1992). In addition, activation during passive rest can be dominated by continuous processing of linguistically-mediated thoughts (whether day dreaming or intense mental processing), thereby effectively reducing the differential activation of language networks between the active and control tasks (McKiernan, D'Angelo, Kaufman, & Binder, 2006; Stark & Squire, 2001).

Finally, the task demands should be adjusted according to the patient's level of performance. For example, shorter and/or easier versions of the tasks may be needed for young children who tend to have a shorter attention span and a different knowledge base. As will be elaborated in the second part of this chapter, an interesting alternative approach to active task paradigms is passive resting-state fMRI. The resting-state paradigm is independent of patient performance, is time efficient, and can therefore serve as an alternative for patients who cannot comply with active task demands.

### 1.3. Comparative evaluation of three fMRI language tasks

To demonstrate the impact of the choice of paradigm on resulting fMRI maps, we compared three language tasks in terms of sensitivity and specificity in regions of interest for language. These tasks are: an auditory semantic word decision task (Binder, et al., 1997), an auditory definition naming task, and a silent word generation task.

The semantic task consists of a dual-criteria go/no-go semantic word decision (SWD) to auditorily presented animal names (i.e., press the keypad if "this animal is found in North America and used by people"), contrasted with a dual-criteria go/no-go auditory decision task (press the keypad if "this tone sequence contains two high-pitch tones"). Sixteen blocks of 8 trials alternating between the tasks are presented in two separate runs. This task has been shown to reliably activate regions in left inferior and middle frontal gyri, left middle temporal gyrus, left fusiform gyrus, and left angular gyrus, involved in phonological and lexico-semantic functions (Binder, et al., 1997). The degree of lateralization of these activated areas has been shown to correspond with Wada language asymmetry in individual epilepsy patients (Binder, et al., 1996) and predicts language and verbal memory outcome after left temporal lobectomy (Binder, et al., 2008; Sabsevitz, et al., 2003).

The auditory definition (or responsive) naming task (DNT) consists of overtly naming (speaking the name of) an object, animal, famous place, or famous person, in response to an auditory description (for example, "a horse with stripes" or "what the king wears on his head") (Hamberger & Seidel, 2003). This task is contrasted with an auditory control task consisting of speaking the number of siren sounds embedded in a sequence of white noise. This task uses an event-related design with 128 naming trials and 128 control trials, presented intermixed in 4 separate runs. Relative to the SWD, the DNT places additional demands on the language system because it involves word retrieval and overt speech. This task is expected to engage stronger, or more extensive activation within language areas, particularly in the left inferior frontal, middle temporal and parietal cortex (Okada & Hickok, 2006; Tomaszewki Farias, Harrington, Broomand, & Seyal, 2005).

The silent word generation (SWG) task consists of covertly finding words that start with certain letters, each displayed on a screen for 5 seconds. The control task consists of visually fixating on letters from foreign alphabets. We compared the SWG task with the SWD and DNT tasks because it is simple to implement, and therefore often used for fMRI language mapping in clinical settings. Nevertheless, a significant drawback of this task is that there is no monitoring of task performance. In addition, the task engages primarily phonological processing, but imposes fewer demands on the semantic system.

The reliability of each of the three fMRI language tasks was examined in eleven right handed neurologically-healthy volunteers, using sensitivity and specificity measures described previously (Hirsch, et al., 2000). Target regions of interest (ROIs) for language (inferior frontal gyrus, IFG; middle temporal gyrus, MTG; and angular gyrus, AG) were defined using a digital atlas based on cytoarchitectonic and macro anatomical labels (Eickhoff, et al., 2005). An adaptive thresholding scheme, consisting of mapping the activation in each subject as a percentage of local excitation, was used as a means to reduce the variability in the extent of activation between subjects (Voyvodic, 2006). The amplitude threshold each ROI was set individually at 40% of the peak positive activation within that ROI. This level of thresholding was selected because it was shown to yield highly reproducible and specific individual motor activation maps in a large cohort of subjects (Voyvodic, et al., 2009). Individual maps were then grouped using a random effects model to account for intersubject variability and capture effects in the whole population. Sensitivity measures across the group for each task were computed based on the individual mean value of the t-statistic in all voxels exceeding the threshold in the target ROIs. Specificity was measured across subjects as the proportion of the above-threshold positive activation volume (computed as the mean t-value weighted by the number of voxels exceeding the threshold) in the target ROI relative to the whole brain. Lateralization indices (LI) were computed for each of the ROIs in the language tasks because of the clinical relevance of language dominance as a predictor of post surgical neurological deficit, and because quantitative measures of laterality show better within-subject reproducibility than quantitative measures of the volume of activation (Harrington, Buonocore, & Farias, 2006). The LI was computed as the ratio of the difference and the sum of the activation in each left and right region of interest (LI=[QLHQRH]/[QLH+QRH]), where the activation in the left and right hemispheres (QLH and QRH, respectively) was represented by the sensitivity or specificity measures described above. In this formulation, LI varies between 1 and-1, with positive values reflecting left hemisphere dominance and negative values reflecting right hemisphere dominance. LI measures incorporating both the magnitude and extent of activation were selected here because they have been shown to be more robust and reproducible (Fernandez et al., 2003; Jansen et al., 2006). Note that the size of the contralateral ROIs defined in the atlas were similar though not identical, but this did not bias the LI comparison between tasks because any ROI asymmetries were consistent across tasks.

The group maps of fMRI activation in the language ROIs for the three language tasks are shown in Figure 1, and the corresponding sensitivity and specificity measures in each ROI and task are shown in Figures 2 and 3. Activation was observed in all ROIs for all tasks. The LI based on the sensitivity measure (Figure 2) was similar for all tasks in IFG. However, it was larger for SWD and DNT in AG, with a similar trend in MTG. LI was largest for DNT when all three regions were combined. The LI based on the specificity measure (Figure 3) was larger for SWG in IFG, and larger for SWD and DNT in AG, with no differences observed in MTG. The LI was largest for DNT when all three regions were combined.

Figure 4 shows an example of presurgical fMRI language maps using the SWD and SWG tasks in a patient with right frontotemporal low-grade glioma. Activation for both the SWD and SWG tasks was left lateralized. Only the SWD task activated the angular gyrus. The SWG task produced stronger activation in IFG and MFG. Figure 5 shows an example of fMRI language maps in a neurologically healthy left handed volunteer. In this subject, the three maps consistently indicate right hemisphere dominance for language. As in previous examples, only the SWD and DNT tasks activated the angular gyrus. The SWG task activated specifically the frontal cortex.

Taken together, these results suggest that an important advantage of the semantic word decision (SWD) and definition naming (DNT) tasks over the silent word generation (SWG) task, is that the former tasks activate the angular gyrus (AG) with high sensitivity and specificity. The AG activation can be used to compute more robust lateralization indices. In contrast, the SWG task activates the inferior frontal gyrus (IFG) with high specificity, such that lateralization patterns in this area are more robust with the SWG compared to the SWD task. Thus, an optimal set of paradigms for presurgical language mapping would consist of a combination of the SWG task with the SWD or DNT tasks.

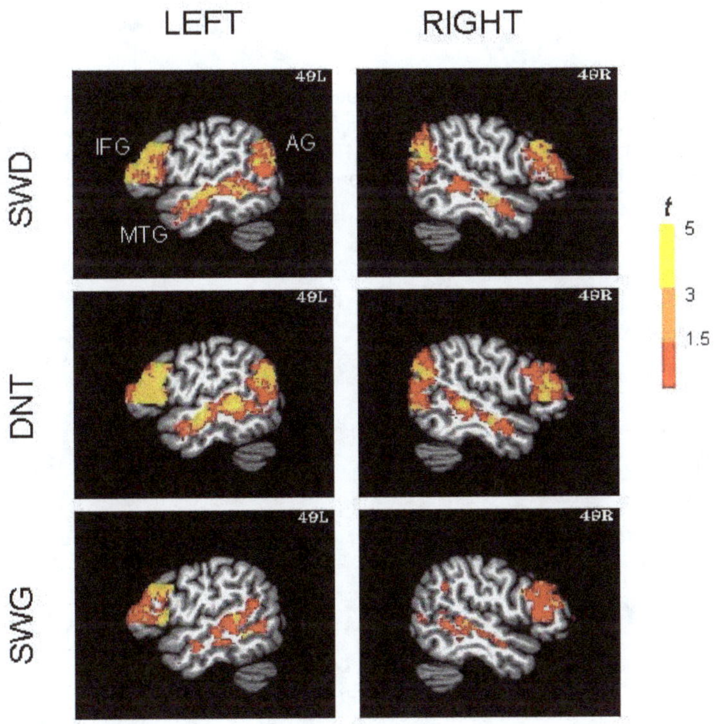


**Figure 1.** FMRI activation within the three language ROIs for a group of right handed, neurologically healthy adults (n=11), during auditory semantic word decision (SWD), auditory definition naming (DNT), and silent word generation (SWG) tasks. The individual activation maps in each task were thresholded at 40% of the maximum activation in each ROI, projected into standard stereotaxic space (Talairach & Tournoux, 1988), and combined across subjects using random effects analysis. The fMRI activity in the three language ROIs is displayed on sagittal slices of a template brain (Colin N27), at 49 mm to the left (49L, left panels) and to the right (49R, right panels) of the midsagittal plane. In this map, t=2.57 corresponds to p<0.01 (orange), and t=3.3 corresponds to p<0.001 (yellow).

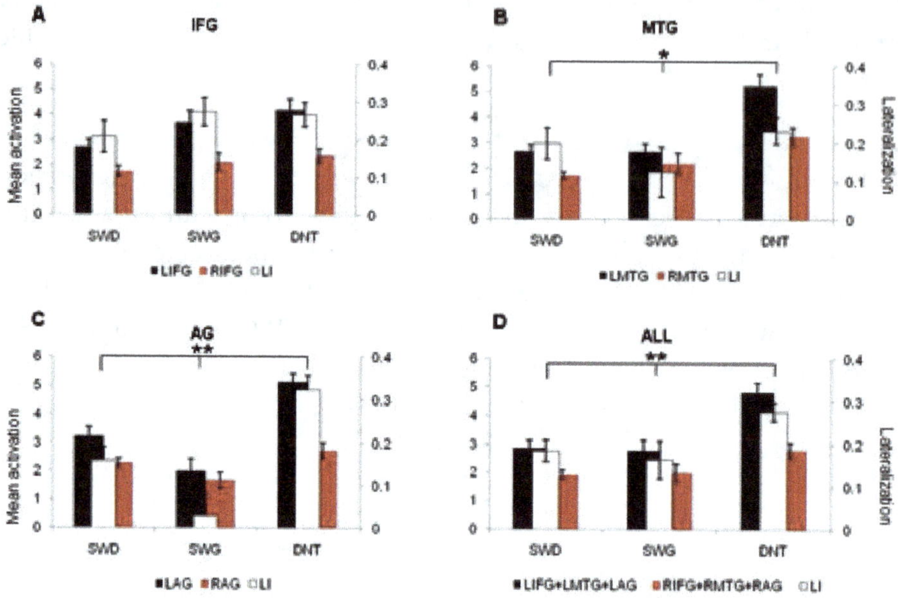


**Figure 2.** The sensitivity measure (expressed as mean *t*-value of supra threshold voxels) and corresponding lateralization index (LI) in the regions of interest for language (A. left and right inferior frontal gyri, B. left and right middle temporal gyri, C. left and right angular gyri – LIFG, RIFG, LMTG, RMTG, LAG, RAG, respectively), during semantic word decision (SWD), silent word generation (SWG), and definition naming (DNT). *p<0.1; **p < 0.05.

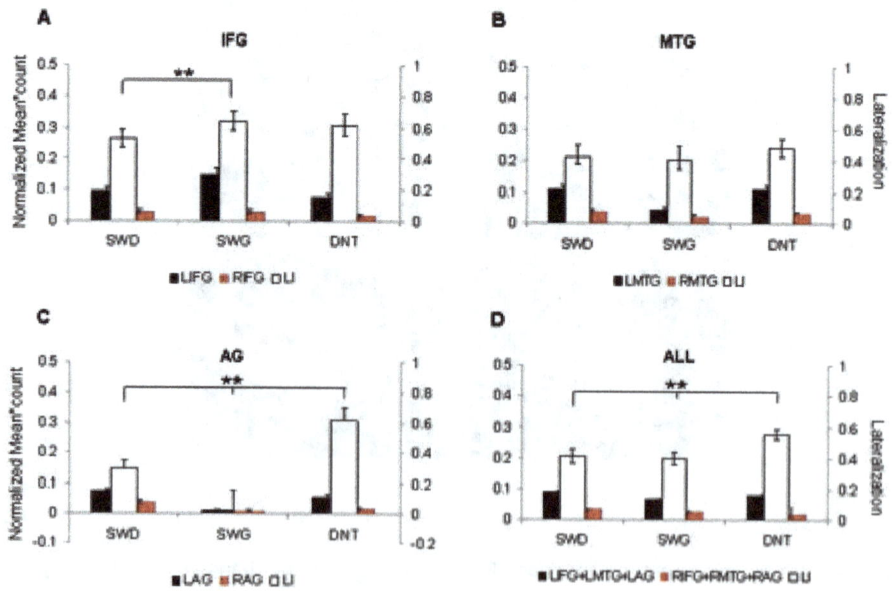


**Figure 3.** The specificity measure (expressed as mean *t*-value of supra threshold voxels weighted by voxel count in each ROI, normalized to the whole brain) and corresponding LI in each language task. Abbreviations as in Figure 2. **p < 0.05.

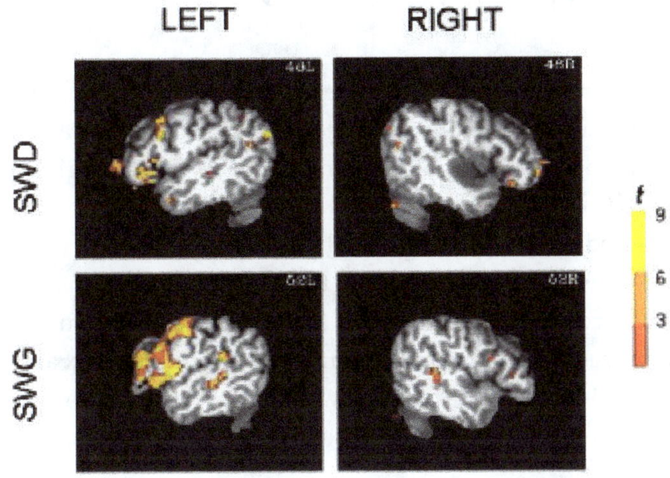


**Figure 4.** Presurgical fMRI language maps for the semantic word decision (SWD) and silent word generation (SWG) tasks, in a patient with right frontotemporal low-grade glioma (37 year old, right handed, female).

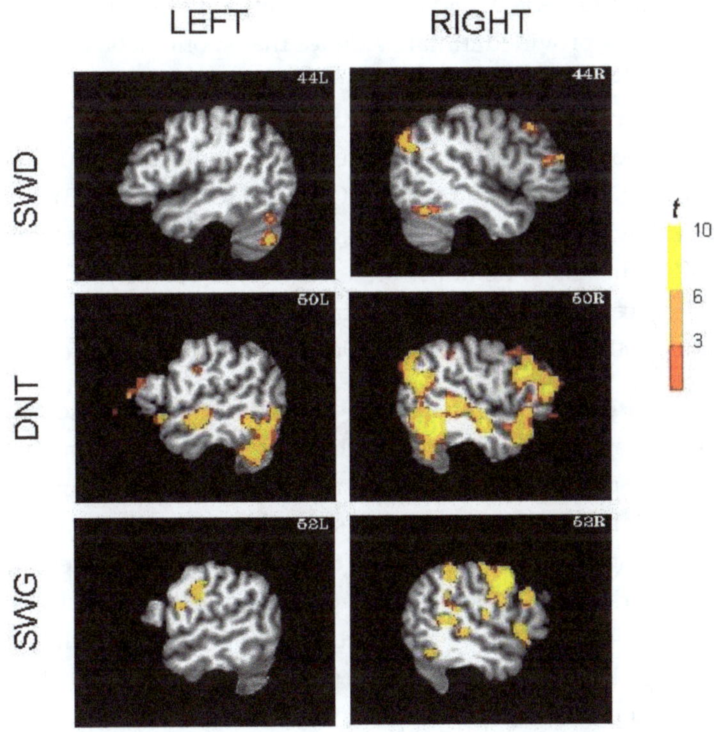


**Figure 5.** FMRI language maps in the three language tasks, in a neurologically healthy, left handed volunteer (Edinburgh Handedness Inventory score=-0.8). In these maps, the activation was thresholded at 40% of the maximal activation in the entire brain. The three maps are consistent with one another in suggesting right hemisphere dominance for language.

## 2. The origins of resting-state fMRI

As with many major scientific advances, the use of fMRI to investigate the resting state of the human brain was discovered essentially by accident. In 1995, Biswal and colleagues (Biswal, Yetkin, Haughton, & Hyde, 1995) initially meant to isolate physiological noise in fMRI data collected from subjects during rest; however, it was observed that a prominent low-frequency signal (< 0.1 Hz) remained after removing the physiological noise. To investigate this further, high frequencies were filtered from all voxels in the brain, and the signal from the left primary sensorimotor cortex was compared to the signal from all other voxels in the brain. A high level of correlation was observed with the right primary sensorimotor cortex and other motor areas. It was thus hypothesized that spontaneous low-frequency fluctuations in the BOLD signal were the result of functional connections between these brain regions.

With fMRI itself still in its infancy and no clear explanation of how the resting-state signal was generated, there remained some controversy as to whether the resting-state signal was neurologically significant. One study found that the strength of left/right inter-hemispheric correlations during the resting state decreased when subjects held their breath, and returned to normal levels once the subjects began breathing again (Biswal, Hudetz, Yetkin, Haughton, & Hyde, 1997). This study provided initial evidence that spontaneous low-frequency fluctuations were indeed blood-oxygenation dependent, like the BOLD signal. It was later observed using voltage sensitive dyes that neurons in the visual cortex exhibit patterns of spontaneous activity similar to the activation patterns elicited in response to stimuli of a specific visual orientation angle (Kenet, Bibitchkov, Tsodyks, Grinvald, & Arieli, 2003). This was one of the first studies to provide evidence that the resting-state signal had a physiological basis. In recent years, a number of studies have demonstrated a link between physiological, electrophysiological, and BOLD processes and the resting-state signal (Laufs, et al., 2003; Leopold, Murayama, & Logothetis, 2003; Mantini, Perrucci, Del Gratta, Romani, & Corbetta, 2007).

Through the validation of the resting-state phenomenon, resting-state fMRI has become a valuable tool to investigate how the brain functions at rest and how brain networks at rest are organized; however, the physiological mechanisms underlying the resting-state signal are still under investigation. Higher field scanners (3 Tesla and above) with improved signal-to-noise ratios, improved imaging sequences and head coils, and a better understanding of fMRI in general, have also contributed to the ubiquity of resting-state research. Many resting-state studies have been published since the first study, investigating a multitude of disease and normal brain states (e.g., Lowe, 2010; van den Heuvel & Hulshoff Pol, 2010). Since resting-state fMRI is still a relatively new concept, appropriate methods of collecting and analyzing resting-state data are still under development. With these advances in methodology, resting-state fMRI will continue to be an invaluable research tool for investigations of normal and pathological human brain function. However, as we will discuss in the remainder of this chapter, resting-state fMRI has the added potential of becoming a powerful diagnostic and assessment tool for individual clinical cases (Freilich & Gaillard, 2010; Sakoglu, et al., 2011).

## 3. Resting-state fMRI: The basics

### 3.1. The resting-state signal

The resting-state fMRI signal resides within a narrow frequency range of 0.01 to 0.1 Hz (De Luca, et al., 2006; Damoiseaux, et al., 2006). The similarity of these low-frequency fluctuations between spatially distinct brain regions implies a functional connection. The degree of similarity, which quantifies the strength of the functional connection, is called *functional connectivity*, and the collection of brain regions identified as connected constitute a *resting-state network*. These resting-state networks are consistent with our knowledge of structural connections via the connective white matter tracts. In a study of patients with multiple sclerosis, a significant correlation was found between the integrity of the white matter tracts (i.e., structural connectivity) within the motor pathway and functional connectivity of the motor network (Lowe, et al., 2008). This suggests that when white matter cannot functional properly, functional connectivity is diminished or even lost in the specific resting-state network. Even in healthy control subjects, the strength of functional connections within resting-state networks seems to be correlated with the strength of anatomical connections in the same area, as measured by diffusion tensor imaging (Skudlarski, et al., 2008). These studies have helped to establish a link between our knowledge of the anatomical connections in the brain and the resting-state fMRI signal.

### 3.2. The procedure

Acquiring resting-state fMRI data is relatively simple because of its non-demanding nature in terms of effort required from the subject. The subject is asked to remain still inside the MR scanner for a period of five to ten minutes, think of nothing in particular, and stare at a fixation cross or keep their eyes closed. It has been demonstrated that when the eyes are open, the functional connections between the thalamus and visual cortex are weakened as opposed to when the eyes are closed (Zou, et al., 2009). Conversely, it has been shown that the functional connections are stronger within the "default mode" network (consisting of the posterior cingulate cortex, precuneus, medial prefrontal cortex, ventral anterior cingulate cortex and lateral parietal cortex) when subjects have their eyes open (Yan, et al., 2009). Taken together, these studies suggest that the benefit of having subjects stare at a fixation cross or keep their eyes closed differs between resting-state networks, and must be taken into account when a study is planned.

Once the data has been collected, it is subjected to a pre-processing pipeline the same as that for task fMRI: motion correction, spatial and temporal smoothing, and spatial normalization to a standard template (i.e., the Montreal Neurological Institute brain or the Talairach atlas). In terms of the analysis of resting-state data, there are two broad categories: model-dependent or model-independent (Joel, Caffo, van Zijl, & Pekar, 2011; Margulies, et al., 2010). A model-dependent analysis assumes *a priori* knowledge of the approximate location of a brain region within the resting-state network under investigation. Using this knowledge, a seed region (consisting of a voxel or voxels) is typically defined either anatomically or by an apposite task. The average time course of this seed region is extracted and compared to the time course of every other voxel in the brain, usually by some variant of the General Linear Model including nuisance signals from cerebral spinal fluid, white matter, the average signal from the whole brain and physiological recordings of cardiac and respiratory signals (Glover, Li, & Ress, 2000; Murphy, Birn, Handwerker, Jones, & Bandettini, 2009). The voxels whose time courses are strongly correlated to the seed region are considered to be functionally connected to the seed region, and constitute a whole-brain map of the resting-state network. In contrast, a model-independent analysis is performed when there is no specific hypothesis about a brain region and its inclusion in a resting-state network. One common example of this approach is independent component analysis (ICA) (Hu, Yang, LaConte, & Weng, 2008). The ICA algorithm identifies groupings of spatial clusters (i.e., components) that are maximally independent and whose BOLD signal fluctuations are similar; however, knowledge of brain networks is still required to select and group the components to form a final map of the desired resting-state network. Whether the approach to resting-state connectivity analysis is ICA or a seed region, there is good agreement as to the number and location of these networks in the healthy human brain across studies (Damoiseaux, et al., 2006; De Luca, Beckmann, De Stefano, Matthews, & Smith, 2006; Kiviniemi, et al., 2009).

The ease of data collection from the subject's perspective is just one of the many reasons why resting-state is becoming a popular brain imaging method. As we will discuss in the next few sections, the resting-state method is being applied to a number of neurological and psychiatric disease states, which could eventually advance resting-state fMRI towards actual clinical use.

### 3.3. Current uses of resting-state fMRI

Because there is no effort required by the subject during imaging, resting-state fMRI is quickly becoming a popular research tool. The majority of resting-state investigations are conducted in tandem with task-related fMRI, to gain complementary information about the brain's functional networks. For some patient populations, however, task-based fMRI may not be possible because patients are non-compliant. Resting-state fMRI may permit the investigation of patients who would otherwise not be studied using fMRI. Thus, resting-state fMRI may be a good candidate for translation into the clinical realm (Freilich & Gaillard, 2010; Sakoglu, et al., 2011). A few of the current uses and techniques of resting-state fMRI will be outlined in this section.

To better understand the nature and mechanisms of functional connectivity, current studies combine resting-state fMRI with diffusion tensor imaging (DTI), an MR technique that provides an anatomical map of white matter tract integrity and quantifies structural connectivity (Skudlarski, et al., 2008). This combination of techniques permits a direct investigation of the relationship between structural and functional connectivity, since white matter tracts may provide the means for distant brain areas to remain functionally connected through correlated fluctuations in the BOLD signal. Studies have shown a strong correlation between structural and functional connectivity in the brain on a whole-brain scale (Skudlarski, et al., 2008) and for individual functional networks (Greicius, Supekar, Menon, & Dougherty, 2009). Hence, these types of studies provide insight into how structure and function are directly related in the human brain.

Resting-state fMRI is also being used to investigate a number of brain diseases and disorders. Disrupted resting-state networks have been identified in neurological disorders such as Alzheimer's disease (Jiang, et al., 2006) and psychopathologies such as schizophrenia (Liu, et al., 2007). One group has even used resting-state fMRI to distinguish patients with major depressive disorder from healthy controls (Craddock, Holtzheimer, Hu, & Mayberg, 2009), demonstrating that resting-state fMRI has the potential for individual patient diagnosis. Studies have also demonstrated changes in resting-state connectivity over the course of mild cognitive impairment (Wang, et al., 2011) and recovery after stroke (Park, et al., 2011). Hence, there is potential for resting-state fMRI in the clinical assessment of disease progression and recovery, as well as in the assessment of treatment strategies.

### 3.4. Advantages of resting-state fMRI

Resting-state fMRI has a number of advantages over task-based fMRI and other imaging modalities. Unlike PET, fMRI in general is noninvasive and unlike EEG, deep-brain activity can be more easily detected. In comparison to task-based fMRI, there are little or no practice effects associated with multiple resting-state sessions. The main advantage of resting-state fMRI, however, is that it requires no effort from the patient. This is especially helpful when studying patients with physical or psychological deficits who cannot perform or understand the required task. For example, most task-based fMRI studies of stroke involving the upper extremities require patients to perform repetitive finger or hand movements (Buma, Lindeman, Ramsey, & Kwakkel, 2010; Calautti & Baron, 2003). For many stroke patients, it is difficult to move a single finger or hand, and often other fingers or body parts move in unison (i.e. mirror movements) (Nelles, et al., 1998). As a result, it is difficult to obtain a reliable anatomical map of brain activity in response to the desired movement. Typically, these patients, who make up a large proportion of stroke patients, are simply not studied, creating a significant patient selection bias in research studies. As a result, this poses severe limits on the translation of task-based fMRI into clinical use. Since resting-state fMRI does not require any movement or action from the patient, this problem can be avoided. All patients, even the most severely impaired, can undergo a resting-state study, thus increasing the likelihood of gaining significant insight into the disease.

### 3.5. Disadvantages of resting-state fMRI

Despite continual advances in resting-state fMRI, there are still some drawbacks to the method. The most significant problem is that the physiological basis of the resting-state signal is still not completely understood. As discussed above, a number of studies support the notion that the resting-state BOLD signal has a neuronal basis (e.g., Lowe, et al., 2008; Skudlarski, et al., 2008). However, because of the inherent difficulty associated with recording neuronal activity from multiple spatially distinct sites, no studies have explicitly established the link between spontaneous fluctuations of the BOLD signal associated with the resting-state signal and neural activity.

Another problem is that although subjects are asked to lie still and not think of anything in particular, it is likely that periods of rest actually possess frequent states of unrest, such as transient cognitive processes and inner monologues. These states interfere with the accurate determination of resting-state networks, especially those that involve the frontal cortices (Squire & Stark, 2001; McKiernan, et al., 2006). Indeed, it is impossible to achieve a state of "language rest". However, as we will demonstrate later in this chapter, this disadvantage can actually be exploited for the purposes of presurgical mapping of language processing.

Unless a seed region for resting-state analysis can be defined easily using an anatomical atlas, like motor cortex (Yousry, et al., 1995), an appropriate task-based experiment designed to activate a particular area of the brain is still required. This becomes more difficult if resting-state maps of higher cognitive functions are desired. A recent study, however, has demonstrated that ROIs can be defined using the resting-state data by selecting the voxels that exhibit the greatest inter-voxel cross-correlation (Goodyear & Golestani, 2011), thus removing the need for the task-based scan.

Of course, there are several disadvantages to fMRI in general. Compared to other brain imaging techniques such as EEG, fMRI possesses relatively low temporal resolution. This is because the hemodynamic response takes approximately two seconds to initiate, 6 to 8 seconds to reach its peak, and tens of seconds to return to baseline. In addition, because the BOLD signal is dependent on blood oxygenation and blood flow, there are many factors that can influence the generated signal such as age, brain pathology, and medications (Haller & Bartsch, 2009).

## 4. Resting-state fMRI for presurgical mapping

The downside to using any functional MRI technique for presurgical mapping, however, is that the brain shifts following tissue resection due to gravity, brain swelling and cerebrospinal fluid drainage (Nimsky, et al., 2000). This complicates the interpretation of functional localization post-surgically. Inaccuracy in brain function localization associated with this brain shift can be avoided using intraoperative MRI to assist in anatomical registration of fMRI data (Nimsky, Ganslandt, Hastreiter, & Fahlbusch, 2001). However, brain shift remains a problem for centers that do not have access to intraoperative MR scanners.

As noted above, resting-state fMRI circumvents the limitations associated with task-based fMRI: no task is necessary to isolate a specific brain region, it can be used on any patient regardless of their level of impairment, and multiple maps can be created from one short scan. This technique may also provide an easy means to track plasticity or recruitment of brain function that may occur following surgery. One advantage specific to epilepsy research is that resting-state fMRI can be used to study epileptogenic networks and foci, potentially assisting presurgical plannning (Guye, et al., 2010; Moeller, et al., 2011).

To date, very few studies have investigated resting-state fMRI for the purposes of presurgical mapping. Therefore, its feasibility and effectiveness as a presurgical tool is yet to be determined. For resting-state fMRI to become a clinically useful tool, it must provide reliable information on a single subject level. One study demonstrated good concordance between resting-state fMRI and ICS of patients with sensorimotor tumors, in terms of the identification of sensorimotor cortex (Zhang, et al., 2009). Another study demonstrated similar findings in patients with tumors or epileptic foci near the motor cortex. The patients that underwent surgery following fMRI mapping showed no new neurological deficits post-surgery (Liu, et al., 2009). Together, these studies provide the necessary framework to help move presurgical planning using resting-state fMRI from research into practice. However, before clinical application can be realized, studies are needed to validate resting-state techniques for presurgical mapping in terms of the brain regions that are identified and the dependence statistical threshold on deciding if brain regions are indeed significantly connected.

## 5. Clinical cases of resting-state fMRI

As an example of a typical case for presurgical motor fMRI, a patient with a right-hemisphere frontal lobe glioma in proximity to the motor cortex was referred to our centre for clinical fMRI. The clinical question was whether the patient exhibited a normal pattern of predominantly right-hemisphere motor activity in response to left hand movements and whether this activity was in close proximity or abutting the glioma. The motor task consisted of sequential finger tapping at a self-regulated pace of approximately 2 Hz. This task is performed easily by most patients and is effective in reliably activating sensorimotor regions, including contralateral primary somatosensory, premotor, and supplementary motor regions and the ipsilateral cerebellum (Gountouna et al., 2009; Yoo et al., 2005). The task was designed as twelve 30-sec blocks alternating between three visually cued conditions, right hand, left hand, and rest. The patient also underwent a 7-minute resting-state scan while staring at a fixation cross.

The results of the task-based fMRI and resting-state fMRI are shown in Figure 6. In response to left hand movement task, a typical pattern of brain activity was observed. A predominance of right hemisphere motor activity was observed within motor and sensorimotor cortices, like that for healthy control subjects. Bilateral premotor activity, however, was also present, and frontal activity associated with the cognitive components of the task was also observed. The conclusions drawn from this clinical fMRI study were that the patient exhibited a normal pattern of motor and sensorimotor activity, with an atypical distribution of bilateral premotor activity, possibly the result of functional compensation in response to the impinging glioma. It was advised that any resection should attempt to avoid the premotor regions lateral to the glioma.

A contralateral pattern of motor activity is associated with strong interhemispheric resting-state correlations in healthy subjects (Damoiseaux, et al., 2006). This was also the case for this patient (Figure 6). Strong intra-and inter-hemispheric correlations were observed, as well as strong correlations with the supplementary motor area (SMA) along the midline. The SMA is associated with the coordination of bimanual and complex movements (Sadato, Yonekura, Waki, Yamada, & Ishii, 1997; Wu, Wang, Hallett, Li, & Chan). Activity within the SMA was not observed for the simple hand movement task. In this case, the conclusions were that the interhemispheric resting-state connections are intact and that care must be taken during resection to avoid the SMA along the medial edge of the glioma. This clinical case is a clear example where task-based fMRI and resting-state fMRI provide complementary and clinically relevant information for the purposes of presurgical planning.

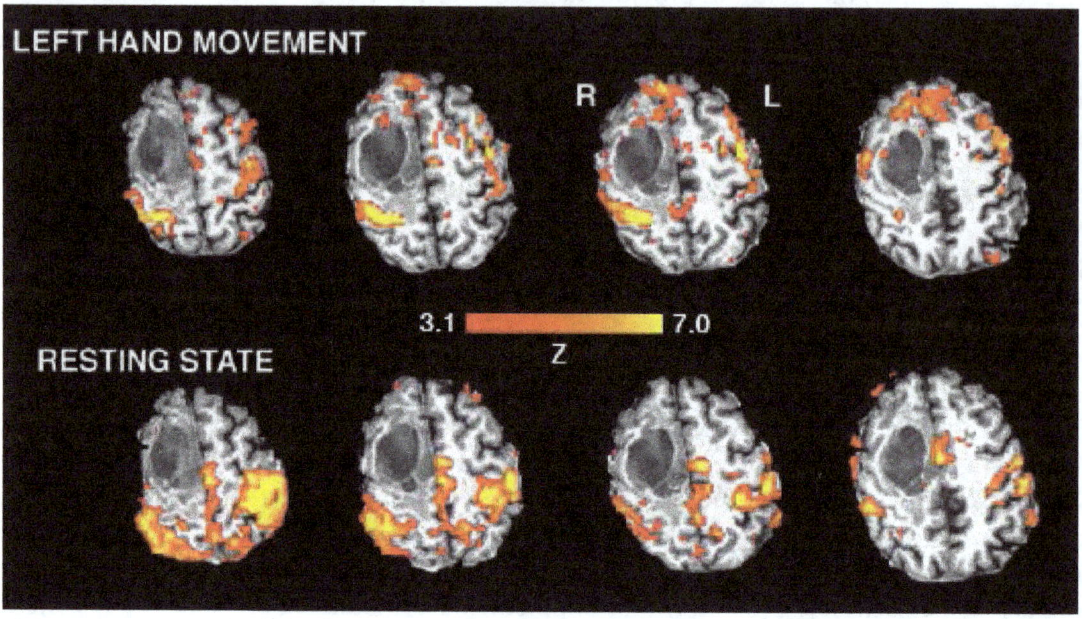


**Figure 6.** Motor task fMRI and resting-state fMRI data from a presurgical patient with a right frontal lobe glioma (clusters corrected to a significance level of α=0.05, using Gaussian Random Fields theory). For the motor task (left hand movement), a typical predominance of brain activity was observed within the right motor and sensorimotor cortices. Some prefrontal and frontal activity was also observed, likely associated with the cognitive components of the task (e.g., self-pacing of movement). In this case, it was concluded that motor activity is not in close proximity to the glioma. Resting-state fMRI using the right motor cortex as the seed region revealed strong correlations with left motor cortex as well as with supplementary motor cortex along the midline in close proximity to the glioma. Red-to-yellow indicates the increasing relative strength of brain activity (for the task) or resting-state correlation (both expressed as a statistical Z-score).

As examples of typical cases for presurgical language fMRI, two patients with left temporal lobe epilepsy were referred to our centre for clinical fMRI. The clinical question was whether the patient exhibited a normal pattern of predominantly left-hemisphere inferior frontal gyrus (i.e., Broca's area) activity in response to language processing. The language task consisted of the SWD task described earlier. The patients also underwent a 5-minute resting-state scan while staring at a fixation cross. Patients were not instructed to try to suppress any internal dialogue, but rather to just let their mind wander.

The results of the task-based fMRI and resting-state fMRI for the first patient are shown in Figure 7. In response to the language tasks, bilateral activity was observed within the inferior frontal gyrus (i.e., Broca's area). It was concluded from the task-related fMRI study that there was an atypical bilateral representation of language processing in this patient. A number of other brain regions were also activated by these tasks, which involved significant cognitive components. Of interest, however, was the lack of left-hemisphere Wernicke's area activity in response to these tasks.

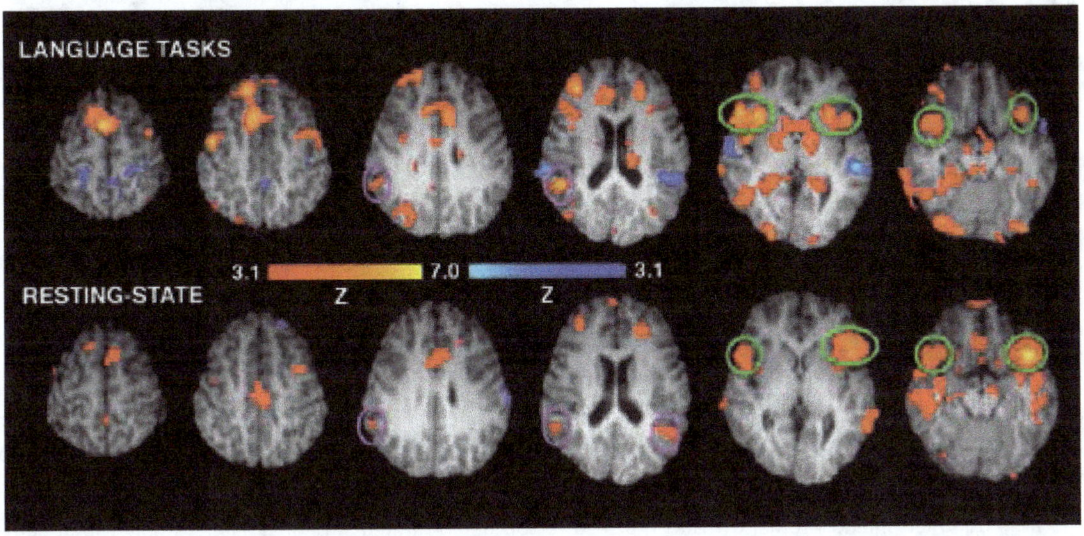


**Figure 7.** Language task fMRI and resting-state fMRI data from a presurgical patient with left temporal lobe epilepsy (clusters corrected to a significance level of α=0.05, using Gaussian Random Fields theory). For the language tasks (verb generation and lexical retrieval), significant bilateral activity within the inferior frontal gyri (green circles) was observed. Other cognitive areas associated with the task were also observed, including the anterior cingulate, caudate, and prefrontal cortex. Language processing was represented bilaterally. Resting-state fMRI using the left inferior frontal gyrus as the seed region demonstrated strong correlations with right inferior frontal gyri as well as bilateral Wernicke's area (purple circles). In this case, the conclusion was also a bilateral representation of language processing. Red-to-yellow indicates the increasing relative strength of brain activity (for the task) or resting-state correlation. Blue-to-light blue indicates the increasing relative strength of negative brain activity (for the task) or negative resting-state correlation (both expressed as a statistical Z-score).

The resting-state fMRI map revealed strong similarities to the language task fMRI; strong inter-hemispheric correlations were observed between the inferior frontal gyri, as well as between left and right Wernicke's areas. These identified regions suggest that the patient was indeed not in a resting-state for language, and in fact these results further suggest that internal dialogue during rest may be sufficient to determine the contribution of each hemisphere to language processing.

The results of the task-based fMRI and resting-state fMRI for the second patient are shown in Figure 8. In response to the language tasks, activity was observed predominantly within the left inferior frontal gyrus. It was concluded from the task-related fMRI study that there was a typical left-hemisphere dominant representation of language processing in this patient. A number of other brain regions were also activated by these tasks, which involved significant cognitive components.

As with the other clinical case, the resting-state fMRI map was similar to the language task fMRI map; weak or absent inter-hemispheric correlations were observed between the inferior frontal gyri, as well as between left and right Wernicke's areas. These results also suggest that

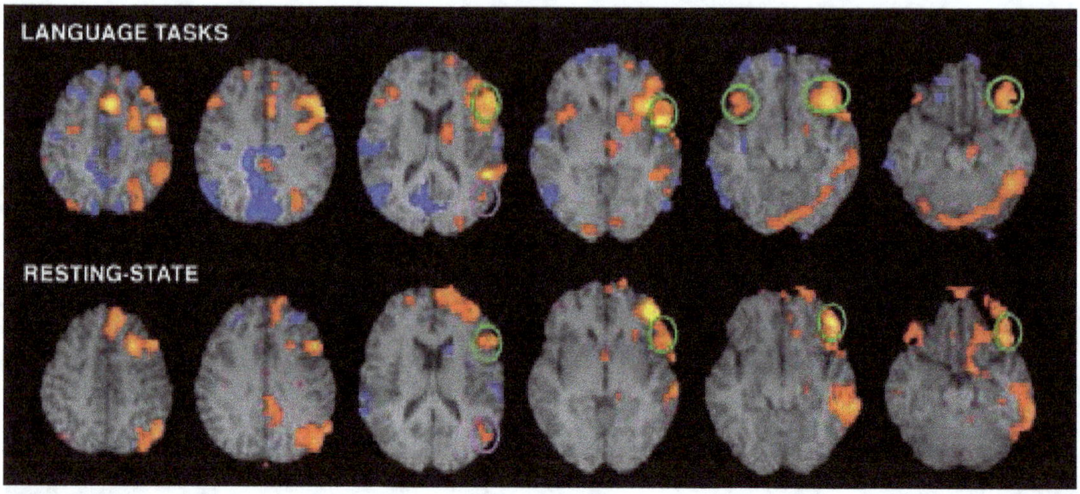


**Figure 8.** Language task fMRI and resting-state fMRI data from another presurgical patient with left temporal lobe epilepsy. For the language tasks (verb generation and lexical retrieval), significant left hemisphere dominant activity within the inferior frontal gyrus (green circles) was observed. Other cognitive areas associated with the task were also observed. In this case, the conclusion was a left hemisphere dominant representation of language processing. Resting-state fMRI using left inferior frontal gyrus as the seed region demonstrated strong correlations only within hemisphere, including left Wernicke's area (purple circles). In this case, the conclusion was also a left hemisphere dominant representation of language processing. Red-to-yellow indicates the increasing relative strength of brain activity (for the task) or resting-state correlation. Blue-to-light blue indicates the increasing relative strength of negative brain activity (for the task) or negative resting-state correlation.

internal dialogue may be sufficient to determine the contribution of each hemisphere to language processing.

## 6. Conclusions

In task-based fMRI, task selection has a critical impact on the resulting maps and their interpretation. In this chapter, we have shown that an important advantage of the semantic word decision and definition naming tasks over the commonly used silent word generation task is that the former tasks activate the angular gyrus with high sensitivity and specificity, allowing for more reliable estimation of hemispheric dominance in semantic processing. In contrast, the silent word generation task activates the inferior frontal gyrus with high specificity, such that estimation of lateralization patterns in this area is more robust with this task. Thus, a comprehensive set of paradigms for presurgical language mapping would consist of a combination of tasks targeting both phonological and semantic processing.

Resting-state fMRI provides a potential alternative to task-based fMRI in cases where patients are unable to comply with task instructions. As we have demonstrated in this chapter, resting-state fMRI of the motor network of individual patients provides important clinically relevant information complementary to task-based fMRI related to motor activity. We have also demonstrated that resting-state fMRI of the language network can also elucidate the laterality of language processing.

In summary, active or passive fMRI can provide a comprehensive delineation (and perhaps overestimation) of somatomotor and language regions surrounding a lesion, and this information can assist in assessing the risks of a surgery and the potential benefit of intrasurgical functional mapping. If the functional regions identified by fMRI are found to be distant from the lesion, this can facilitate a decision for radical tumor resection. If fMRI activation associated with vital sensory, motor or cognitive functions is demonstrated near the radiological tumor boundary and partial resection is suggested, ICS mapping can be used to identify the precise resection margin during the surgery itself. In this case, the presurgical information can be useful in speeding up the ICS procedure and in guiding the extent of the craniotomy (Bartos, et al., 2009; Rutten, et al., 2002).

## Author details

Victoria A.L. Mosher[1], Einat Liebenthal[1,3] and Bradley G. Goodyear[1]

1 University of Calgary, Canada

University of Manitoba, Canada

2 Medical College of Wisconsin, USA

## References

[1] Acharya, J. N., Dinner, D. S. (1997). Use of the intracarotid amobarbital procedure in the evaluation of memory. *J Clin Neurophysiol, 14*(4), 311-325.

[2] Bandettini, P. A., Wong, E. C., Hinks, R. S., Tikofsky, R. S., & Hyde, J. S. (1992). Time course EPI of human brain function during task activation. *Magn Reson Med, 25*(2), 390-397.

[3] Bartos, R., Jech, R., Vymazal, J., Petrovicky, P., Vachata, P., Hejcl, A., et al. (2009). Validity of primary motor area localization with fMRI versus electric cortical stimulation: a comparative study. *Acta Neurochir (Wien), 151*(9), 1071-1080.

[4] Binder, J. R., Frost, J. A., Hammeke, T. A., Cox, R. W., Rao, S. M., & Prieto, T. (1997). Human brain language areas identified by functional magnetic resonance imaging. *J Neurosci, 17*(1), 353-362.

[5] Binder, J. R., Sabsevitz, D. S., Swanson, S. J., Hammeke, T. A., Raghavan, M., & Mueller, W. M. (2008). Use of preoperative functional MRI to predict verbal memory decline after temporal lobe epilepsy surgery. *Epilepsia, 49*(8), 1377-1394.

[6] Binder, J. R., Swanson, S. J., Hammeke, T. A., Morris, G. L., Mueller, W. M., Fischer, M., et al. (1996). Determination of language dominance using functional MRI: a comparison with the Wada test. *Neurology, 46*(4), 978-984.

[7] Binder, J. R., Swanson, S. J., Hammeke, T. A., & Sabsevitz, D. S. (2008). A comparison of five fMRI protocols for mapping speech comprehension systems. *Epilepsia, 49*(12), 1980-1997.

[8] Binder, J. R. (2011). Functional MRI is a valid noninvasive alternative to Wada testing. *Epilepsy Behav, 20*(2), 214-222.

[9] Biswal, B., Hudetz, A. G., Yetkin, F. Z., Haughton, V. M., & Hyde, J. S. (1997). Hypercapnia reversibly suppresses low-frequency fluctuations in the human motor cortex during rest using echo-planar MRI. *J Cereb Blood Flow Metab, 17*(3), 301-308.

[10] Biswal, B., Yetkin, F. Z., Haughton, V. M., & Hyde, J. S. (1995). Functional connectivity in the motor cortex of resting human brain using echo-planar MRI. *Magn Reson Med, 34*(4), 537-541.

[11] Bookheimer, S. (2007). Pre-surgical language mapping with functional magnetic resonance imaging. *Neuropsychology Review, 17*(2), 145-155.

[12] Buma, F. E., Lindeman, E., Ramsey, N. F., & Kwakkel, G. (2010). Functional neuroimaging studies of early upper limb recovery after stroke: a systematic review of the literature. *Neurorehabil Neural Repair, 24*(7), 589-608.

[13] Calautti, C., & Baron, J. C. (2003). Functional neuroimaging studies of motor recovery after stroke in adults: a review. *Stroke, 34*(6), 1553-1566.

[14] Craddock, R. C., Holtzheimer, P. E., Hu, X. P. P., & Mayberg, H. S. (2009). Disease State Prediction From Resting State Functional Connectivity. *Magnetic Resonance in Medicine, 62*(6), 1619-1628.

[15] Damoiseaux, J. S., Rombouts, S. A., Barkhof, F., Scheltens, P., Stam, C. J., Smith, S. M., et al. (2006). Consistent resting-state networks across healthy subjects. *Proc Natl Acad Sci U S A, 103*(37), 13848-13853.

[16] De Luca, M., Beckmann, C. F., De Stefano, N., Matthews, P. M., & Smith, S. M. (2006). fMRI resting state networks define distinct modes of long-distance interactions in the human brain. *Neuroimage, 29*(4), 1359-1367.

[17] De Luca, M., Beckmann, C. F., De Stefano, N., Matthews, P. M., & Smith, S. M. (2006). fMRI resting state networks define distinct modes of long-distance interactions in the human brain. *Neuroimage, 29*(4), 1359-1367.

[18] Demonet, J. F., Chollet, F., Ramsay, S., Cardebat, D., Nespoulous, J. L., Wise, R., et al. (1992). The anatomy of phonological and semantic processing in normal subjects. *Brain, 115 ( Pt 6)*, 1753-1768.

[19] Desmond, J. E., & Annabel Chen, S. H. (2002). Ethical issues in the clinical application of fMRI: factors affecting the validity and interpretation of activations. *Brain Cogn, 50*(3), 482-497.

[20] Eickhoff, S. B., Stephan, K. E., Mohlberg, H., Grefkes, C., Fink, G. R., Amunts, K., et al. (2005). A new SPM toolbox for combining probabilistic cytoarchitectonic maps and functional imaging data. *Neuroimage, 25*(4), 1325-1335.

[21] Fernandez, G., Specht, K., Weis, S., Tendolkar, I., Reuber, M., Fell, J. (2003). Intrasubject reproducibility of presurgical language lateralization and mapping using fMRI. *Neurology, 60*, 969-975.

[22] FitzGerald, D. B., Cosgrove, G. R., Ronner, S., Jiang, H., Buchbinder, B. R., Belliveau, J. W., et al. (1997). Location of language in the cortex: a comparison between functional MR imaging and electrocortical stimulation. *AJNR Am J Neuroradiol, 18*(8), 1529-1539.

[23] Freilich, E. R., Gaillard, W. D. (2010). Utility of functional MRI in pediatric neurology. *Curr Neurol Neurosci Rep, 10*(1), 40-46.

[24] Glover, G. H., Li, T. Q., & Ress, D. (2000). Image-based method for retrospective correction of physiological motion effects in fMRI: RETROICOR. *Magn Reson Med, 44*(1), 162-167.

[25] Goodyear, B. G., & Golestani, A. M. (2011). Regions of interest for resting-state fMRI analysis determined by inter-voxel cross-correlation. *Neuroimage, 56*(1), 246-251.

[26] Greicius, M. D., Supekar, K., Menon, V., & Dougherty, R. F. (2009). Resting-State Functional Connectivity Reflects Structural Connectivity in the Default Mode Network. *Cerebral Cortex, 19*(1), 72-78.

[27] Guye, M., Bettus, G., Bartolomei, F., Confort-Gouny, S., Guedj, E., Chauvel, P., et al. (2010). Role of resting state functional connectivity MRI in presurgical investigation of mesial temporal lobe epilepsy. *Journal of Neurology Neurosurgery and Psychiatry, 81*(10), 1147-1154.

[28] Haberg, A., Kvistad, K. A., Unsgard, G., & Haraldseth, O. (2004). Preoperative blood oxygen level-dependent functional magnetic resonance imaging in patients with primary brain tumors: Clinical application and outcome. *Neurosurgery, 54*(4), 902-914.

[29] Hall, W. A., & Truwit, C. L. (2008). Intraoperative MR-guided neurosurgery. *J Magn Reson Imaging, 27*(2), 368-375.

[30] Haller, S., & Bartsch, A. J. (2009). Pitfalls in FMRI. *Eur Radiol, 19*(11), 2689-2706.

[31] Hamberger, M. J., & Seidel, W. T. (2003). Auditory and visual naming tests: normative and patient data for accuracy, response time, and tip-of-the-tongue. *J Int Neuropsychol Soc, 9*(3), 479-489.

[32] Harrington, G. S., Buonocore, M. H., & Farias, S. T. (2006). Intrasubject reproducibility of functional MR imaging activation in language tasks. *AJNR Am J Neuroradiol, 27*(4), 938-944.

[33] Hirsch, J., Ruge, M. I., Kim, K. H., Correa, D. D., Victor, J. D., Relkin, N. R., et al. (2000). An integrated functional magnetic resonance imaging procedure for preoperative mapping of cortical areas associated with tactile, motor, language, and visual functions. *Neurosurgery, 47*(3), 711-721; discussion 721-712.

[34] Holodny, A. I., Schulder, M., Liu, W. C., Wolko, J., Maldjian, J. A., & Kalnin, A. J. (2000). The effect of brain tumors on BOLD functional MR imaging activation in the adjacent motor cortex: implications for image-guided neurosurgery. *AJNR Am J Neuroradiol, 21*(8), 1415-1422.

[35] Hu, X. P., Yang, Z., LaConte, S., & Weng, X. C. (2008). Ranking and averaging independent component analysis by reproducibility (RAICAR). *Human Brain Mapping, 29*(6), 711-725.

[36] Jack, C. R., Jr., Thompson, R. M., Butts, R. K., Sharbrough, F. W., Kelly, P. J., Hanson, D. P., et al. (1994). Sensory motor cortex: correlation of presurgical mapping with functional MR imaging and invasive cortical mapping. *Radiology, 190*(1), 85-92.

[37] Jansen, A., Deppe, M., Schwindt, W., Mohammadi, S., Sehlmeyer, C., Knecht, S. (2006). Interhemispheric dissociation of language regions in a healthy subject. *Arch Neurol, 63*, 1344-1346.

[38] Jiang, T. Z., Wang, L., Zang, Y. F., He, Y., Liang, M., Zhang, X. Q., et al. (2006). Changes in hippocampal connectivity in the early stages of Alzheimer's disease: Evidence from resting state fMRI. *Neuroimage, 31*(2), 496-504.

[39] Joel, S. E., Caffo, B. S., van Zijl, P. C., & Pekar, J. J. (2011). On the relationship between seed-based and ICA-based measures of functional connectivity. *Magn Reson Med.*

[40] Kenet, T., Bibitchkov, D., Tsodyks, M., Grinvald, A., & Arieli, A. (2003). Spontaneously emerging cortical representations of visual attributes. *Nature, 425*(6961), 954-956.

[41] Kiviniemi, V., Starck, T., Remes, J., Long, X., Nikkinen, J., Haapea, M., et al. (2009). Functional segmentation of the brain cortex using high model order group PICA. *Hum Brain Mapp, 30*(12), 3865-3886.

[42] Krings, T., Reinges, M. H., Erberich, S., Kemeny, S., Rohde, V., Spetzger, U., et al. (2001). Functional MRI for presurgical planning: problems, artefacts, and solution strategies. *J Neurol Neurosurg Psychiatry, 70*(6), 749-760.

[43] Krishnan, R., Raabe, A., Hattingen, E., Szelenyi, A., Yahya, H., Hermann, E., et al. (2004). Functional magnetic resonance imaging-integrated neuronavigation: correlation between lesion-to-motor cortex distance and outcome. *Neurosurgery, 55*(4), 904-914; discusssion 914-905.

[44] Kwong, K. K., Belliveau, J. W., Chesler, D. A., Goldberg, I. E., Weisskoff, R. M., Poncelet, B. P., et al. (1992). Dynamic magnetic resonance imaging of human brain activity during primary sensory stimulation. *Proc Natl Acad Sci U S A, 89*(12), 5675-5679.

[45] Laufs, H., Krakow, K., Sterzer, P., Eger, E., Beyerle, A., Salek-Haddadi, A., et al. (2003). Electroencephalographic signatures of attentional and cognitive default modes in spontaneous brain activity fluctuations at rest. *Proc Natl Acad Sci U S A, 100*(19), 11053-11058.

[46] Lee, C. C., Jack, C. R., Jr., & Riederer, S. J. (1998). Mapping of the central sulcus with functional MR: active versus passive activation tasks. *AJNR Am J Neuroradiol, 19*(5), 847-852.

[47] Lee, C. C., Ward, H. A., Sharbrough, F. W., Meyer, F. B., Marsh, W. R., Raffel, C., et al. (1999). Assessment of functional MR imaging in neurosurgical planning. *AJNR Am J Neuroradiol, 20*(8), 1511-1519.

[48] Lehericy, S., Cohen, L., Bazin, B., Samson, S., Giacomini, E., Rougetet, R., et al. (2000). Functional MR evaluation of temporal and frontal language dominance compared with the Wada test. *Neurology, 54*(8), 1625-1633.

[49] Lehericy, S., Duffau, H., Cornu, P., Capelle, L., Pidoux, B., Carpentier, A., et al. (2000). Correspondence between functional magnetic resonance imaging somatotopy and individual brain anatomy of the central region: comparison with intraoperative stimulation in patients with brain tumors. *J Neurosurg, 92*(4), 589-598.

[50] Leopold, D. A., Murayama, Y., & Logothetis, N. K. (2003). Very slow activity fluctuations in monkey visual cortex: implications for functional brain imaging. *Cereb Cortex, 13*(4), 422-433.

[51] Liebenthal, E. (2011). Introduction to Brain Imaging. In: Biomechanics of the brain (Miller K, ed), pp 41-68. Springer Science+Business Media, LLC.

[52] Liegeois, F., Connelly, A., Salmond, C. H., Gadian, D. G., Vargha-Khadem, F., & Baldeweg, T. (2002). A direct test for lateralization of language activation using fMRI: comparison with invasive assessments in children with epilepsy. *Neuroimage, 17*(4), 1861-1867.

[53] Liu, H., Buckner, R. L., Talukdar, T., Tanaka, N., Madsen, J. R., & Stufflebeam, S. M. (2009). Task-free presurgical mapping using functional magnetic resonance imaging intrinsic activity. *J Neurosurg, 111*(4), 746-754.

[54] Liu, Z. N., Zhou, Y., Liang, M., Tian, L. X., Wang, K., Hao, Y. H., et al. (2007). Functional disintegration in paranoid schizophrenia using resting-state fMRI. *Schizophrenia Research, 97*(1-3), 194-205.

[55] Lowe, M. J. (2010). A historical perspective on the evolution of resting-state functional connectivity with MRI. *MAGMA, 23*(5-6), 279-288.

[56] Lowe, M. J., Beall, E. B., Sakaie, K. E., Koenig, K. A., Stone, L., Marrie, R. A., et al. (2008). Resting state sensorimotor functional connectivity in multiple sclerosis inversely correlates with transcallosal motor pathway transverse diffusivity. *Hum Brain Mapp, 29*(7), 818-827.

[57] Mantini, D., Perrucci, M. G., Del Gratta, C., Romani, G. L., & Corbetta, M. (2007). Electrophysiological signatures of resting state networks in the human brain. *Proc Natl Acad Sci U S A, 104*(32), 13170-13175.

[58] Margulies, D. S., Bottger, J., Long, X., Lv, Y., Kelly, C., Schafer, A., et al. (2010). Resting developments: a review of fMRI post-processing methodologies for spontaneous brain activity. *MAGMA, 23*(5-6), 289-307.

[59] McKiernan, K. A., D'Angelo, B. R., Kaufman, J. N., & Binder, J. R. (2006). Interrupting the "stream of consciousness": an fMRI investigation. *Neuroimage, 29*(4), 1185-1191.

[60] Medina, L., Aguirre, E., Bernal, B., Altman, N. R. (2004). Functional MR inaging versus Wada test for evaulation of language laterlaization: cost analysis. *Radiology, 230,* 49-54.

[61] Moeller, F., Maneshi, M., Pittau, F., Gholipour, T., Bellec, P., Dubeau, F., et al. (2011). Functional connectivity in patients with idiopathic generalized epilepsy. *Epilepsia, 52*(3), 515-522.

[62] Murphy, K., Birn, R. M., Handwerker, D. A., Jones, T. B., & Bandettini, P. A. (2009). The impact of global signal regression on resting state correlations: are anti-correlated networks introduced? *Neuroimage, 44*(3), 893-905.

[63] Nelles, G., Cramer, S. C., Schaechter, J. D., Kaplan, J. D., Finklestein, S. P. (1998). Quantitative assessment of mirroe movements after stroke. *Stroke, 29*(6), 1187-1187.

[64] Nimsky, C., Ganslandt, O., Cerny, S., Hastreiter, P., Greiner, G., & Fahlbusch, R. (2000). Quantification of, visualization of, and compensation for brain shift using intraoperative magnetic resonance imaging. *Neurosurgery, 47*(5), 1070-1079.

[65] Nimsky, C., Ganslandt, O., Hastreiter, P., & Fahlbusch, R. (2001). Intraoperative compensation for brain shift. *Surgical Neurology, 56*(6), 357-364.

[66] Ogawa, S., Lee, T. M., Kay, A. R., & Tank, D. W. (1990). Brain magnetic resonance imaging with contrast dependent on blood oxygenation. *Proc Natl Acad Sci U S A, 87*(24), 9868-9872.

[67] Okada, K., & Hickok, G. (2006). Identification of lexical-phonological networks in the superior temporal sulcus using functional magnetic resonance imaging. *Neuroreport, 17*(12), 1293-1296.

[68] Park, C. H., Chang, W. H., Ohn, S. H., Kim, S. T., Bang, O. Y., Pascual-Leone, A., et al. (2011). Longitudinal changes of resting-state functional connectivity during motor recovery after stroke. *Stroke, 42*(5), 1357-1362.

[69] Pouratian, N., Bookheimer, S. Y., Rex, D. E., Martin, N. A., & Toga, A. W. (2002). Utility of preoperative functional magnetic resonance imaging for identifying language cortices in patients with vascular malformations. *J Neurosurg, 97*(1), 21-32.

[70] Pujol, J., Conesa, G., Deus, J., Vendrell, P., Isamat, F., Zannoli, G., et al. (1996). Presurgical identification of the primary sensorimotor cortex by functional magnetic resonance imaging. *J Neurosurg, 84*(1), 7-13.

[71] Rutten, G. J., Ramsey, N. F., van Rijen, P. C., Noordmans, H. J., & van Veelen, C. W. (2002). Development of a functional magnetic resonance imaging protocol for intraoperative localization of critical temporoparietal language areas. *Ann Neurol, 51*(3), 350-360.

[72] Sabsevitz, D. S., Swanson, S. J., Hammeke, T. A., Spanaki, M. V., Possing, E. T., Morris, G. L., 3rd, et al. (2003). Use of preoperative functional neuroimaging to predict language deficits from epilepsy surgery. *Neurology, 60*(11), 1788-1792.

[73] Sadato, N., Yonekura, Y., Waki, A., Yamada, H., & Ishii, Y. (1997). Role of the supplementary motor area and the right premotor cortex in the coordination of bimanual finger movements. *J Neurosci, 17*(24), 9667-9674.

[74] Sakoglu, U., Upadhyay, J., Chin, C. L., Chandran, P., Baker, S. J., Cole, T. B., Fox, G. B., Day, M., Luo, F. (2011). *Biochem Pharmacol, 81*(12), 1374-1387.

[75] Skudlarski, P., Jagannathan, K., Calhoun, V. D., Hampson, M., Skudlarska, B. A., & Pearlson, G. (2008). Measuring brain connectivity: Diffusion tensor imaging validates resting state temporal correlations. *Neuroimage, 43*(3), 554-561.

[76] Squire, L. R., & Stark, C. E. L. (2001). When zero is not zero: The problem of ambiguous baseline conditions in fMRI. *Proceedings of the National Academy of Sciences of the United States of America, 98*(22), 12760-12765.

[77] Stark, C. E., & Squire, L. R. (2001). When zero is not zero: the problem of ambiguous baseline conditions in fMRI. *Proc Natl Acad Sci U S A, 98*(22), 12760-12766.

[78] Talairach, J., Tournoux, P. (1998). Co-planar stereotaxic atals of the human brain. New York: Thieme Medical Publishers,

[79] Tomaszewki Farias, S., Harrington, G., Broomand, C., & Seyal, M. (2005). Differences in functional MR imaging activation patterns associated with confrontation naming and responsive naming. *AJNR Am J Neuroradiol, 26*(10), 2492-2499.

[80] van den Heuvel, M. P., & Hulshoff Pol, H. E. (2010). Exploring the brain network: a review on resting-state fMRI functional connectivity. *Eur Neuropsychopharmacol, 20*(8), 519-534.

[81] Van Westen, D., Skagerberg, G., Olsrud, J., Fransson, P., & Larsson, E. M. (2005). Functional magnetic resonance imaging at 3T as a clinical tool in patients with intracranial tumors. *Acta Radiol, 46*(6), 599-609.

[82] Voyvodic, J. T. (2006). Activation mapping as a percentage of local excitation: fMRI stability within scans, between scans and across field strengths. *Magn Reson Imaging, 24*(9), 1249-1261.

[83] Voyvodic, J. T., Petrella, J. R., Friedman, A. H. (2009). fMRI activation mapping as a percentage of local excitation: consistent presurgical motor maps without threshold adjustment. *J Magn Reson Imaging, 29*, 751-759.

[84] Wada, J., Rasmussen, T. (1960). Intracarotid injection of Sodium Amytal for the lateralization of cerebral speech dominance. Experimental and clinical observations. *J Neurosurg, 17*, 266-282.

[85] Wang, Z., Liang, P., Jia, X., Qi, Z., Yu, L., Yang, Y., et al. (2011). Baseline and longitudinal patterns of hippocampal connectivity in mild cognitive impairment: Evidence from resting state fMRI. *J Neurol Sci, 309*, 79-85.

[86] Wu, T., Wang, L., Hallett, M., Li, K., & Chan, P. Neural correlates of bimanual antiphase and in-phase movements in Parkinson's disease. *Brain, 133*(Pt 8), 2394-2409.

[87] Yan, C., Liu, D., He, Y., Zou, Q., Zhu, C., Zuo, X., et al. (2009). Spontaneous brain activity in the default mode network is sensitive to different resting-state conditions with limited cognitive load. *PLoS One, 4*(5), e5743.

[88] Yetkin, F. Z., Mueller, W. M., Morris, G. L., McAuliffe, T. L., Ulmer, J. L., Cox, R. W., et al. (1997). Functional MR activation correlated with intraoperative cortical mapping. *AJNR Am J Neuroradiol, 18*(7), 1311-1315.

[89] Yousry, T. A., Schmid, U. D., Jassoy, A. G., Schmidt, D., Eisner, W. E., Reulen, H. J., et al. (1995). Topography of the cortical motor hand area: prospective study with functional MR imaging and direct motor mapping at surgery. *Radiology, 195*(1), 23-29.

[90] Zhang, D. Y., Johnston, J. M., Fox, M. D., Leuthardt, E. C., Grubb, R. L., Chicoine, M. R., et al. (2009). Preoperative Sensorimotor Mapping in Brain Tumor Patients Using Spontaneous Fluctuations in Neuronal Activity Imaged with Functional Magnetic Resonance Imaging: Initial Experience. *Neurosurgery, 65*(6), 226-236.

[91] Zou, Q., Long, X., Zuo, X., Yan, C., Zhu, C., Yang, Y., et al. (2009). Functional connectivity between the thalamus and visual cortex under eyes closed and eyes open conditions: a resting-state fMRI study. Hum Brain Mapp, 30(9), 3066-3078.

7

# Structural and Functional Magnetic Resonance Imaging in Hepatic Encephalopathy

Long Jiang Zhang, Guang Ming Lu and Hui Mao

## 1. Introduction

Hepatic encephalopathy (HE) is a neuropsychiatric syndrome that develops in patients with severe liver diseases and/or portal-systemic shunting. HE is characterized by a wide spectrum of clinical manifestations, ranging from alterations of psychometric performance to stupor and coma (Rovira et al., 2008; Cordoba J., 2011). Several non-invasive neuroimaging techniques, such as particularly magnetic resonance imaging (MRI) and magnetic resonance spectroscopy (MRS), are used for the diagnosis and prognosis of HE. These MR techniques can identify and measure the abnormal accumulation and increase of metabolite, such as glutamine and glutamate (Glx) as a result of HE in the central nervous system (CNS). Under normal circumstances, these substances are efficiently metabolized by the liver. This chapter will review the pathophysiology of HE and its conventional MRI, MRS and functional MRI findings.

## 2. Pathophysiology of hepatic encephalopathy

Various hypotheses have been proposed to explain the complex neuropsychiatric syndrome seen in HE. Imbalance between inhibitory and excitatory neurotransmission and hyperammonemia is the primary and most widely accepted hypothesis for HE (Rovira et al., 2008; Butterth et al., 2003; Cordoba J., 2011; Cordoba & Minguczb., 2008). Downregulation of glutamate receptors and an increase in inhibitory neurotransmission result in clinical manifestations of HE. In addition, patients with liver failure or portal-systemic shunt surgery have elevated levels of circulating ammonia, which enters the brain through the blood-brain barrier, and increases the ammonia concentration in the cerebral blood up to four fold (normally in the order of two) in liver failure. Hyperammonemia disease leads to profound astrocyte changes, including astrocyte swelling in acute HE and Alzheimer type II astrocyte changes in chronic HE (Matsusue et al., 2005).

## 3. Clinical features of hepatic encephalopathy

The Working Party at the 11th World Congresses of Gastroenterology, held in Vienna in 1998, recommended the nomenclature and types of HE (Table 1) (Ferenci et al., 2002). The West Haven criteria for semi-quantitative grading of HE are summarized in Table 2. HE can be classified in three main groups: episodic, chronic, and minimal, based on duration and characteristics of the clinical manifestations. Episodic HE is characterized by the development of an impaired mental state, neuromuscular abnormalities, asterixis (tremor, jerking movement of the wrist), fetor hepaticus (metcarpans pass into the lungs resulting in the presence of ammonia and ketones in the breath), and hyperventilation, which develops during a short period of time and fluctuates in severity. Chronic HE can be further classified into subgroups: relapsing HE and persistent HE. Relapsing HE manifests itself as frequent episodes of acute HE, while persistent HE refers to manifestations that do not reverse despite adequate treatment. Characteristic manifestations of severe persistent HE are dementia, Parkinsonism, or myelopathy in combination with neurologic involvement, such as ataxia, gait abnormalities, tremor (Rovira et al., 2008). Minimal HE refers to those patients HE type with cirrhosis or portal-systemic shunts who have subtly abnormal cognitive and/or neurophysiologic functions. These abnormalities cannot be detected by the standard clinical examination and can only be determined by a detailed assessment of the patient's history and a comprehensive neurologic evaluation of cognitive performance and motor functions. The neuropsychological features of the minimal HE type include abnormalities in executive functions, particularly in selective attention and psychomotor speed (Amodio et al., 2004). However, other abnormalities, such as memory impairments, are also seen (Amodio et al., 2004). A complete psychometric assessment by a neuropsychologist is the best way to determine the extent of the attention-related cognitive impairment of a HE patient. A large number of neuropsychologic tests, such as the number connection test (NCT), the line-tracing, and inhibitory control test have been developed and are applied to describe cognitive abnormalities in patients without any clinical evidence of HE (Ferenci et al., 2002; Amodio et al., 2010). Testing across various neuropsychological domains is probably the optimal approach in order to identify cognitive and motor system abnormalities, such as attention and fine motion control. A standardized test battery, including the NCT type A and NCT type B, the line-tracing, the serial-dotting, and the digit-symbol tests (PSE-Syndrome-Test) has a high specificity for HE as compared with other metabolic encephalopathies (Ferenci et al., 2002). Changes in EEG/evoked responses and neuroimaging findings are non-specific and may not be able to provide sufficient information for the diagnosis of minimal HE.

| HE type | Nomenclature | Subcategory | Subdivisions |
|---|---|---|---|
| A | Encephalopathy associated with acute liver failure | | |
| B | Encephalopathy associated with portal-systemic bypass and no intrinsic hepatocellular disease | | |
| C | Encephalopathy associated with cirrhosis and portal cirrhosis and portal hypertension/ or portal-systemic shunts | Episodic HE | Precipitated, spontaneous, recurrent |
| | | Persistent HE | Mild, severe, treatment-dependent |
| | | Minimal HE | |

**Table 1.** The nomenclature of HE

| Grade | Criteria |
|---|---|
| 1 | Trivial lack of awareness, euphoria or anxiety, shortened attention span, impaired performance of addition |
| 2 | Lethargy or apathy, minimal disorientation for time or place, subtle personality change, inappropriate behaviour, impaired performance of subtraction |
| 3 | Somnolence to semi stupor, but responsive to verbal stimuli; confusion; gross disorientation |
| 4 | Coma (unresponsive to verbal or noxious stimuli) |

**Table 2.** West Haven criteria for semiquantitative grading of HE

# 4. Conventional MRI findings

In MRI exam of HE, bilateral hyperintensities at basal ganglia in T1 weighted images but without the corresponding abnormal T2 weighted signal intensity is a typical imaging feature of HE (Figure 1A).This imaging characteristic is attributed to hypermanganesemia (Gover et al., 2006; Mcphail & Taylor-Robinson., 2010).

The observed hyperintensities in bilateral basal ganglia on T1 weighted images can be reduced, or even disappear, after liver transplantation (Figure 1B and 1C) (Naegele et al., 2000; Cordoba et al., 2001; Long et al., 2009). However, no correlation between signal intensities on T2 weighted images in basal ganglia and the clinical encephalopathy or neuropsychological test performance was found, after a number of studies (Spahr et al., 2002; Thuluvath et al., 1995). Although mild brain oedema has been reported in the studies using other advanced MR sequences, no mild abnormalities can be detected in the conventional T1 and T2 weighted images, in addition to basal ganglia hyperintensity. Some studies reported high signal intensity at the centrum semiovale or corticospinal tract (along the hemispheric white matter in or around the corticospinal tract) on fast fluid attenuated inversion recovery (FLAIR) T2-

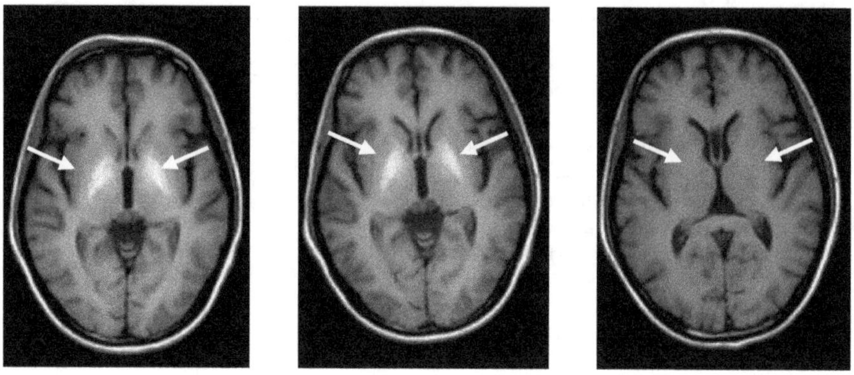

A B C

**Figure 1.** T1 weighted spin echo images of a selected axial brain section from a patient before and after receiving liver transplantation A) An axial T1 weighted image shows the symmetrical areas with high intensity in bilateral basal ganglia (arrows) before liver transplantation; B) 1 week after liver transplantation; and C) 4 months after liver transplantation, noticing that the symmetrical high intensity in bilateral basal ganglia shown in A, B, has disappeared.

weighted images (Figure 2) (Mínguez et al., 2007; Rovira et al., 2008). This is strikingly similar to signalintensity abnormalities noted in cases of amyotrophic lateral sclerosis, a neurodegenerative disease that affects motor neurons. The progressive normalization of the abnormal high signal-intensity in patients with cirrhosis can be found after the successful liver transplantation or effective treatment. (Mínguez et al., 2007; Rovira et al., 2008). Therefore, observation of FLAIR white matter hyperintensities without additional imaging sequences, such as T2 weighted images cannot be used to diagnose HE.

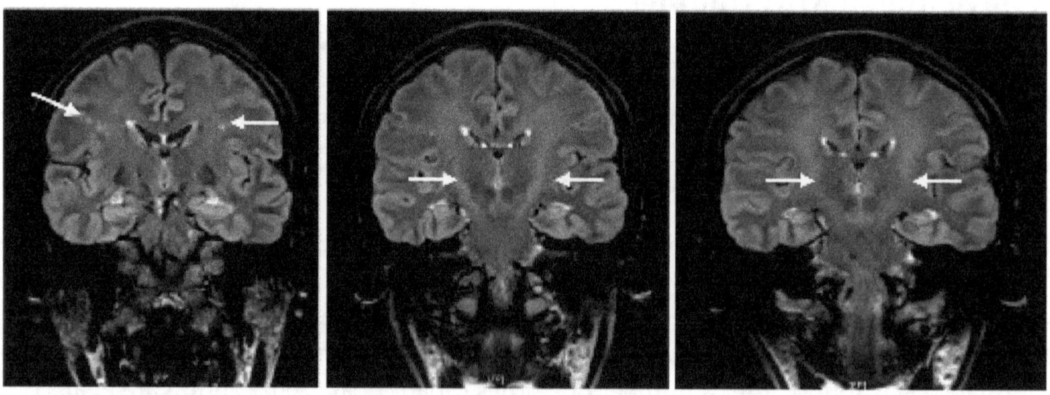

A B C

**Figure 2.** Coronal FLAIR images of a cirrhotic patient A to C. Coronal FLAIR images show the areas with abnormal high signal intensity in or around the corticospinal tract (arrows).

## 5. Magnetic transfer imaging (MTI)

Magnetic transfer imaging (MTI) is a singular MRI technique that has been shown to be useful in the diagnosis of HE. It is mainly based on the interaction (cross-relaxation) between protons in a relatively free environment and those in which motion is restricted (immobile water). Exchange of the saturated magnetization with free water reduces the signal intensity observed in the subsequent MR images. The degree of the signal-intensity loss depends on the attenuation of the macromolecules in a given tissue. MTI allows the measurement of magnetic transfer ratios (MTR), which reflect brain parenchymal changes that may not be visible using the standard MR techniques (Mcphail & Taylor-Robinson., 2010; Grover et al., 2006). Lower MTR can be the result of pathologies that alter the structural integrity and the relative macromolecular-water composition of brain parenchyma, such as in multiple sclerosis plaques (Rovira et al., 1999) or in end-stage cirrhosis (Rovira et al., 2001). Severe MTR decrease may be attributed to the demyelination and axonal loss, but a less severe decrease can be the result of inflammation and moderate demyelination.

All studies using MTI in HE found reduced MTR values in the examined brain regions of HE patients compared to those of controls (Miese et al., 2006; Miese et al., 2009; Poveda et al., 2010). Observed MTR decrease is mild (approximately 10%) and is not accompanied by significant abnormalities on conventional T1-and T2-weighted images, compared with the other metabolic and neurodegenerative diseases, such as experimental autoimmune encephalomyelitis, toxic demyelination, progressive multifocal leukoencephalopathy, human immunodeficiency virus encephalitis, and multiple sclerosis. The MTR reduction seems to have a temporal process in HE, an early involvement of basal ganglia and white matter has been shown (Miese et al., 2009). The MTR decrease almost returns to normal values after liver transplantation, thus supporting the hypothesis that the reduced MTR values reflect mild reversible brain edema.

## 6. Diffusion weighted imaging and diffusion tensor imaging

Diffusion weighted imaging (DWI) is an MRI method that generates brain images based on the image contrast that is dependent on the mobility of H2O molecules in the different tissue compartments (Thoeny & De Keyzer, 2011). Water molecule motion follows the principles of Brownian motion (Provenzale et al., 2006). In a container of water, molecules undergo free, thermally agitated diffusion, which is also called isotropic (means equal in all directions). However, limited diffusion is observed since the movement of water molecules is restricted by their interactions with cell membranes and macromolecules, causing the directional specific motion of water molecules in environments, which is called anisotropic diffusion (Figure 3). DWI derives its image contrast on the basis of differences in the mobility of protons (primarily associated with water) between tissues (Thoeny & De Keyzer., 2011). Apparent diffusion coefficient (ADC) is a measurement obtained from DWI that provides estimation of water motion. DWI has a potential to locate the compartment where the increase of mobility of water molecules is more prominent. Therefore, it can be applied to differentiate cytotoxic oedema from vasogenic oedema in HE patients (Lodi et al., 2004; Mies et al., 2006; Sugimoto et al., 2008). Brain oedema refers to excess water accumulation in the intracellular and extracellular spaces of the brain. In cytotoxic oedema, there is shift of water from extracellular to intracellular compartments producing cellular swelling expressing low ADC, while in vasogenic oedema the reverse happens, producing increased ADC (Schaefer et al., 2000). Recent studies on the application of mean diffusivity measurements within normal-appearing white matter of chronic cirrhotic patients have shown significant increase in brain water diffusivity, which is more pronounced with increased severity of HE (Lodi et al., 2004). These diffusivity values correlated with neuropsychological impairment (Kumar et al., 2008) and increased venous ammonia (Lodi et al., 2004). These findings suggest an accumulation of water in the extracellular compartment and a hypothesis of cortical astrocytic swelling is not supported, but rather increased interstitial fluid or chronic demyelination (Lodi et al., 2004; Sugimoto et al., 2008; Miese et al., 2006) due to glutamine accumulation is cited as the cause of diffuse brain oedema in chronic liver failure (Lodi et al., 2004; Sugimoto et al., 2008; Miese et al., 2006).

On the other hand, the morphology and structure of tissues vary in different organs and pathologic states. Water motion occurs preferentially in some directions in certain tissues due to the presence of obstacles that limit molecular movement in some directions. Diffusion-tensor imaging (DTI) can be used to obtain anisotropy information about water diffusion in tissues when specific diffusion weighted gradients in at least six directions are applied. The most commonly used invariant indices for the measurement of anisotropic diffusions by DTI are; the relative anisotropy (RA), the fractional anisotropy (FA), and the volume ratio (VR) indices (Figure 4A). In brain imaging applications, these indices provide a quantitative measurement of the changes of white matter integrity in different brain regions that are affected by HE. Using DTI together with advanced fibre-tracking algorithms based on the obtained diffusion tensors, white matter tractography can be derived from DTI data. Therefore, it is possible to noninvasively construct 3D trajectories of neural tracts, allowing the modelling of white matter neural connectivity (Figure 4B) (Mukherjee et al., 2008a; Mukherjee et al., 2008).

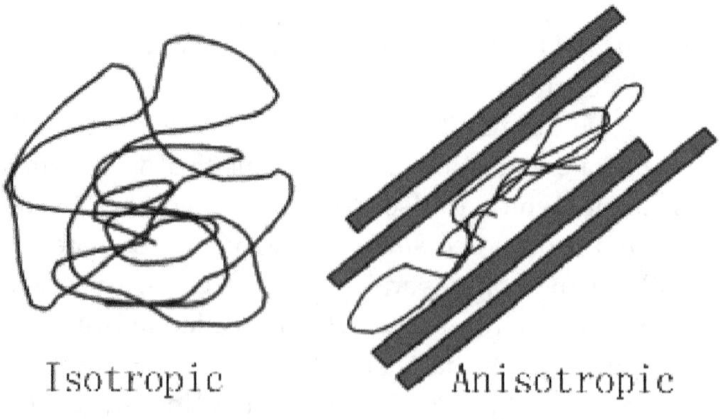


**Figure 3.** Schematic illustrations describe the isotropic diffusion and anisotropic restricted diffusion

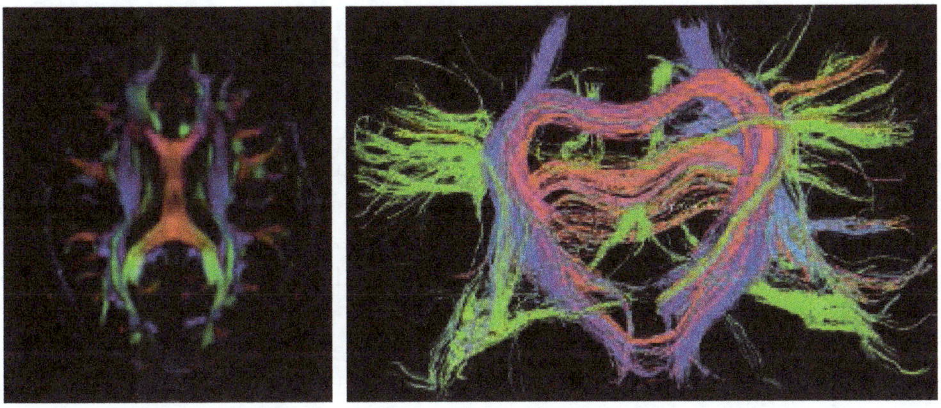

A B

**Figure 4.** Presentations of diffusion tensor images of a cirrhotic patient acquired at a 3T MR scanner A. FA image, B. tractography of the brain derived from diffusion tensor imaging

FA, an index reflecting the white matter integrity, shows no significant changes in patients with chronic HE compared with normal subjects, indicating an absence of microstructural damage in these patients (Kale et al., 2006). Recently, a study by Chavarria et al. (Chavarria et al., 2010) into a rat model of acute liver failure provided experimental evidence to support the cytotoxic origin of brain oedema. Their results suggested that the metabolism of ammonia in astrocytes induces an increase of glutamine and lactate, which may mediate cortical cellular swelling. Saksena et al. (Saksena et al., 2007) also found decreased mean diffusivity values in patients with acute liver failure, suggesting an increase in the intracellular brain water content. Other studies also found decreased ADC value and high cortical signal intensity in patients with acute HE (McKinney et al., 2010; Toru et al., 2011). Therefore, it appears that two different types of brain oedema, intracellular in acute forms and probably interstitial in chronic forms, may exist in liver failure.

## 7. Magnetic Resonance Spectroscopy (MRS)

MRS is a non-invasive analytical method for analysing brain metabolites, often accompanied by MRI in neuroradiology practices. MR spectroscopic analysis offers a tool to interrogate the molecular process within body tissue and fluids in vivo and in vitro. In clinical application, MRS is capable of identifying and measuring the individual chemicals in the brain regions localized and sampled from MR images. 1H MRS can provide information about brain metabolites such as choline (Cho), creatine (Cr), N-acetyl aspartate (NAA), glutamine and glutamate (Glx), as well as osmolytes, such as myoinositol (mI) and taurine (Ross et al., 1994; Kreis R et al., 1992; Cordoba et al., 2002; Mcphail & Taylor-Robinson. 2010). NAA is a derivative of an amino acid found mostly in neurons; therefore, it is commonly considered as a measure of neuronal density. The peak at 3.19-3.24 ppm of MR spectra obtained in vivo represents a total Cho, including soluble membrane phospholipids: phosphorylcholine (PCho), glycerophosphocholine (GPC) and a relatively small amount of free choline. PCho is involved in the synthesis of the insoluble membrane phospholipids (Vance DE,1996), while GPC is a product of membrane degradation and free choline is involved in synthesis of the neurotransmitter, acetylcholine, as well as of membrane synthesis (Michel et al., 2006). An increase in the total Cho peak is associated with an increase in membrane breakdown or turnover, myelination or inflammation (Astley et al., 2009). The peak of Cr spectrum is assigned at 3.02 ppm. This peak represents a combination of molecules containing creatine and phosphocreatine. When energy supply is insufficient from the Kreb's cycle, ATP is produced from adenosine diphosphate (ADP) instead of glucose. This reaction is buffered by the phosphocreatine–creatine (PCr-Cr) system, where PCr donates a phosphate group to become Cr. It is assumed that the Cr peak reflects energy use. Glutamine and glutamate (Glx) are amino acids. Glutamate is the most abundant amino acid in the brain and is released by approximately 90% of excitatory neurons. The spectral peaks of these molecules are often grouped together as Glx in the spectra obtained at the low field, because their overlap makes it hard to resolve them separately. Two compounds become increasingly separated in the higher magnetic fields; therefore, with the increasing clinical availability of stronger magnets, there is growing importance and interests in studying these compounds. Myo-inositol (mI), a simple sugar-alcohol compound, and precursor for inositol lipid synthesis, is a putative glial cell marker because it is located primarily in glial cells and not in neurons. Astrocytes, microglia, and macrophages have been shown to increase their levels of the Na+/mI cotransporter (SMIT) in response to stress or injury and an accumulation of mI, suggesting a role of this compound in inflammation and a marker for astrogliosis and microglia activity (Gupta et al., 2010).

1H MRS has been extensively used in HE studies and has consensus findings on the intracellular metabolite changes in HE. Typical 1H MRS findings of HE include: lower Cho/Cr and mI/Cr and higher Glx/Cr in all examined brain regions compared with controls (Figure 5) (Taraow et al., 2003; Weissenborn et al., 2004; Stewart et al., 2005; Mechtcheriakov et al., 2005; Miese et al., 2006; Weissenborn et al.,2007; Verma et al., 2008). Ammonia plays an important role in the series of metabolite changes in patients with cirrhosis. The increase in brain glutamine during HE increases intracellular osmolality. To maintain osmotic equilibrium, the astrocytes lose osmolytes such as mI and Cho, and a large amount of water enters the astrocyte and results in cellular swelling and impairment of cellular metabolism, further influencing neuronal and astrocyte function and the interaction between them. MRS measurable metabolite changes have been shown to correlate with improved psychometric performance (Binesh et al., 2006) following treatment (Haseler et al., 1998) and following liver transplantation (Naegele et al., 2000; Córdoba et al., 2001; Long et al., 2009). Recent pilot studies on in vitro 1H MRS of human blood or urine in acute liver failure have demonstrated significant metabolite abnormalities between survivors and nonsurvivors (Saxena et al., 2006). They found glutamine in serum and the urine glutamine: creatinine ratio was higher in non-surviving patients compared with surviving patients [serum glutamine, 3.08 (1.68-7.11) vs. 0.56 (0.34-0.99) mM, median and range; P=0.0001 and urine glutamine:creatinine ratio, 1.72 (0.24-7.76) vs. 0.39 (0.1-0.84), P=0.1], and urine urea:creatinine ratio was higher in surviving patients compared with non-surviving patients [10.83 (0.2-22.6) vs. 2.09 (0.96-4.0), P=0.002]. Their study indicated MRS had a potential use for clinical decision making about the need for advanced therapeutic intervention, such as artificial liver support or emergency liver transplantation in acute liver failure. Of these available MRS measurements, mI seems to be a more sensitive biomarker than Cho to detect HE. mI levels were negatively related to the Child-Pugh score and degree of HE (Lee et al., 1999; Zhang et al., 2010). However, values in a normal range have not been established and the diagnostic accuracy of 1H-MRS remains uncertain.

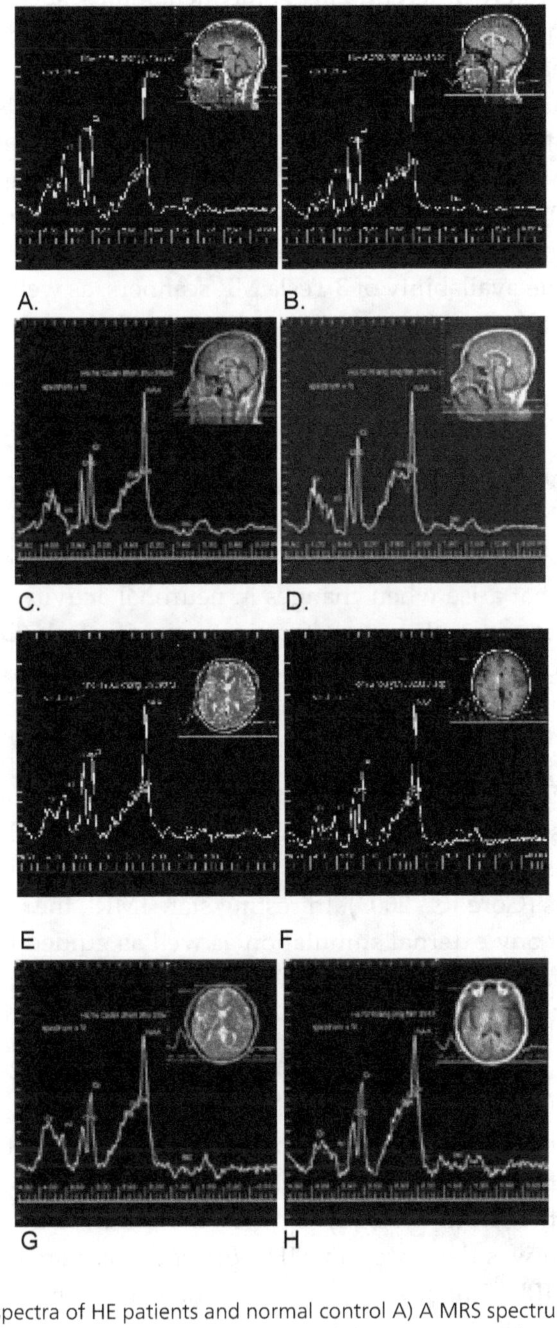


**Figure 5.** A set of brain MR spectra of HE patients and normal control A) A MRS spectrum obtained from the anterior cingulate cortex (ACC) of a healthy adult. B) A MRS spectrum of the anterior cingulate cortex from a 25-year-old fe-

male cirrhotic patient. C) MRS of the anterior cingulate cortex of a 44-year-old minimal hepatic encephalopathy (MHE) patient shows decreased mI and increased Glx. D) MRS of anterior cingulate cortex of a 70-year-old HE patient shows decreased mI and Cho and increased Glx. E) MRS of right basal ganglia of the same subject as in A). F) MRS of right basal ganglia in the same patient as in B) shows decreased mI and Cho. G) MRS of right basal ganglia of the same patient as in (C) shows decreased mI and Cho and increased Glx. H) MRS of right basal ganglia of the same patient in (D) shows decreased mI and Cho and increased Glx. The spectra were collected using single voxel PRESS sequence at 1.5T scanner.

In clinical practice, accurately differentiating some metabolites, such as Glx and taurine, can be challenging with the clinical MR scanners currently available. Two-dimensional MR spectroscopy may enhance the spectral resolution to distinguish metabolites based on Jcoupling patterns of individual molecules. On the other hand, more sophisticated statistical techniques, such as principal components analysis (PCA), enable assessment of the variation in individual metabolites based on the data obtained from MRS measurements (Barba et al., 2008; Singhal et al., 2010). These techniques can provide quantitative information of metabolic processes and changes in the diseased tissue, and therefore can be helpful in the understanding of HE pathogenesis. Wide availability of 3 Tesla MR scanners, as well as short TE acquisition, can improve the spectral resolution and thus, allow the differentiation of Glx from NAA (Sawara et al., 2004).

## 8. Blood oxygen level dependent functional MRI

Functional magnetic resonance imaging (fMRI) detects blood oxygen level-dependent (BOLD) changes in MRI signal that arise when changes in neuronal activity occur in a region of the brain after responding to a stimulus or performing a specific task (Ogawa et al., 1992). The BOLD signal is the ratio of oxy-haemoglobin to deoxy-haemoglobin during brain activation (Gore JC., 2003).

According to experimental paradigms, fMRI can be classified to task-related and resting state fMRI. In task-related fMRI design, a subject is placed in the magnet of an MRI machine, where various different kinds of stimulus are administered in a controlled fashion. Two main experimental paradigms are commonly used in task-related fMRI studies: block design and event-related paradigms (Gore JC., 2003). In resting state fMRI, the participants are required to rest in the absence of any external stimulation as well as guided to avoid reiterating any goal-directed thought pattern in their heads (Damoiseaux et al., 2006).

Many behavioural studies have claimed the existence of attention alterations in cirrhotic patients without overt HE (Zhang et al., 2007a; Randolph et al., 2009; Bajaj et al., 2009). There are only a few fMRI studies into HE. Zafiris et al. (Zafiris et al., 2004) first analysed the pathologically impaired neural mechanisms of cirrhotic patients using fMRI. Nine subjects with minimal HE (MHE) and 10 controls underwent scanning while they indicated the apparent transition from a steady light to the onset of a flicker light. Judgment-related BOLD activation was decreased in MHE patients compared to controls in the right inferior parietal cortex (IPL). Impaired neural interaction between the IPL and the parietooccipital cortex (Poc), the intraparietal sulcus, the anterior cingulate cortex (ACC), the right

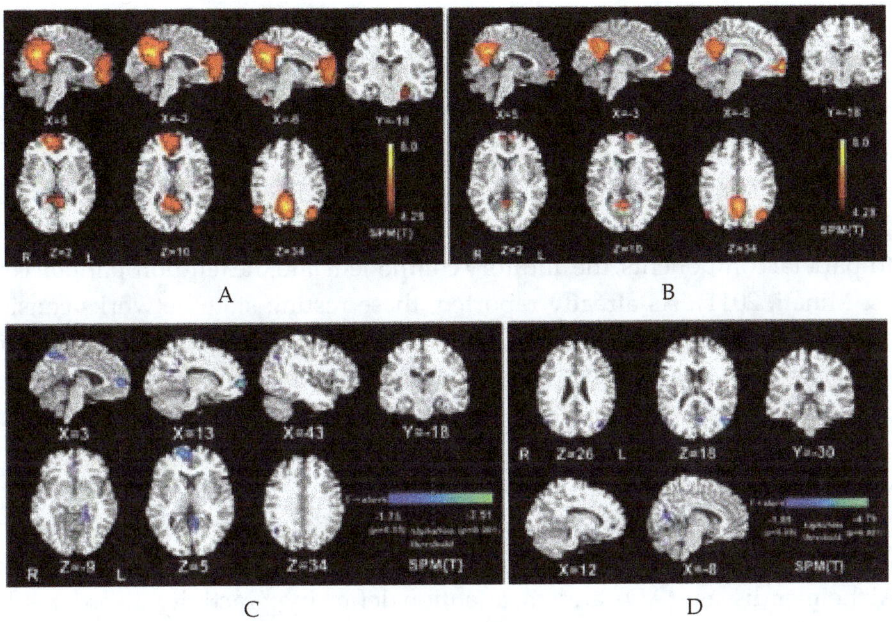

**Figure 6.** Default mode network changes of HE patients A) DMN of the controls consists of bilateral precuneus/posterior cingulate cortex, medial prefrontal cortex, anterior cingulate cortex, angular gyri, and temporal pole ($P < 0.05$, FDR corrected). B) DMN of HE patients consists of bilateral precuneus/posterior cingulate cortex, medial prefrontal cortex, anterior cingulate cortex, angular gyri, and temporal pole ($P < 0.05$, FDR corrected). Patterns in the HE patients are similar but with a reduced size compared to the ones of normal subjects in (A). C) Differences between the DMN of the HE patients and the controls are noted in the left posterior cingulate cortex and bilateral precuneus, right angular gyrus, bilateral middle frontal cortex, and left parahippocampus ($P<0.05$ for all, uncorrected) and in the right middle frontal gyrus and left posterior cingulate cortex ($P<0.05$ corrected, combined height threshold $P < 0.01$ and a minimum cluster size of 24 voxels). D) Statistical t-maps of the vein blood ammonia against z-scores in ICA in the HE group. The right middle frontal gyrus, left posterior cingulate cortex, left parahippocampus, bilateral angular gyri ($P<0.05$ for all, uncorrected) and the left angular gyrus colour-coded bright blue ($P<0.05$ corrected, combined height threshold $P<0.01$ and a minimum cluster size of 24 voxels) had a negative correlation with venous blood ammonia. From Zhang et al., Brain default-mode network abnormalities in hepatic encephalopathy: a resting-state functional MRI study. Hum Brain Mapp, 2011, DOI:10.1002/hbm.21295, with permission

prefrontal cortex (PFC), the medial temporal lobe, and the extrastriate cortex V5 and an enhanced coupling between IPL and the postcentral cortex were found in MHE patients. This study demonstrated an impaired and compensatory neural mechanism during visual judgment in the earliest stages of HE. Zhang et al. (Zhang et al., 2007a) used a Chinese character Stroop task as the target stimulus to investigate the neural mechanism of the cognitive control impairment in cirrhotic patients using fMRI. This study showed that simple tasks (incongruous word-reading tasks) increased the activity of the precentral and postcentral gyri in cirrhotic patients, and harder tasks (incongruous colour-naming tasks) decrease the activity of bilateral SFG, MFG, IFG, medial wall frontal gyrus, anterior cingulate cortex (ACC), temporal cortex, and parietal cortex. This study provides suggests that the abnormal anterior cingulate cortex–prefrontal cortex–parietal "fusiform" cortex circuit could be the neural substrarte responsible for this impaired cognitive control. However, the task-induced fMRI is better suited to the patients with low-grade or minimal HE who can perform the test tasks (Mcphail and Taylor-Robinson, 2010).

Recently, increasing attention has been given to detecting brain activities during resting state (Greicius et al., 2003; Greicius et al., 2004; Zhang et al., 2007b; Zhang et al., 2011). Most reported resting-state network components include; the default mode network (DMN), the sensorimotor component, the executive control component, up to three visual components, two lateralized fronto-parietal components, the auditory component and the temporoparietal component (Rosazza & Minati, 2011). As already reported, these resting-state networks consist of anatomically distinct, but functionally connected regions, which display a high level of correlated BOLD signal activity. Nowadays the DMN is the most studied network in comparison to task-induced brain networks. DMN includes the medial prefrontal cortex, rostral anterior cingulate, posterior cingulated cortex (PCC), and precuneus (Greicius et al., 2003; Greicius et al., 2004). The DMN is described by increased activity during rest, while decreased activation suppressed during cognitively demanding tasks, such as visual and auditory attention, language processing, memory, and motor activities. Abnormal default function network has been known to relate to Alzheimer disease (AD), autism, attention deficit hyperactivity disorder, schizophrenia, epilepsy, and other diseases (et al., 2005; Rombouts et al., 2005; Kennedy et al., 2006; Liang M, et al., 2006; Tian et al., 2006). In a study by Zhang et al. (Zhang et al., 2007), the DMN of the cirrhotic patients was investigated using a block-design in which a modified Chinese Stroop task was used as the target stimulus.

In this study, a subtraction method was used to study the resting-state network in patients with hepatic cirrhosis. The functional data suggest that cirrhotic patients may have a deactivated DMN. The absence of deactivation in the PCC and precuneus may be a sensitive, rather than specific, marker in patients with hepatic cirrhosis. Recently, in a resting state fMRI study (Zhang et al., 2011), a significantly reduced functional connectivity in the right middle frontal gyrus, left precuneus, and left PCC in the HE patients was observed when compared to the controls. A negative correlation was shown between left angular gyrus and left PCC activation and venous blood ammonia levels, suggesting this can be an important biomarker for HE (Figure 6).

## 9. Conclusion

In conclusion, HE appears as diffuse mild brain oedema, and is associated with cognition functional changes such as attention, and functional brain area changes, such as default mode brain areas. HE-associated functional and physiological abnormalities have been demonstrated by a variety of MR techniques. MRI offers a range of capabilities for investigating HE in clinical diagnosis. The recent development of fMRI and MRS expands the applications of the study of HE with the capability of assessing functional changes in brain affected by HE. These advances opens up the opportunities to better understand the pathopsychological mechanisms of HE.

## Acknowledgements

We express our thanks for the grants from Natural Scientific Foundation of China (30700194 and 81230032 to L.Z.) and Natural Scientific Foundation of Jiangsu Province of China (BK2007572 to L. Z.).

## Author details

Long Jiang Zhang[1], Guang Ming Lu[2] and Hui Mao[2]

1 Department of Medical Imaging, Nanjing University College of Clinical Medicine, Nanjing, China

2 Department of Radiology, Emory University School of Medicine, Atlanta, Georgia, USA

## References

[1] Amodio P, Montagnese S, Gatta A, Morgan MY (2004) Characteristics of minimal hepatic encephalopathy. Metab Brain Dis 19:253-26

[2] Amodio P, Ridola L, Schiff S, et al. (2010) Improving the inhibitory control task to detect minimal hepatic encephalopathy. Gastroenterology 139:510-51

[3] Astley SJ, Richards T, Aylward EH, et al. (2009) Magnetic resonance spectroscopy outcomes from a comprehensive magnetic resonance study of children with fetal alcohol spectrum disorders. Magn Reson Imaging 27:760-77

[4] Bajaj JS, Wade JB, Sanyal AJ (2009) Spectrum of neurocognitive impairment in cirrhosis Implications for the assessment of hepatic encephalopathy. Hepatology 50:2014-202

[5] Barba I, Chatauret N, Garcia-Dorado D, Cordoba J (2008) A 1H nuclear magnetic resonancebased metabonomic approach for grading hepatic encephalopathy and monitoring the effects of therapeutic hypothermia in rats. Liver Int 28:1141–114

[6] Binesh N, Huda A, Thomas MA, et al. (2006) Hepatic encephalopathy: a neurochemical, neuroanatomical, and neuropsychological study. J Appl Clin Med Phys 7:86-9

[7] Butterworth RF (2003) Pathogenesis of hepatic encephalopathy: new insights from neuroimaging and molecular studies. J Hepatol 39:278-28

[8] Chavarria L, Oria M, Romero-Gimenez J, Alonso J, Lope-Piedrafita S, Cordoba J (2010) Diffusion tensor imaging supports the cytotoxic origin of brain edema in a rat model of acute liver failure. Gastroenterology 138:1566-157

[9] Córdoba J (2011) New assessment of hepatic encephalopathy. J Hepatol 54:1030-104

[10] Córdoba J, Alonso J, Rovira A, et al. (2001) The development of low-grade cerebral edema in cirrhosis is supported by the evolution of (1)H-magnetic resonance abnormalities after liver transplantation. J Hepatol 35:598-60

[11] Córdoba J, Mínguez B (2008) Hepatic encephalopathy. Semin Liver Dis 28:70-8

[12] Córdoba J, Sanpedro F, Alonso J, Rovira A (2002) 1H magnetic resonance in the study of hepatic encephalopathy in humans. Metab Brain Dis 17:415-42

[13] Damoiseaux JS, Rombouts SA, Barkhof F, et al. (2006) Consistent resting-state networks across healthy subjects. Proc Natl Acad Sci U S A 103:13848-1385

[14] Dupont S, Duron E, Samson S, et al. (2010) Functional MR imaging or Wada test: which is the better predictor of individual postoperative memory outcome? Radiology 255:128-13

[15] Ferenci P, Lockwood A, Mullen K, Tarter R, Weissenborn K, Blei AT (2002) Hepatic encephalopathy--definition, nomenclature, diagnosis, and quantification: final report of the working party at the 11th World Congresses of Gastroenterology, Vienna, 1998. Hepatology 35:716-72

[16] Gore JC (2003) Principles and practice of functional MRI of the human brain. J Clin Invest 112:4–

[17] Gotman J, Grova C, Bagshaw A, Kobayashi E, Aghakhani Y, Dubeau F (2005) Generalized epileptic discharges show thalamocortical activation and suspension of the default state of the brain. Proc Natl Acad Sci U S A 102:15236–1524

[18] Greicius MD, Krasnow B, Reiss AL, Menon V (2003) Functional connectivity in the resting brain: a network analysis of the default mode hypothesis. Proc Natl Acad Sci U S A 100:253-25

[19] Greicius MD, Srivastava G, Reiss AL, Menon V (2004) Default-mode network activity distinguishes Alzheimer's disease from healthy aging: evidence from functional MRI. Proc Natl Acad Sci U S A 101:4637-464

[20] Grover VP, Dresner MA, Forton DM, et al. (2006) Current and future applications of magnetic resonance imaging and spectroscopy of the brain in hepatic encephalopathy. World J Gastroenterol 12:2969-297

[21] Gupta RK, Yadav SK, Rangan M, et al. (2010) Serum proinflammatory cytokines correlate with diffusion tensor imaging derived metrics and (1)H-MR spectroscopy in patients with acute liver failure. Metab Brain Dis 25:355-36

[22] Haseler LJ, Sibbitt WL Jr, Mojtahedzadeh HN, Reddy S, Agarwal VP, McCarthy DM (1998) Proton MR spectroscopic measurement of neurometabolites in hepatic encephalopathy during oral lactulose therapy. AJNR Am J Neuroradiol 19:1681- 168

[23] Kale RA, Gupta RK, Saraswat VA, et al. (2006) Demonstration of interstitial cerebral edema with diffusion tensor MR imaging in type C hepatic encephalopathy. Hepatology 43:698-70

[24] Kennedy DP, Redcay E, Courchesne E (2006) Failing to deactivate: resting functional abnormalities in autism. Proc Natl Acad Sci U S A 103:8275–828

[25] Kreis R, Ross BD, Farrow NA, Ackerman Z (1992) Metabolic disorders of the brain in chronic hepatic encephalopathy detected with H-1 MR spectroscopy. Radiology 182:19-2

[26] Kumar R, Gupta RK, Elderkin-Thompson V, et al. (2008) Voxel-based diffusion tensor magnetic resonance imaging evaluation of low-grade hepatic encephalopathy. J Magn Reson Imaging 27:1061-106

[27] Lee JH, Seo DW, Lee YS, et al. (1999) Proton magnetic resonance spectroscopy (1H-MRS) findings for the brain in patients with liver cirrhosis reflect the hepatic functional reserve. Am J Gastroenterol 94:2206-221

[28] Liang M, Zhou Y, Jiang T, et al. (2006) Widespread functional disconnectivity in schizophrenia with resting-state functional magnetic resonance imaging. Neuroreport 17:209–21

[29] Lodi R, Tonon C, Stracciari A, et al. (2004) Diffusion MRI shows increased water apparent diffusion coefficient in the brains of cirrhotics. Neurology 62:762-76

[30] Long LL, Li XR, Huang ZK, Jiang YM, Fu SX, Zheng W (2009) Relationship between changes in brain MRI and (1)H-MRS, severity of chronic liver damage, and recovery after liver transplantation. Exp Biol Med (Maywood) 234:1075-108

[31] Matsusue E, Kinoshita T, Ohama E, Ogawa T (2005) Cerebral cortical and white matter lesions in chronic hepatic encephalopathy: MR-pathologic correlations. AJNR Am J Neuroradiol 26:347-35

[32] McKinney AM, Lohman BD, Sarikaya B, et al. (2010) Acute hepatic encephalopathy: diffusion-weighted and fluid-attenuated inversion recovery findings, and correlation with plasma ammonia level and clinical outcome. AJNR Am J Neuroradiol 31:1471-147

[33] McPhail MJ, Taylor-Robinson SD (2010) The role of magnetic resonance imaging and spectroscopy in hepatic encephalopathy. Metab Brain Dis 25:65-7

[34] Mechtcheriakov S, Schocke M, Kugener A, et al. (2005) Chemical shift magnetic resonance spectroscopy of cingulate grey matter in patients with minimal hepatic encephalopathy. Neuroradiology 47:27-3

[35] Michel V, Yuan Z, Ramsubir S, Bakovic M (2006) Choline transport for phospholipid synthesis. Exp Biol Med (Maywood) 231:490-50

[36] Miese F, Kircheis G, Wittsack HJ, et al. (2006) 1H-MR spectroscopy, magnetization transfer, and diffusion-weighted imaging in alcoholic and nonalcoholic patients with cirrhosis with hepatic encephalopathy. AJNR Am J Neuroradiol 27:1019-102

[37] Miese FR, Wittsack HJ, Kircheis G, et al. (2009) Voxel-based analyses of magnetization transfer imaging of the brain in hepatic encephalopathy. World J Gastroenterol 15:5157-516

[38] Mínguez B, Rovira A, Alonso J, Córdoba J (2007) Decrease in the volume of white matter lesions with improvement of hepatic encephalopathy. AJNR Am J Neuroradiol 28:1499-50

[39] Mukherjee P, Berman JI, Chung SW, Hess CP, Henry RG (2008) Diffusion tensor MR imaging and fiber tractography: theoretic underpinnings. AJNR Am J Neuroradiol 29:632-64

[40] Mukherjee P, Chung SW, Berman JI, Hess CP, Henry RG (2008) Diffusion tensor MR imaging and fiber tractography: technical considerations. AJNR Am J Neuroradiol 29:843-85

[41] Naegele T, Grodd W, Viebahn R, et al. (2000) MR imaging and (1)H spectroscopy of brain metabolites in hepatic encephalopathy: time-course of renormalization after liver transplantation. Radiology 216:683-69

[42] Ogawa S, Tank DW, Menon R, et al. (1992) Intrinsic signal changes accompanying sensory stimulation: functional brain mapping with magnetic resonance imaging. Proc Natl Acad Sci U S A 89:5951–595

[43] Poveda MJ, Bernabeu A, Concepción L, et al. (2010) Brain edema dynamics in patients with overt hepatic encephalopathy A magnetic resonance imaging study. Neuroimage 52:481-48

[44] Provenzale JM, Mukundan S, Barboriak DP (2006) Diffusion-weighted and perfusion MR imaging for brain tumor characterization and assessment of treatment response. Radiology 239:632-64

[45] Randolph C, Hilsabeck R, Kato A, et al. (2009) Neuropsychological assessment of hepatic encephalopathy: ISHEN practice guidelines. Liver Int 29:629-63

[46] Rombouts SA, Barkhof F, Goekoop R, Stam CJ, Scheltens P (2005) Altered resting state networks in mild cognitive impairment and mild Alzheimer's disease: an fMRI study. Hum Brain Mapp 26:231–23

[47] Rosazza C, Minati L (2011) Resting-state brain networks: literature review and clinical applications. Neurol Sci 2011; DOI 10.1007/s10072-011-0636-y

[48] Ross BD, Jacobson S, Villamil F, et al. (1994) Subclinical hepatic encephalopathy: proton MR spectroscopic abnormalities. Radiology 193:457-46

[49] Rovira A, Alonso J, Cordoba J (2008) MR imaging findings in hepatic encephalopathy. AJNR Am J Neroradiol 29:1612–162

[50] Rovira A, Alonso J, Cucurella G, et al. (1999) Evolution of multiple sclerosis lesions on serial contrast-enhanced T1-weighted and magnetization-transfer MR images. AJNR Am J Neuroradiol 20:1939– 4

[51] Rovira A, Grive′ E, Pedraza S, et al. (2001) Magnetization transfer ratio values and proton MR spectroscopy of normal-appearing cerebral white matter in patients with liver cirrhosis. AJNR Am J Neuroradiol 22:1137– 114

[52] Rovira A, Mínguez B, Aymerich FX, et al. (2007) Decreased white matter lesion volume and improved cognitive function after liver transplantation. Hepatology 46:1485-149

[53] Saksena S, Rai V, Saraswat VA, et al. (2008) Cerebral diffusion tensor imaging and in vivo proton magnetic resonance spectroscopy in patients with fulminant hepatic failure. J Gastroenterol Hepatol 23:e111-11

[54] Sawara K, Kato A, Yoshioka Y, Suzuki K (2004) Brain glutamine and glutamate levels in patients with liver cirrhosis: assessed by 3.0-T MRS. Hepatol Res 30:18-2

[55] Saxena V, Gupta A, Nagana Gowda GA, Saxena R, Yachha SK, Khetrapal CL (2006) 1H NMR spectroscopy for the prediction of therapeutic outcome in patients with fulminant hepatic failure. NMR Biomed 19:521–52

[56] Schaefer PW, Grant PE, Gonzalez RG (2000) Diffusion-weighted MR imaging of the brain. Radiology 217:331-34

[57] Singhal A, Nagarajan R, Hinkin CH, et al. (2010) Two-dimensional MR spectroscopy of minimal hepatic encephalopathy and neuropsychological correlates in vivo. J Magn Reson Imaging 32:35-4

[58] Spahr L, Burkhard PR, Grötzsch H, Hadengue A (2002) Clinical significance of basal ganglia alterations at brain MRI and 1H MRS in cirrhosis and role in the pathogenesis of hepatic encephalopathy. Metab Brain Dis 17:399-41

[59] Stewart CA, Reivich M, Lucey MR, Gores GJ (2005) Neuroimaging in hepatic encephalopathy. Clin Gastroenterol Hepatol 3:197-20

[60] Sugimoto R, Iwasa M, Maeda M, et al. (2008) Value of the apparent diffusion coefficient for quantification of low-grade hepatic encephalopathy. Am J Gastroenterol 103:1413- 142

[61] Tarasów E, Panasiuk A, Siergiejczyk L, et al. (2003) MR and 1H MR spectroscopy of the brain in patients with liver cirrhosis and early stages of hepatic encephalopathy. Hepatogastroenterology 50:2149-215

[62] Thoeny HC, De Keyzer F (2011) Diffusion-weighted MR imaging of native and transplanted kidneys. Radiology 259:25-3

[63] Thuluvath PJ, Edwin D, Yue NC, deVilliers C, Hochman S, Klein A (1995) Increased signals seen in globus pallidus in T1-weighted magnetic resonance imaging in cirrhotics are not suggestive of chronic hepatic encephalopathy. Hepatology 21:440-44

[64] Tian L, Jiang T, Wang Y, et al. (2006) Altered resting-state functional connectivity patterns of anterior cingulate cortex in adolescents with attention deficit hyperactivity disorder. Neurosci Letters 400:39–4

[65] Toru S, Matumura K, Kawaguchi R, Kobayashi T, Irie T (2011) Widespread cortical lesions on diffusion-weighted imaging in acute portal systemic shunt encephalopathy caused by primary biliary cirrhosis. AJNR Am J Neuroradiol 32:E55-5

[66] Vance DE: Phospholipid biosynthesis. In: Biochemistry of Lipids, Lipoproteins and Membranes. Vance DE and Vance J (eds.). Amsterdam, Elsevier Science Publishers B. V., pp. 153-181, 199

[67] Verma A, Saraswat VA, Radha Krishna Y, Nath K, Thomas MA, Gupta RK (2008). In vivo 1H magnetic resonance spectroscopy-derived metabolite variations between acuteon- chronic liver failure and acute liver failure. Liver Int 28:1095-110

[68] Weissenborn K, Ahl B, Fischer-Wasels D, et al. (2007) Correlations between magnetic resonance spectroscopy alterations and cerebral ammonia and glucose metabolism in cirrhotic patients with and without hepatic encephalopathy. Gut 56:1736-174

[69] Weissenborn K, Bokemeyer M, Ahl B, et al. (2004) Functional imaging of the brain in patients with liver cirrhosis. Metab Brain Dis 19:269-28

[70] Zafiris O, Kircheis G, Rood HA, Boers F, Haussinger D, Zilles K (2004) Neural mechanism underlying impaired visual judgement in the dysmetabolic brain: an fMRI study. Neuroimage 22:541–55

[71] Zhang L, Qi R, Wu SY, et al. (2011) Brain default-mode network abnormalities in hepatic encephalopathy: a resting-state functional MRI study. Human Brain Mapping DOI: 10.1002/hbm.2129

[72] Zhang LJ, Yang G, Yin J, Liu Y, Qi J (2007a) Neural mechanism of cognitive control impairment in patients with hepatic cirrhosis: a functional magnetic resonance imaging study. Acta Radiol 48:577-58

[73] Zhang LJ, Yang G, Yin J, Liu Y, Qi J (2007b) Abnormal default-mode network activation in cirrhotic patients: a functional magnetic resonance imaging study. Acta Radiol 48:781-78

[74] Zhang LJ, Yin JZ, Qi J, Lu GM (2010) Metabolic changes of anterior cingulate cortex in patients with hepatic cirrhosis: a magnetic resonance spectroscopy study. Hepatol Res 40:777-78

# 8

# Neuroimaging of Epilepsy: EEG-fMRI in the Presurgical Evaluation of Focal Epilepsy

Mirko Avesani, Silvia Giacopuzzi and
Antonio Fiaschi

## 1. Introduction

Epilepsies of surgical interest are focal and drug-resistant forms associated with various different conditions (malformations, stroke, tumors, infectious and/or inflammatory processes, brain injuries). There is mounting evidence that early resective surgery can achieve seizure-free status or reduce seizure frequency. The main challenge in the presurgical assessment of patients with epilepsy is to localize the area of seizure onset (the epileptogenic zone) and to distinguish it from lesional and interictal foci (the irritative zone) because it is only by treating the epileptogenic zone that seizure freedom or a reduction in events may be attained (Thorton, 2010).

This is explained by the fact that since the interictal focus is larger than the epileptogenic zone, the epileptogenic zone does not always overlap the lesional area and the epileptogenic focus is often larger than lesional area (Avesani, 2008/a; Manganotti, 2008; Thorton, 2010). In general, interictal epileptic discharges may affect brain areas well beyond the presumed region in which they are generated (Gotman, 2008). While resection of the lesional area alone is not sufficient, neither can the entire interictal focus be removed due to the high risk of cognitive, motor, sensitive or language deficits.

Presurgical evaluation involves invasive investigation by stereoelectroencephalography (SEEG) performed after other routine exams (standard EEG, video-EEG, functional neuroimaging) to identify the interictal focus within the epileptogenic zone. The lesional area, instead, is nowadays studied with advanced MRI techniques developed to better identify the interictal focus.

## 2. Functional imaging in epilepsy

Functional imaging refers to noninvasive methods to identify the interictal focus and the epileptogenic zone which, in a subsequent step, is studied with an invasive technique (SEEG, electrocortical mapping). The most widely used are:

- positron-emission tomography (PET)
- single-photon-emission computed tomography (SPECT)
- magnetic resonance spectroscopy (MRS)
- functional magnetic imaging (fMRI)

These techniques allow the study of a specific area of the brain, obviating the need for invasive studies of the entire brain. PET and SPECT were initially utilized for this purpose. While both provide a better knowledge of the brain's functional anatomy, they rarely allow for a precise localization of an epileptogenic focus, making them less useful for surgical planning (Marks, 1992; Henry, 1993; Newton, 1995).

The rationale for SPECT is based on its ability to reveal, in vivo, the volume distribution of a radiotracer after intravenous injection, and to evaluate, quantitatively and qualitatively, regional brain perfusion (Devous, 2005). The application of SPECT in epilepsy derives from a known association between an electrical event and brain perfusion: brain perfusion increases during the ictal phase and decreases during the interictal phase. Studies using dynamic and static SPECT have demonstrated interictal temporal hypoperfusion in 50% patients with temporal-lobe epilepsy (TLE). Nevertheless, the limitation of this technique is that 5-10% of patients demonstrate contralateral hypoperfusion, which raises the risk of false localization (Krausz, 1991). The localization power of SPECT during the interictal phase is, therefore, variable, with a sensitivity of 36% and a specificity of 95% (Engel, 1982). For this reason, SPECT is useful as a comparative study of ictal and interictal perfusion in selected patients. When applied during a seizure, it demonstrates the dynamic aspect of the seizure during its development. Unlike interictal studies, ictal SPECT, in both temporal and extratemporal epilepsy, is accurate in localizing an epileptogenic focus. During the ictal phase it can reveal, with a sensitivity of 70-95%, hyperperfusion in an area activated by seizures (Engel, 1983; Lee, 1994).

PET is a powerful imaging technique to quantify, in vivo and noninvasively, cerebral blood flow, metabolism and receptorial links. Its main application derives from the need to identify epileptogenic foci in patients with drug-resistant epilepsy, potential candidates for surgical treatment to control or abolish drug-resistant focal seizures. In up to 20-30% of such patients, who are candidates for surgical treatment, the MRI exam is negative (Duncan, 1997) because microscopic structural malformations, identifiable only by histological study, are not detectable with conventional MRI (Kuzniecky, 1991). Using [11C]flumazenil positron-emission tomography ([11C]FMZ-PET), Hammers studied 18 patients with TLE and normal MRI: 16 demonstrated abnormalities in the binding of $^{11}$C-FMZ in the temporal lobe; 7 of these were concordant with clinical and standard EEG data; 3 patients underwent surgical treatment of the anterior temporal lobe, with marked clinical improvement. The neuropathological data revealed microdysgenesis not detected by MRI (Hammers, 2002).

In patients with focal seizures, glucose metabolism and cerebral blood flow in a particular focal region are increased during an ictal event (Engel, 1983). In the postictal phase, hyperperfusion gradually returns to the basal level, but glucose metabolism remains elevated for 24-48 hours after seizure termination (Leiderman, 1994). In the interictal phase, PET demonstrates a decrease in glucose metabolism and cerebral blood flow in the epileptogenic focus. Studies using *18*-fluoro-2-deoxy-glucose-positron emission tomography (*18F-FDG-PET*) demonstrated hypometabolism in the temporal lobe in 60-90% of patients with interictal spikes (Duncan, 1997). Nevertheless, an area with abnormal cerebral blood flow and metabolism, as detected with PET, is larger than the real structural anomaly generating an epileptogenic focus probably because of deafferentation phenomena in the surrounding neurons in areas of seizure propagation (Duncan, 1997). Since this carries the risk of false localization, PET is regarded as being more suitable for studying lateralization than localization (Tai, 2004).

MR spectroscopy can be utilized in the noninvasive assessment of specific cerebral metabolites. In epilepsy the aim is to determine a focal change in the main metabolites deriving from focal brain dysfunction. The initial aim of the method was to delimit the epileptogenic focus and to analyze the distant repercussions of the lesion and the focus. For example, spectroscopy can reveal bilateral hippocampal abnormalities in unilateral mesial temporal sclerosis (MTS). The technique has demonstrated its utility in identifying metabolic dysfunction in patients with TLE. Nevertheless, owing to its high sensitivity, metabolic abnormalities may be revealed in regions without an epileptogenic focus, making it difficult to distinguish the causal abnormalities from their consequences (Ruben, 2005).

In patients with drug-resistant TLE, spectroscopy demonstrated a lower N-acetyl aspartate/creatine (NAA/Cr) ratio, a reliable marker of neuronal integrity, in the ipsi- and contralateral lobes, and this finding correlated negatively with seizure duration (Bernasconi, 2002). Patients with frequent generalized seizures were noted to have a lower NAA/Cr ratio than those with rare or no seizures. Another interesting finding was the demonstration of reversible dysfunction in the cortical area after surgical treatment (Hugg, 1996). What all this suggests is that seizures may induce additional neuronal damage that will progress with the duration of epilepsy. From this point of view, spectroscopy may be useful as a metabolic marker of disease progression. In the future, it may be possible to decide whether evidence of disease progression on spectroscopy may be sufficient to suggest a change of therapy (Petroff, 2002).

Functional MRI (fMRI) provides high-resolution images using the classical principles of MRI, with the difference that signal recording exploits the paramagnetic properties of hemoglobin when its iron atom changes from $Fe^{3+}$ (oxygenated hemoglobin) to $Fe^{2+}$ (deoxygenated hemoglobin). Only $Fe^{2+}$ has the ability to locally modify the magnetic state of cerebral tissues (Berns, 1999). Activation of a cerebral area causes both oxidative metabolism and local cerebral blood flow to increase, leading to greater oxygen extraction by the tissues. This results in a local increase of deoxyhemoglobin. Functional MRI reveals the activation of a cerebral area from the higher level of deoxyhemoglobin compared to the basal condition. And it does this indirectly by measuring the vascular response to activation of the cerebral area under study.

The response has a variable latency (from 3-5 to 10 seconds), which is why this kind of information is defined as "functional", and the recorded signal, related to hemoglobin oxygenation, is defined as BOLD (Blood Oxygen Level Dependent) (Ogawa, 1990; Prichard, 1994).

fMRI works by comparing the images obtained in rest condition with those acquired during a task. Whether and to what extent physiological correlates match different BOLD phases (Menon, 2001) continues to fuel debate, though studies suggest that the fMRI signal is closely related to neuronal activation (Logothetis, 2001). The method was first applied to localize areas associated with motor, sensory and cognitive functions in epileptic patients and to obtain a precise localization of these functions in the presurgical evaluation of epilepsy (Puce, 1995; Binder, 1996; Dupon, 2002).

## 3. EEG-fMRI

This noninvasive technique provides reliable information to localize cerebral regions generating interictal epileptic activity. It involves the simultaneous recording of EEG and fMRI. With ongoing refinement of the technology (first of all removal of magnetic field artifact on EEG), initial technical limitations have been overcome (Ives, 1993). EEG-fMRI permits the study cerebral activation and deactivation related to infra-clinical spikes by comparing EEG with spiked activity against EEG without abnormalities (Krakow, 1999 and 2001; Lazeyras 2000; Archer, 2003).

Research to date has investigated lesional epilepsy in the temporal region in particular, the most frequent cause of epilepsy of surgical interest. Up until several years ago, triggered EEG-fMRI was used. EEG was recorded during a scanning session, and fMRI acquisition was performed when a neurologist identified, on line, interictal (spikes, polyspikes, spike waves) activity on EEG. Acquisition was performed after a fixed latency (3-5 seconds) from detected interictal activity, which was decided before starting acquisition. The technique had several limitations: it was based on the concept of standardized cerebral hemodynamic activity, even if we know that such activity varies widely (from 3 up to 10 seconds); analysis had to be performed offline using, as a task, spikes with different morphology; and the temporal dynamics of hemodynamic responses could not be identified. Owing to these limitations, early studies with triggered EEG-fMRI (Krakow, 1999 and 2001) showed low sensitivity (60%) in detecting hemodynamic activation related to interictal activity.

Later studies (Lazeyras, 2001; Lemieux, 2001; Al-Asmi, 2003) demonstrated the superiority of continuous EEG-fMRI based on offline analysis after simultaneous EEG recording during a fMRI scanning session and following artifact removal. This development brought about clear advantages: since it was no longer necessary to decide beforehand which abnormal events were to be studied (and recorded) during a single acquisition, the temporal evolution of activations (after 1 to 10 seconds) could be identified and pathophysiological hypotheses about their propagation postulated. Continuous EEG-fMRI detects activation with a sensitivity of 80%.

Numerous studies have applied continuous EEG-fMRI to investigate various different epileptic syndromes (Boor, 2003; Salek-Haddadi, 2003 and 2006; Bagshaw, 2004 and 2006; Aghakhani, 2004 and 2005; Gotman, 2004 and 2005; Kobayashi, 2005 and 2006; Laufs, 2006; Di Bonaventura, 2006; Vaudano, 2009). Some studied focal epilepsies, while others examined idiopathic generalized forms underlying absence seizures.

## 4. EEG-fMRI in absence seizures

The application of EEG-fMRI in idiopathic generalized epilepsy (IGE), for evident technical problems, is limited to absence seizures or nonconvulsive status, to analyze the network underlying impaired consciousness related to generalized spike wave (GSW) discharges. Clinically, absences are characterized by a blank stare and impaired consciousness. Activities requiring vigilant attention have been coupled with a lesser likelihood of absences, whereas an increased frequency of seizures during relaxation is well established (Andermann, 2000; Guey, 1969). These findings suggest a causal link between changes in the level of awareness and the occurrence of GSW discharges.

Recent functional imaging studies have revealed the existence of a set of brain regions which show increased functional and metabolic activity during rest, compared to attention-demanding tasks (Raichle, 2000; Mazoyer, 2001). Involved brain areas (the posterior cingulated cortex, the precuneus, the medial prefrontal cortex, the mid-dorsolateral prefrontal and the anterior temporal cortices) have been hypothesized to constitute the so-called default mode network (DMN) (Raichle, 2000). Decreased DMN activity during cognitive tasks indicates that the network sustains spontaneous thought processes or self-oriented mental activity that characterizes the brain's resting state.

Additionally, the precuneus/posterior cingulate node has been recently demonstrated to have the highest degree of interactions (as shown by a partial correlation approach to fMRI data) with the rest of the DMN (Frasson, 2008), suggesting a pivotal role of this area within the network. This interpretation is in line with evidence from previous PET studies that this brain region, and the precuneus in particular, has the highest metabolic rate, consuming 35% more glucose than any other area of the cerebral cortex at rest (Gusnard, 2001).

The DMN shows decreased activity during both attention-demanding tasks and states of reduced vigilance and, especially in the posteromedial cortical regions, during altered states of consciousness (Laureys, 2004; Faymonville, 2006). From these observations, several authors (Cavanna, 2006 and 2007; Boly, 2008) suggested a pivotal role of the posteromedial cortical region in self-consciousness inside the DMN.

EEG-correlated functional magnetic resonance imaging (EEG-fMRI) studies have shown a common pattern of BOLD signal decrease in the precuneus and other DMN areas, together with an increase in the thalamic BOLD signal, during ictal and interictal GSW discharges (Aghakhani, 2004; Archer, 2003; Gotman, 2005; Hamandi, 2006; Laufs, 2006; Salek-Haddadi, 2003; De Tiège, 2007; Labate, 2005). Decreased cerebral blood flow consistent with a decrease in neuronal activity was demonstrated in DMN regions during GSW discharges (Hamandi, 2008). Therefore, these relative BOLD signal decreases can be interpreted as a transitory suspension of the brain's "default state" which occurs in association with an altered level of awareness observed during GSW discharges and absences, respectively (Gotman, 2005; Hamandi, 2006; Laufs, 2006; Salek-Haddadi, 2003).

The pathophysiological substrate of GSW remains enigmatic. Studies in animals and humans have tried to answer persistent questions about the putative role of the thalamus and cortex as generators. Data from invasive recordings and manipulations in well-validated genetic models of absence epilepsy have lent support to the hypothesis that absence seizures are of cortical origin (Steriade, 1998; Meeren, 2002 and 2005; Polack, 2007; Holmes, 2004; Tucker, 2007).

Following on the suggestion of the involvement of dorsal cortical regions (particularly the posterior-medial cortical regions) in GSW discharges from neuroimaging studies (Gotman, 2005; Hamandi, 2006; Laufs, 2006; Salek-Haddadi, 2003) and their role in conscious awareness (Faymonville, 2006; Boly, 2008), a recent work (Vaudano, 2009) attempted to elucidate the interaction between these areas and the (frontal)cortical-thalamic loop by means of dynamic causal modeling (DCM) to study effective connectivity based on simultaneously recorded EEG-fMRI data in 7 patients with GSW discharges.

The results of this study are consistent with the concept of the precuneus as a key region that changes its activity with altered states of vigilance, thus influencing the occurrence of generalized seizures: changes in the precuneus state (an increase or decrease in its neuronal activity), which reflects spontaneous fluctuations in awareness, act on the thalamic-(frontal) cortical network, facilitating the development of GSW. This contrasts with previous observations (Gotman, 2005; Hamandi, 2006; Laufs, 2006) that decreases in precuneal activity reflect the semiology of impaired consciousness and are a consequence of GSW.

A similar hypothesis was advanced by Archer et al. (Archer, 2003) who observed a significant posterior cingulate negative BOLD response in 5 IGE patients with interictal GSW discharges but no BOLD signal changes in the thalamus or prefrontal cortex. The authors suggested that decreases in posterior cingulate activity and associated regions may be involved in the initiation of GSW activity.

Additionally, a fMRI study showed a BOLD signal decrease in the posterior cingulate in IGE subjects following photic stimulation whether or not GSW activity occurred, while the control subjects showed no change in this region (Hill, 1999). Such changes would be consistent with a decrease in posterior cingulate activity being a precursor (or facilitator) of GSW activity rather than a secondary phenomenon. The posterior cingulate cortex is adjacent to the precuneus and some authors would define it as part of the precuneal cortical area (Frackowiak, 1997; Frasson, 2008).

Current thinking about the pathophysiology of GSW has it that the neuronal state of the precuneus, and the level of awareness, may reflect a "physiological initiator" of generalized synchronous discharges. In this connection, EEG-fMRI adds electrophysiological data to GSW generation and precuneal involvement where, besides the scant evidence for a strict consequentiality between a particular state of vigilance and the occurrence of GSW discharges, there is a notable lack of studies on the possible role of cortical structures (particularly the precuneus) other than the thalamus and frontal cortex in GSW.

Unlike surface electrophysiological recordings, fMRI studies with concurrent EEG in patients with GSW discharges have shown common hemodynamic changes not only in the thalamus and frontal cortex, but also in the precuneus and other brain regions (including the fronto-parietal association cortices) of the DMN (Aghakhani, 2004; Archer, 2003; Gotman, 2005; Laufs, 2007). Moreover, fMRI's relatively homogeneous sensitivity across the brain compared to that of scalp EEG may explain why recent EEG-fMRI studies have been able to reveal precuneal involvement in epilepsies characterized by impaired consciousness and associated with GSW (Gotman, 2005; Hamandi, 2006; Laufs, 2006).

In brief, there is an active role in generalized epilepsy for the precuneus, a region previously neglected in electrophysiological studies of GSW. DCM based on EEG-fMRI data has shown that the precuneus is not only strongly connected with the frontal cortex and the thalamus but also that the neuronal activity in this area may facilitate epileptic activity within a thalamo-cortical loop, the existence of which is well established. These findings suggest that GSW may arise through the direct influence of the neuronal state of the precuneus associated with spontaneous changes in the level of awareness.

## 5. EEG-fMRI in focal seizures: Introduction

### 5.1. Interictal focal spiked activity correlated BOLD signal changes: Aims and results

EEG-fMRI provides insight into the pathophysiology of changes in the level of awareness during GSW discharges in absence seizures; however, the practical usefulness of technique resides in the study of focal epilepsy, especially if drug resistant and associated with a condition which, if amenable to removal, could achieve seizure freedom or a reduction of frequency. Numerous studies have applied EEG-fMRI to focal seizures to identify the interictal focus and the ictal onset zone (Krakow 1999 and 2001; Boor, 2003; Salek Haddadi, 2006; Bagshaw, 2004 and 2006; Aghakani, 2005; Kobayashi, 2005 and 2006). Some also applied SEEG and electrocortical mapping to study areas previously identified with EEG-fMRI and confirmed co-localization between interictal events (IEDs) and hemodynamic activation detected on fMRI (Krakow, 1999; Kobayashi, 2006; Benar, 2006).

All these studies analyzed patients with spiked activity on focal EEG (spikes, spikes and waves, polyspikes) that differed in frequency. It was then suggested that a limiting factor to obtain sufficient BOLD activation is IED frequency. Two studies (Krakow, 1999 and 2001) proposed 1 IED/minute as the minimum value to obtain sufficient activation. But because a lower frequency does not have sufficient power to stimulate an IED-correlated BOLD signal change, the sensitivity of the technique is very low. More recent studies applied EEG-fMRI to compare the location of IED-correlated BOLD signal change with the resected area and postoperative outcome (Thorton, 2010). Seven out of 10 surgically treated patients were seizure-free following surgery and the area of maximal BOLD signal change was concordant with resection in 6 out of 7 patients. In the remaining 3 patients with reduced seizure frequency post-surgically, the areas of significant IED-correlated BOLD signal change lay outside the resection, thus confirming that the epileptogenic zone (to be removed) is different from the lesional area.

### 5.2. Interictal focal slow wave activity correlated BOLD changes: The first case reports

Although some studies analyzed focal epilepsies (Liu, 2008), focal slow-wave activity as a marker of activation of cerebral blood flow was initially studied in only two single case reports (Laufs, 2006/a; Avesani 2008/a-b). The one additionally used SEEG to demonstrate co-localization between IEDs and fMRI activation. The second, our case report (Avesani 2008/a), involved a patient with temporal lobe epilepsy (TLE) due to a cavernoma, who had undergone surgical treatment without attaining freedom of seizures. This woman had no medical history of note until the age of 24 years (1975), when symptoms characterized by painful sensations including a lightening stabbing pain developed in the left parietal region of the head, preceded by absence attacks lasting 30 seconds. After seizures she always experienced profound weakness. Her seizures recurred at a variable rate, ranging from more than one a day to one every 10-15 days. During the seizure-free periods she remained healthy. The EEG at that time was negative for an interictal focus. In 1986, when the patient was 35 years old, the EEG disclosed an interictal focus in left temporal regions, characterized by very frequent, and polymorphous, theta-delta activity in association with sharp waves, blocked by eye opening and without contralateral diffusion. Subsequent EEG confirmed the irritative focus in the left fronto-temporal region. When the patient was 37-year-old she began therapy with phenobarbitone (PB) and carbamazepine (CBZ), benefiting from a decrease in seizure intensity (but not frequency). A computed tomographic (CT) brain scan disclosed a mild, non-homogeneous, subcortical hyperdensity on the mesial side of the left temporal lobe, containing rough calcifications with no contrast enhancement. An MRI scan revealed two small lesions in the left temporal lobe, similar to cavernomas (one anterior, in the Sylvian fissure and another posterior, in the paratrigonal region). The patient underwent surgery but the partial seizures remained unchanged. Treatment with PB and CBZ was therefore continued. Twelve years later (2002), another MRI scan revealed three small independent cavernomas in the left temporal lobe (left temporo-basal, left temporo-mesial, and in the left post-central gyrus). A year later (2003), bleeding of the large lesion (localized in the left temporo-basal region) caused the patient to be re-admitted to the neurosurgical ward to undergo a second operation. Despite repeat surgery the seizures continued so she needed further therapy. A following MRI scan (2005), confirmed the presence of the previous cavernomas without bleeding.

Using interictal focus of slow waves recorded in the left temporal region as a trigger of activation (Fig. 1), we obtained activation in the left posterior cortical region around the poro-encephalic cavity (residual of previous surgical treatment) (Fig. 2). Our findings confirmed observations by Thorton of 3 patients in whom surgical treatment failed to achieve seizure freedom: in these situations areas of significant IED correlated BOLD signal change lay outside the resection (Thorton, 2010).

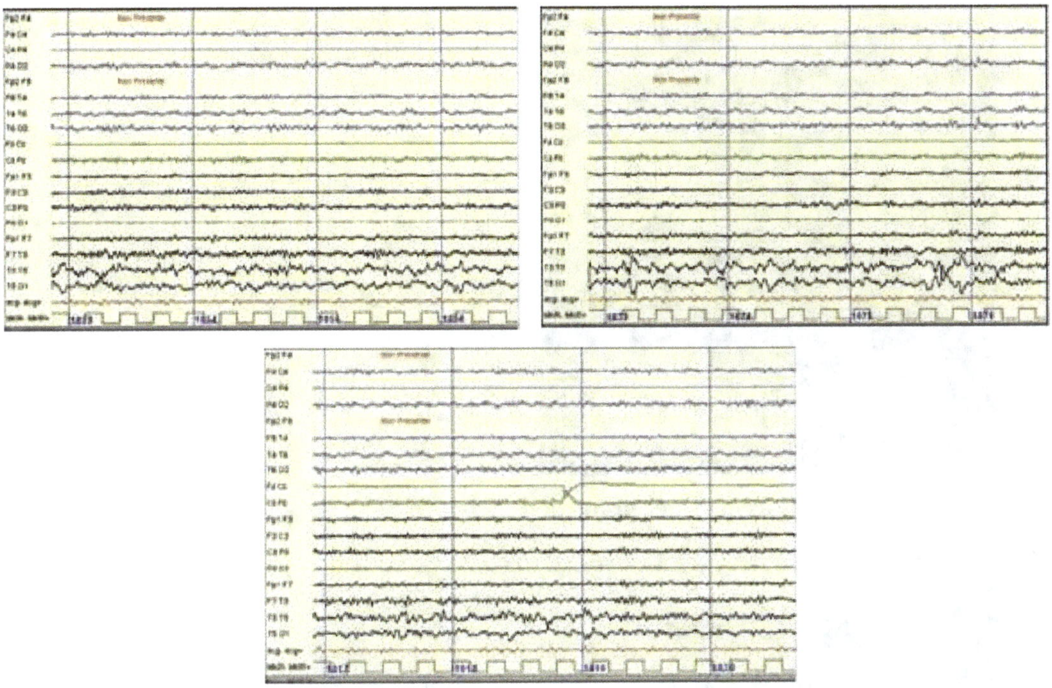

**Figure 1.** Interictal EEG of patient affected by cavernosa. Focal IEDs in left temporal region

## 6. EEG fMRI in focal seizures: The first study of interictal slow wave activity correlated bold changes

### 6.1. Patients enrolled in the study

In a previous study involving 8 patients with focal slow-wave interictal discharges on EEG (Manganotti, 2008), we suggested that an IED-correlated BOLD change triggered by interictal slow-wave activity could be obtained if the focal activity is frequent (about 2 IEDs/min). The study was primarily designed to verify whether the interictal slow waves originating from an EEG interictal focus were sufficient to increase cerebral blood flow in a spatially related brain area. To do so, using EEG-fMRI, we investigated BOLD responses to IEDs characterized by focal interictal slow-wave activity in patients with partial epilepsy.

We also wanted to understand whether, in patients with lesional epilepsy, fMRI-BOLD activation areas were correlated with lesions previously identified with standard MRI. We then investigated whether EEG-fMRI could document the spatial relationship between the interictal zone and the ictal onset zone in patients with interictal focal slow-wave discharges arising from a known epileptogenic lesion (i.e., the lesional area).

To obtain a homogeneous study sample, 8 patients with focal epilepsy were selected from among patients hospitalized in our epilepsy ward whose routine EEG recordings showed frequent focal IEDs manifesting as 5-6 Hz focal EEG activity (slow waves, slow spike waves, high-amplitude slow waves), over a few lateralized electrodes. Three of the 8 patients selected

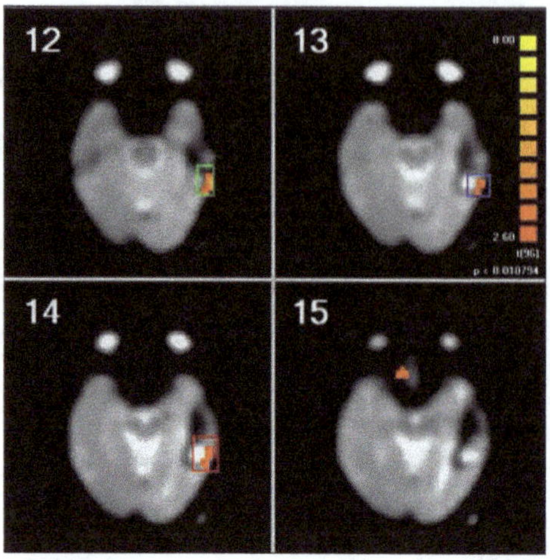


Results of data analysis in 2D reconstruction

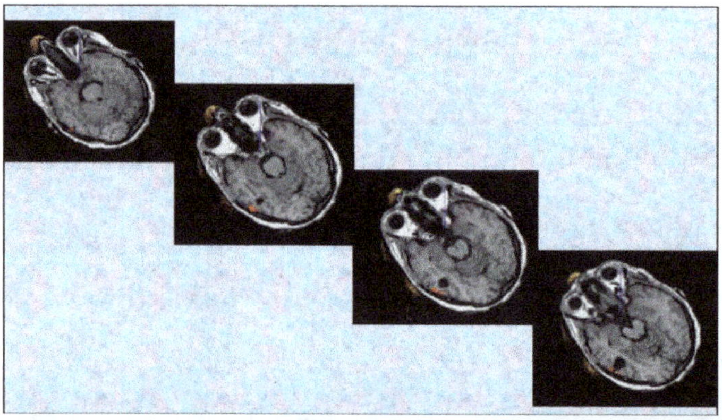

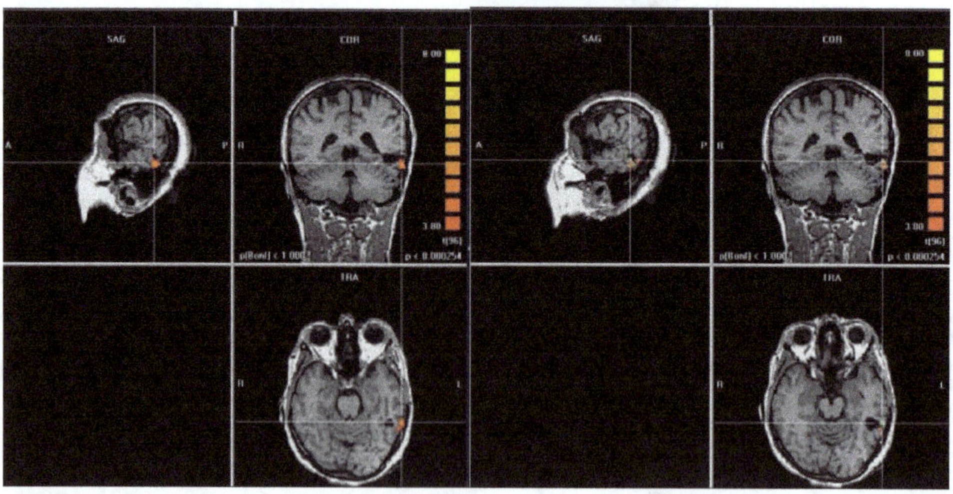


Results of data analysis in 3D recontruction

**Figure 2.** Interitcal focal slow wave activity correlated BOLD activation in patient affected by cavernoma: results of data analysis both in 2D and in 3D recontruction

for study had a structural lesion on MRI: 2 patients with hippocampal atrophy secondary to mesial temporal sclerosis (MTS) and 1 patient with a cavernous angioma. Among the remaining 5 patients, 1 patient had cryptogenic epilepsy and 4 patients had nonlesional (idiopathic) epilepsy. Routine EEG showed slow-wave activity in 1 patient with MTS (P4), the patient with cryptogenic epilepsy (P2) and the one with idiopathic epilepsy (P7); slow spike waves were observed in the patient with a cavernoma (P3) and the 2 patients with idiopathic epilepsy (P5 and P8); high-amplitude slow-waves (> 130 μV) were noted in 1 patient with idiopathic epilepsy (P6) and the second patient with MTS (P1) (Table 1).

| Patients | Type of Epilepsy | Standard MRI findings | IED morphology | Irritative focus |
|---|---|---|---|---|
| 1 | Lesional | MTS | HASW | T3-T5 |
| 2 | Cryptogenic | Negative | SW | T3-T5 |
| 3 | Lesional | Cavernoma | SPSW | T5 |
| 4 | Lesional | MTS | SW | T4-T6 |
| 5 | Idiopathic | Negative | SPSW | O1 |
| 6 | Idiopathic | Negative | HASW | T4-T6 |
| 7 | Idiopathic | Negative | SW | F7 |
| 8 | Idiopathic | Negative | HASPSW | T4-T6 |

MTS denotes mesial temporal sclerosis; SW slow waves; HASW high-amplitude slow waves; SPSW spiked slow waves; HASPSW high- amplitude spiked slow waves.

**Table 1.** Patients enrolled in the first study (Manganotti, 2008).

The good results we obtained (BOLD activations correlated to IEDs in 8/8 patients) allowed us to extend the study to 8 other patients (for a total of 16 patients), all with the same characteristics: focal epilepsy in which routine EEG recordings showed frequent focal IEDs manifesting as 5-6 Hz focal EEG activity (slow waves, slow spike waves, high-amplitude slow waves) over a few lateralized electrodes. The results did not change. MRI revealed a structural lesion in 4 patients: MTS in 2, tuberose sclerosis (TS) in 1; and hypothalamic hamartoma (HH) in 1. Three patients had cryptogenic and one nonlesional (idiopathic) epilepsy.

Standard EEG showed: focal sharp-wave activity in 1 patient (P15) with idiopathic epilepsy; high-amplitude slow-wave activity (or high-amplitude sharp waves) in 1 with TS (P12) and in 1 with HH (P14); spiked sharp waves in 1 with MTS (P10) and in 2 patients with cryptogenic epilepsy (P13 and P16); and high-amplitude spiked waves in 1 with MTS (P9) and in 1 with cryptogenic epilepsy (P11) (Table 2).

| Patient | Type of epilepsy | Standard MRI findings | IED morphology | Irritative focus |
|---|---|---|---|---|
| 9 | Lesional | MTS | HASPSW | T8 |
| 10 | Lesional | MTS | SPSW | F7-T3 |
| 11 | Cryptogenic | Negative | HASPSW | F7-T3 |
| 12 | Lesional | TS | HASW | P4 |
| 13 | Cryptogenic | Negative | SPSW | T6 |
| 14 | Lesional | HH | HASW | T4-T6 |
| 15 | Idiopathic | Negative | SW | T3-T5 |
| 16 | Cryptogenic | Negative | SPSW | F8-T4 |

**Table 2.** Characteristics of the 8 additional patients. MTS denotes mesial temporal sclerosis; TS tuberose sclerosis; HH: hypothalamic hamartoma.

## 6.2. Matherials and methods

### *6.2.1. EEG recordings and analysis*

The EEG was acquired using a MR compatible EEG amplifier (SD MRI 32, Micromed, Treviso, Italy) and a cap providing 32 Ag/AgCl electrodes positioned according to a 10/20 system (impedance was kept below 10 kΩ). To remove pulse and movement artifacts during scanning two of these electrodes were used to record the electrocardiogram (ECG) and electromyogram (EMG). The EMG electrode was placed on the right abductor pollicis brevis (APB) muscle and the other (ECG) on the precordial area.

The reference was placed anterior to Fz, and the ground posterior to Fz as in other studies (Gonçalves et al. 2006; Avesani et al. 2008/a; Formaggio et al., 2008; Manganotti et al. 2008) using the same system. To ensure subjects' safety, the wires were carefully arranged to avoid loops and physical contact with the subject. To minimize the variability in the EEG artifacts due to the MR sequence and avoid wire movement caused by mechanical vibration the wires rested on foam pads.

EEG data were acquired at the rate of 1024 Hz using the software package SystemPlus (Micromed, Treviso, Italy). To avoid saturation, the EEG amplifier had a resolution of 22 bits with a range of ±25.6 mV. An anti-aliasing hardware band-pass filter was applied with a bandwidth between 0.15 and 269.5 Hz. Details of the EEG recording method are given in Bènar (Bènar et al, 2003). The EEG artifact induced by the gradient magnetic field was digitally removed off-line by an adaptive filter (Micromed). EEG artifacts associated with pulsatile blood flow were digitally removed off-line using a simple averaging procedure (Allen, 1998-2000). Subsequently a single electroencephalographer visually reviewed the filtered EEGs, and marked the time of onset and duration of each IED.

### *6.2.2. fMRI acquisition and analysis*

Images were acquired on a 1.5 T MR scanner (Symphony, Siemens, Erlangen, Germany) equipped with EPI capability and a standard transient/receive (TR) head coil. At the start of each study, a T1-weighted anatomical MRI was acquired (192 slices; FOV = 256X256; scanning matrix 512X512; slice thickness 1 mm; sagittal slice orientation; echo time (TE) = 3ms; repetition time (TR) = 1990 ms).

All patients then underwent a 24-min fMRI recording session, after giving informed consent. BOLD fMRI data were acquired, using a standard gradient-echo (EPI) sequence, on the axial orientation, in 1 run of 8 minutes with the patient in the resting state, as described by the Kobayashi team (Kobayashi,2006) (voxel dimension 3x3x3 mm; 36 slices; matrix 64x64; TE = 50 ms, TR = 3.7 s; and slice thickness = 3 mm). At the onset of each fMRI acquisition, the scanner provided a trigger signal that was recorded by the EEG system and used as a volume marker.

For image processing and statistical analysis of the fMRI time series data we used BrainVoyager QX 1.9 software (*Brain Innovation, Maastricht, Netherlands*) running in windows VISTA enviroment. Pre-processing of the functional MRI included three-dimensional motion correction, slice scan time correction (linear interpolation), linear trend removal by temporal high-pass filtering (3 cycles in time course) and transformation into the Talairach coordinate space. Neither spatial nor temporal smoothing was used.

In each subject, activated voxels were identified with a single-subject general linear model (GLM) approach for time series data (Friston, 1995). To account for the hemodynamic delay, the boxcar waveform representing the rest and task conditions was convolved with an empirical hemodynamic response function (Friston, 1998).

A t statistic was used to determine significance on a voxel-by-voxel basis and correlation values were transformed into a normal distribution (Z statistic). The results were displayed on parametric statistical maps in which the pixel Z value is expressed on a colorimetric scale. We identified the single region of condition-associated BOLD signal changes with a statistical threshold based on the amplitude ($p<0.05$) and extent of the regions of activation. The location of voxels with maximal signal increase was expressed in terms of x, y, and z in the Talairach space, and activation volumes were expressed in terms of number of activated voxels. Positive BOLD-fMRI responses were defined as activations. Significant responses were defined as almost five contiguous voxels with $p<0.05$ over at least two contiguous slices (Krakow 1999 and 2001; Salek-Haddadi 2006) in 2D-reconstruction. The anatomic localization of BOLD responses was determined by co-registration of the anatomic data and statistical t maps.

We analyzed the extent and maximum fMRI response for each study, considering all areas with significative activations. We also determined the locations of maximum activation based on the maximum peak response (maximum t value).

### 6.3. Results

In all patients, EEG showed unilateral focal activity during the EEG-fMRI session. IEDs recorded inside the scanner had a localization, amplitude and morphology similar to those seen in the previous routine EEG recordings. EEG recordings showed focal high-amplitude slow waves in 4 patients (P1, P6, P12 and P14), and slow-wave discharges over the temporal electrodes in the other 3 patients (P2, P4 and P15). In 1 patient (P7) slow-wave activity was detected in the extratemporal (F7) region. In the patient with a cavernoma (P3), in 1 with MTS

(P10), and in 2 patients with cryptogenic epilepsy (P13 and P16), focal EEG activity was characterized by focal slow-spiked wave activity, reaching maximal amplitude over the left temporal electrodes (T5). In 1 patient (P5) slow-spiked waves were detected in the extratemporal region (left occipital region). The EEG tracings also showed high-amplitude spiked slow-wave activity in 3 patients (P8, P9 and P11): in the right temporal region in 2 (P8 and P9) and in the left fronto-temporal region in 1 patient (P11).

The mean frequency was 2.4 IEDs per minute (SD 0.17) for the first 8 patients and 2.495 for the second 8 patients, thus confirming sample homogeneity.

In all 8 patients from the first study and in 7/8 from the second study, fMRI analysis showed, in 2-D reconstruction, significant focal BOLD activation in a single activated area related to the EEG irritative focus (Tables 3 and 4). This activation was considered significant (Krakow, 1999) because it was identified in two contiguous MRI slices.

| Patient | IEDs/24 min | IEDs/min | BOLD activation in 2D reconstruction | No. of slices |
|---|---|---|---|---|
| 1 | **61** | **2.54** | Left mesial temporal lobe | 2 |
| 2 | **55** | **2.29** | Left mesial temporal lobe | 2 |
| 3 | **54** | **2.25** | Left superior temporal lobe – neocortical region | 3 |
| 4 | **58** | **2.41** | Right mesial temporal lobe | 2 |
| 5 | **64** | **2.66** | Left occipital lobe-calcarin cortex | 2 |
| 6 | **51** | **2.13** | Right superior temporal lobe | 2 |
| 7 | **58** | **2.41** | Left frontal lobe | 2 |
| 8 | **62** | **2.58** | Right superior temporal lobe | 2 |

**Table 3.** Number of IEDs revealed on EEG during recording and BOLD activation in 2D reconstruction of fMRI, with number of contiguous activated slices.

| Patient | IEDs/24 min | IEDs/min | BOLD activation in 2D reconstruction | No. of slices |
|---|---|---|---|---|
| 9 | **57** | **2.38** | Left mesial temporal lobe | 3 |
| 10 | **57** | **2.38** | Left mesial temporal lobe | 3 |
| 11 | **59** | **2.45** | Left supplementary motor cortex | 5 |
| 12 | **62** | **2.59** | Right parietal lobe | 3 |
| 13 | **64** | **2.66** | Right mesial temporal lobe | 2 |
| 14 | **65** | **2.70** | Right mesial temporal lobe | 2 |
| 15 | **53** | **2.20** | ==== | 0 |
| 16 | **63** | **2.60** | Left mesial temporal lobe | 2 |

**Table 4.** Number of IEDs revealed on EEG during recording and BOLD activation in 2D reconstruction of fMRI, with number of contiguous activated slices, in the second study of 8 patients.

This result was confirmed with analysis of 3D reconstruction of fMRI: in all 8 patients from the first study (Manganotti, 2008) and in 7/8 from the second study, fMRI BOLD activation corresponded to the irritative focus on standard EEG recordings (Tables 5 and 6).

| Patient | No of voxels | Corresponding area in 3D reconstruction |
|---|---|---|
| 1 | 177 | Left cerebrum, limbic lobe, parahippocampal gyrus, **Brodmann area 34** |
| 2 | 522 | Left cerebrum, limbic lobe, parahippocampal gyrus, **Brodmann area 30** |
| 3 | 540 | Left cerebrum, temporal lobe, inferior temporal gyrus, **Brodmann area 20** |
| 4 | 175 | Right cerebrum, limbic lobe, parahippocampal gyrus, **Brodmann area 28** |
| 5 | 1227 | Left cerebrum occipital lobe, lingual gyrus, **Brodmann area 18** |
| 6 | 364 | Right cerebrum, temporal lobe, transverse temporal gyrus, **Brodmann area 42** |
| 7 | 442 | Left cerebrum, frontal lobe, precentral gyrus, **Brodmann area 6** |
| 8 | 422 | Right cerebrum, temporal lobe, middle temporal gyrus, **Brodmann area 21** |

**Table 5.** Number of activated voxels, and localization, according to the Talairach system, of activated regions in 3D reconstruction, of the 8 patients from the first study (Manganotti, 2008).

| Patient | No. of voxels | Activation in 3D reconstruction |
|---|---|---|
| 9 | 368 | 1) Right cerebrum, temporal lobe, superior temporal gyrus **Brodmann area 38** 2) Right cerebrum, frontal lobe, mesial frontal region **Brodman area 10** |
| 10 | 350 | Left cerebrum, temporal lobe, fusiform gyrus **Brodmann area 20** |
| 11 | 322 | Left cerebrum, frontal lobe, supplementary motor cortex **Brodmann area 6** |
| 12 | 52 | Right cerebrum, parietal lobe, precuneus **Brodmann area 7** |
| 13 | 256 | Right cerebrum, temporal lobe, superior temporal gyrus **Brodmann area 38** |
| 14 | 200 | Right cerebrum, anterior cingulate, limbic lobe **Brodmann area 32** |
| 15 | 0 | ===== |
| 16 | 150 | Right cerebrum, parahippocampal gyrus, limbic lobe **Brodmann area 34** |

**Table 6.** Number of activated voxels, and localization, according to the Talairach system, of activated regions in 3D reconstruction, of the 8 patients from the second study.

### *6.3.1. Temporal lobe activation*

Focal BOLD signal changes in 11 patients reached statistical significance in the temporal regions. In 10 patients (4 of which with MTS [P1, P4, P9, and P10]; 1 with HH [P14]; 3 with cryptogenic epilepsy [P2, P13, and P16]; in 2 of the 4 with idiopathic epilepsy [P6 and P8]), the significant BOLD changes were located in the mesial temporal lobe and in the neocortical regions (laterally and posteriorly to the resection margins) in the 1 patient with a cavernoma (P3).

An interesting case of surgically treated mesial temporal sclerosis involved P9. Of Moroccan origin, he has suffered from focal seizures since the age of 6 years, with loss of consciousness and oral and motor automatisms of the legs (pedaling) and arms, preceded by an epigastric aura, lasting 1 minute and resistant to therapy. On MRI, right mesial temporal sclerosis (MTS) was detected (fig.3). Standard EEG demonstrated an interictal focus in the right temporal region. The seizures first occurred rarely but then increased in frequency with time, eventually manifesting in "clusters" of 10-15 seizures every 1 to 2 months. Auras occurred every 2 weeks. Video-EEG demonstrated the same abnormal activity in the right temporal region, with an ictal event manifesting with the same characteristics. The hypothesis was that the seizures arose in an epileptogenic area related to the known MTS and then spread anteriorly to the right mesial frontal region (cause of motor manifestation). EEG-fMRI recording session identified an interictal slow wave activity in right temporal region (T4-T6), with a following diffusion both to contralateral region and to right frontal region (fig. 4). Two significant activations were detected (figg. 5-6): one in the right mesial temporal region (Brodmann area 38) and one in the right mesial frontal region (Brodmann area 10). Also in this case, BOLD activations were concordant with focal IEDs and with clinical syndrome. On subsequent analysis with invasive techniques (SEEG), the origin of seizure in an epileptogenic zone correlated with MTS was confirmed, with spread to the right mesial frontal region. The study also confirmed the co-localization between EEG and fMRI data. He was surgically treated and is now seizure free.

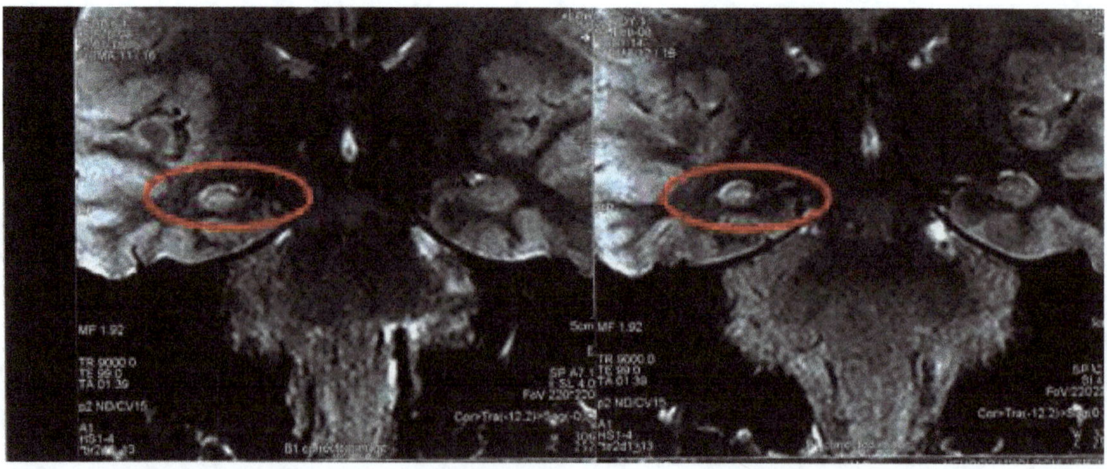

**Figure 3.** Right mesial temporal sclerosis (MTS) in Patient n. 9

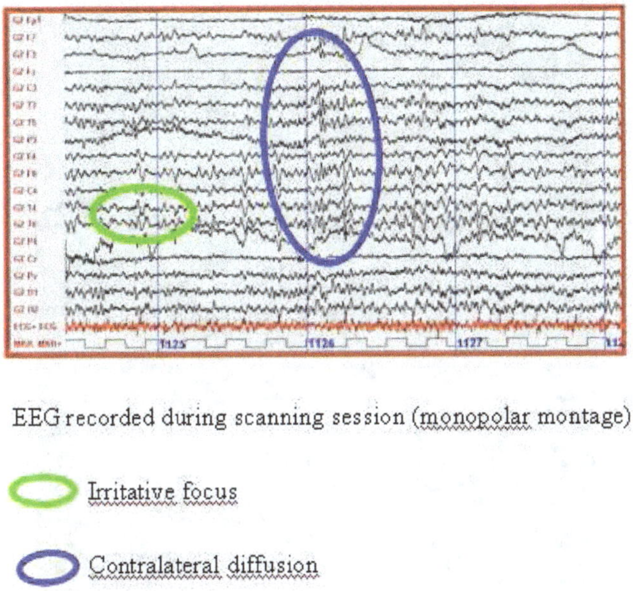


**Figure 4.** Patient n. 9. Focal IEDs in right temporal region, with following diffusion both to contralateral region and to right frontal region

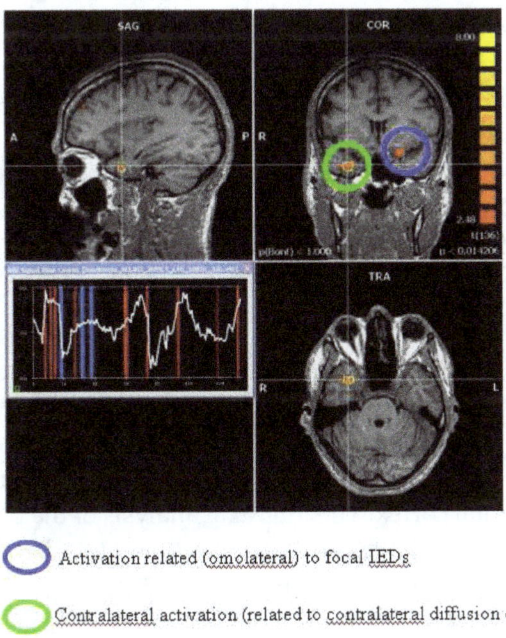


**Figure 5.** Patient n. 9. Focal IEDs correlated BOLD activations in mesial right temporal region, with following diffusion to contralateral region

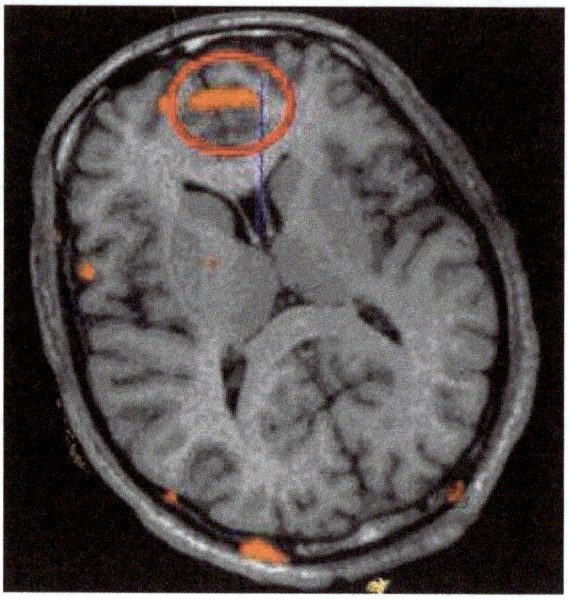

**Figure 6.** Patient n. 9. Focal IEDs correlated BOLD activation in right mesial frontal region

Another case involved a young man (P14) affected with gelastic seizures due to a hypothalamic hamartoma and manifesting since he was 2 years old. They were well defined: dissociated deviation of the eyes (the left eye toward the right and the right eye upwards) or associated deviation of both eyes upwards, followed by right head deviation, absent facial expression, and asymmetric smile. Often, an aura (tingling in the left temporal region) would precede the seizures, with concurrent rubor. The patient attempted to speak but was impeded by fixed smiling. The episode frequency was very high (up to 5 seizures/day). Over time, the syndrome worsened, with falls and subsequent injuries. SEEG confirmed an epileptogenic zone inside the hamartoma, with spread to the right mesial temporal region during the seizures. EEG-fMRI detected a significant BOLD activation in the limbic lobe (anterior cingulate), substantiating the anatomic-clinical correlation suggested by seizures and EEG.

This case parallels recently published findings on the networks involved in seizure generation in hypothalamic hamartoma (Kokkinos, 2012). EEG-fMRI was performed in 2 adult patients with hypothalamic hamartoma, the one with predominantly gelastic seizures and the other with complex partial but no typical gelastic seizures. Ictal and interictal analysis of the patient with gelastic seizures revealed involvement of the hypothalamic hamartoma, the cingulate gyrus, the precuneus and prefrontal cortex. The interictal analysis of the patient with complex partial seizures showed BOLD signal changes over the temporal lobes, the base of the frontal lobe, the precuneus and prefrontal cortex but not the hypothalamic hamartoma. It was presumed that the differences in the neural networks implicated may have accounted for the differences in the clinical manifestation of seizures owing to the tumor.

Other interesting cases are cryptogenic (P2, P13) and idiophatic forms (P6, P8, P15), all characterized by atypical absences and vagal symptomatology. In patient n. 2, focal IEDs (fig.

7) were recorded in left temporal region and focal IEDs correlated BOLD activation (fig. 8) was detected in mesial left temporal region, in limbic lobe. In patient n. 6 focal IEDs were recorded in right temporal region, with a characteristic phase reversal in T4 (fig. 9), and focal IEDs correlated BOLD activation was detected in Brodam area 42 (fig. 10). In patient n. 8, focal IEDs were recorded in right temporal region (fig. 11) and focal IEDs correlated BOLD activation was detected in Brodman area 21 (fig. 12).

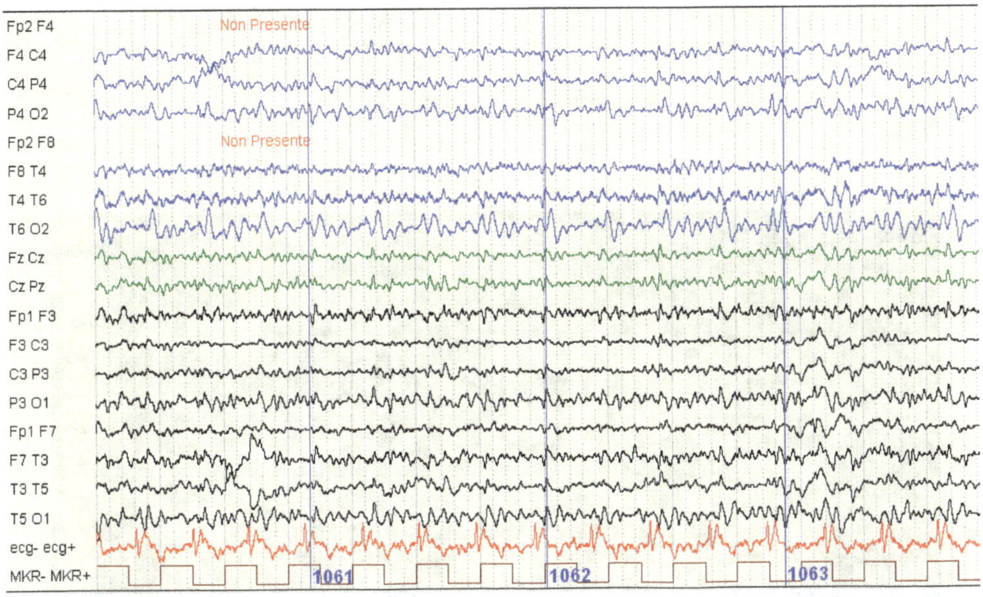


**Figure 7.** Patient n. 2 (cryptogenic epilepsy). Focal IEDs in left temporal region during scanning session

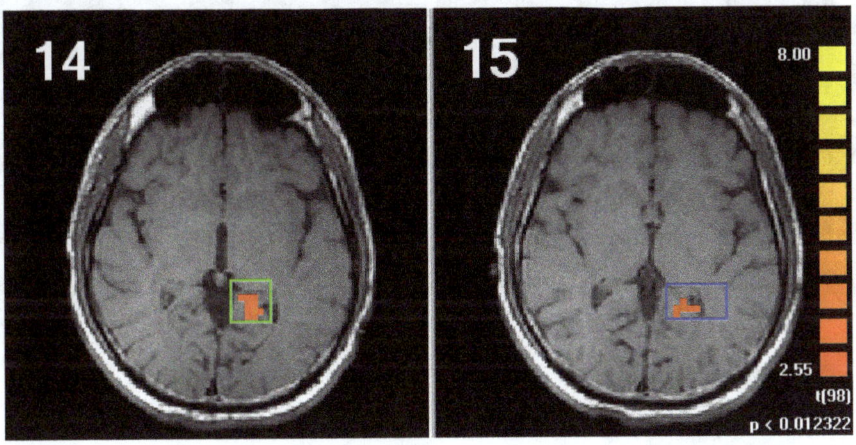


**Figure 8.** Patient n. 2. Focal IEDs correlated BOLD activations in left mesial temporal lobe

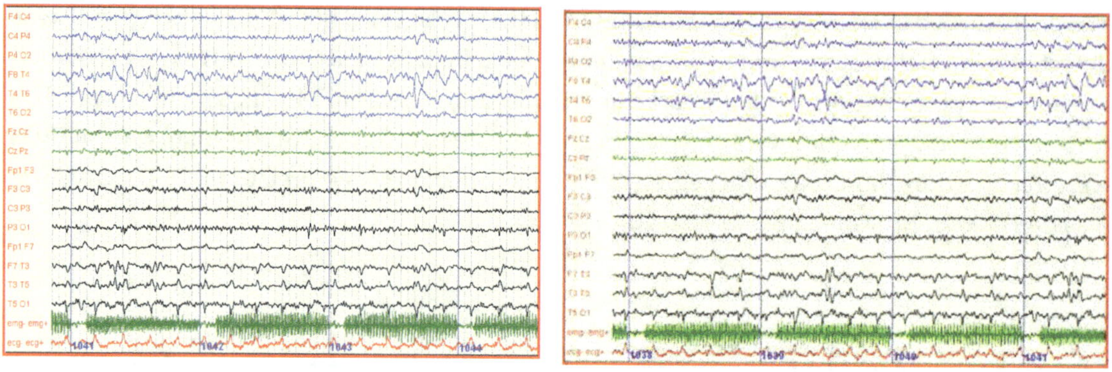

**Figure 9.** Patient n. 6. Focal IEDs in right temporal lobe with phase reversal in T4

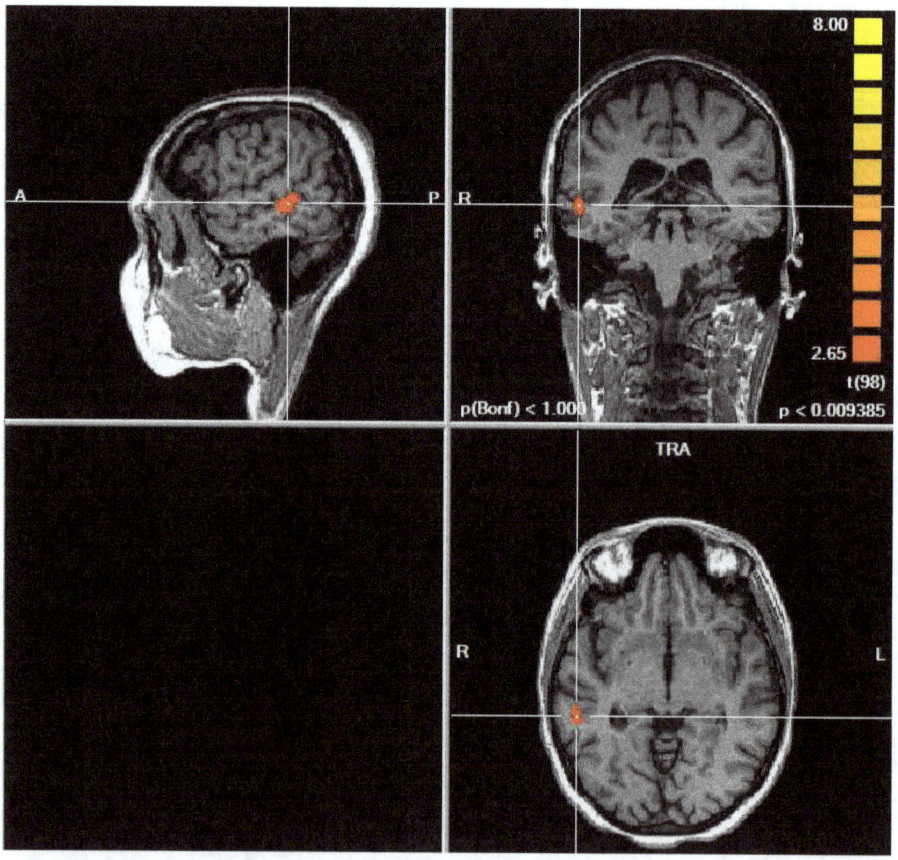


**Figure 10.** Patient n. 6. Focal IEDs correlated activation in transverse temporal gyrus, Brodmann area 42

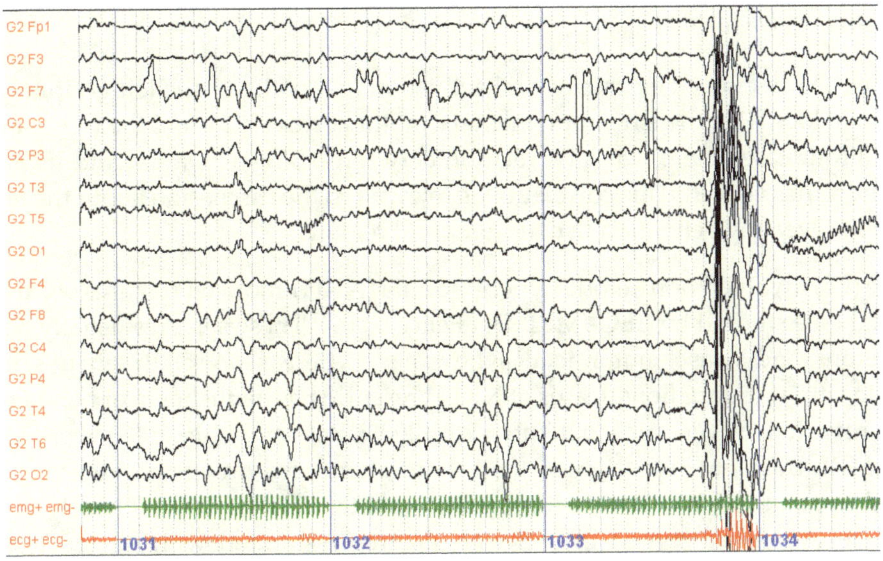


**Figure 11.** Patient n. 8. Focal IEDs in right temporal region

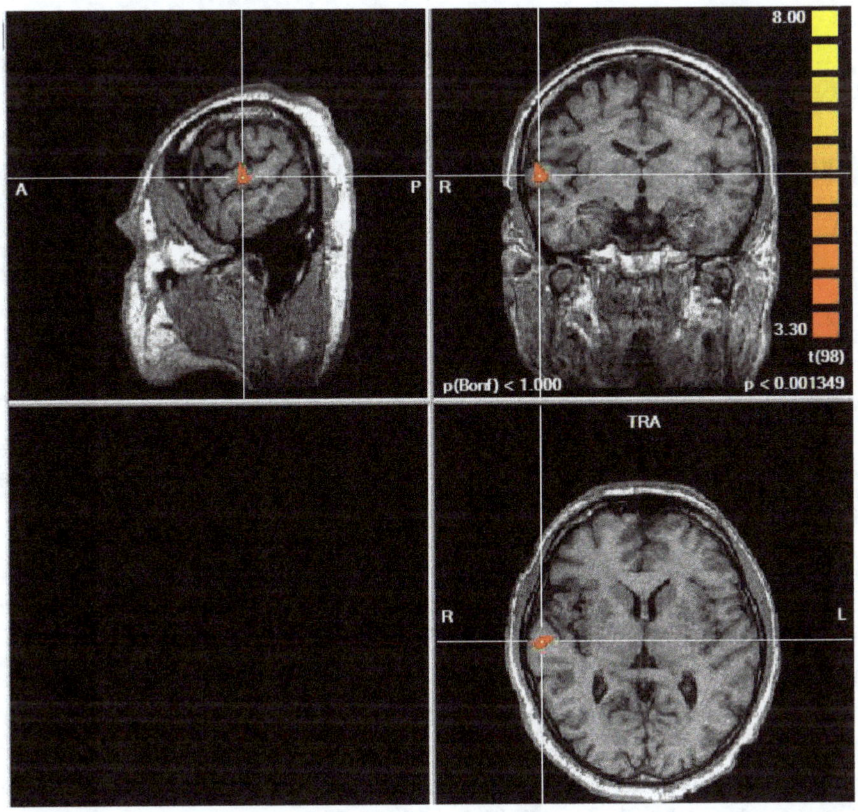


**Figure 12.** Patient n.8. Focal IEDs correlated BOLD activation in middle temporal gyrus, Brodmann area 21

*6.3.2. Extratemporal activation*

In our series, fMRI showed extratemporal activation in 4 patients: the left occipital lobe (P5); the left frontal lobe (P7); the left supplementary motor cortex (P11); and the right parietal lobe (P12). In all four cases there was a correlation between BOLD activation and IEDs and with clinical syndromes as well. This correlation is relevant to the discussion about the technique's sensitivity in revealing activation in extratemporal regions.

A rare case (P5) involved non ketotic hyperglycemia (NKH)-induced seizures occurring in the left occipital lobe studied by EEG-fMRI (Del Felice, 2009). These seizures usually occur in the frontal regions and cause motor ictal syndromes, whereas occipital seizures have been described in very rare situations. Cases of NKH presenting as hemichorea or hemianopia have also been reported. Seven such patients (Seo, 2003; Raghavendra, 2007) were studied by standard MRI transient $T_2$-weighted and fluid-attenuated inversion recovery (FLAIR). Subcortical hypointensity with or without abnormalities in the occipital overlying cortex or striatal nuclei was documented in occipital seizures associated with NKH. A single case investigated by Tc-99m HMPAO SPECT (Wang, 2005) showed occipital hyperperfusion during seizure recurrence and hypoperfusion during the interictal state.

Our patient (P5) was a 50-year-old woman admitted to hospital after repeated emergency room visits because of visual disturbances and left-sided headache. On clinical examination, she was obese and had a right-sided homonymous hemianopia. Her medical history was unremarkable, except for hypertension and a 15-kg weight gain during the past 12 months. She had no history of migraine, epilepsy or neurological disorders. Two days before admission she reported a short-lasting episode of visual disturbance (distortion). A few hours later, she noted diplopia when looking to the right, with image distortion in the right visual field and intermittent right-sided hemianopia, lasting several minutes, elicited by looking to the right or by fixation. The episodes were accompanied by a left-sided throbbing headache but no other autonomic symptoms (i.e., nausea or vomiting). No language disturbance was reported. She was presented to the emergency room.

On neurological examination, a right-sided homonymous hemianopia was noted. A standard computed tomography (CT) scan of the brain and an ophthalmologic exam were negative. She was discharged with a diagnosis of migraine with aura and started on antiplatelet therapy, with the recommendation to undergo out-patient visual field analysis.

Two days later, she was admitted to our ward owing to the persistence of symptoms, including a transient conjugated deviation of the eyes and the head to the right. On that occasion, which lasted less than 1 minute, the patient did not lose consciousness and referred seeing red flashing lights in her right visual field. Standard EEG performed immediately thereafter showed multiple clinical-EEG seizures during a prolonged recording, with spiked slow waves originating from the left posterior region, and with bilateral diffusion (fig. 13). Laboratory data on admission revealed hyperglycemia (14.5 mm/L to 261 mg/dL) with a serum osmolarity of 333 mmol/kg, and glycosilated hemoglobin of 10.5%. Urine analysis was negative for ketone bodies but was strongly positive for glycosuria (>1 g/dL) and microalbuminuria (up to 6 mg/24 h). A brain MRI scan with and without gadolinium, an MR angiography, and a 3T brain

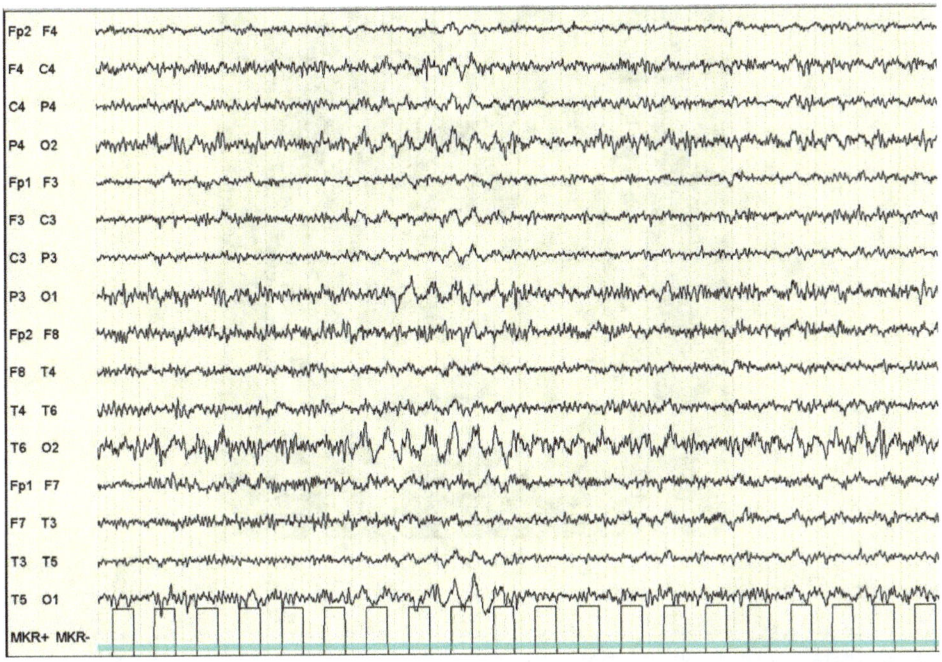


**Figure 13.** Patient n. 5. Standard EEG tracing during clinical seizures. Spiked slow waves on posterior regions (O1 and O2).

MRI were normal. Tc-99m hexamethylpropylene amine oxime (HMPAO) single-photon-emission computed tomography (SPECT), during which no clinical seizures were reported, showed non-significant hypocaptation over the posterior regions bilaterally.

On continuous EEG-fMRI a few days later, no clinical or EEG manifestations of ictal events occurred, but interictal spiked slow wave discharges (IEDs) with localization, amplitude and morphology similar to those previously recorded on routine EEG (fig. 13) were noted. A slow-spiked wave on the left occipital (O1) channel was detected. The mean frequency was 2.4 IEDs per minute. Functional MRI analysis showed significant focal BOLD activation in a single area related to the EEG paroxysmal activity. In a 3D reconstruction using the Talairach system (fig. 14), focal significant BOLD activation based on the EEG-related protocol was identified in Brodmann area 18 (grey matter of the left cerebrum occipital lobe and lingual gyrus). During her hospital stay, she was started on carbamazepine (200 mg/daily, up to 800 mg t. d.), with only partial benefit in frequency and intensity of symptoms. Since her glycemia was still uncontrolled (250 mg/dL), she was started on insulin therapy. Over the following 2 weeks, seizures and hyperglycemia both progressively decreased. On the basis of a possible diagnosis of NKH-induced seizures, carbamazepine was tapered, without the reappearance of symptoms. Serial EEG showed a decrease in epileptic activity (sharp waves) with persistent bilateral slowing. A few weeks later, insulin therapy was replaced with oral antidiabetics. One year later, the patient was seizure free, with a normal EEG. Following the loss of 18 kg, the oral antidiabetics were tapered, with good control of serum glucose and HbA1 values.

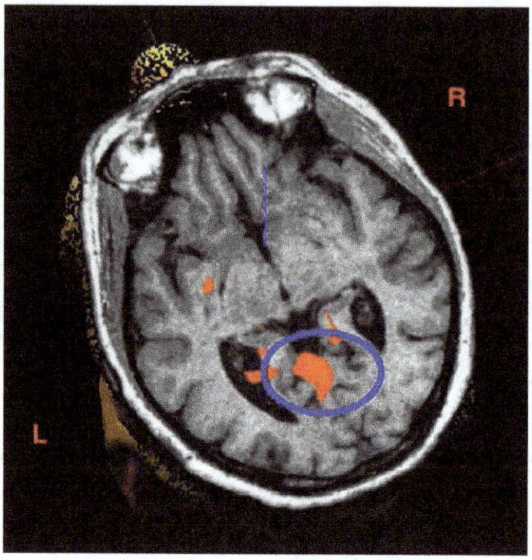


**Figure 14.** Patient n. 5. 3D fMRI-BOLD activation in Brodmann area 18.

A BOLD occipital activation in patients referring visual symptoms has been reported, confirming the involvement of visual functional areas in the occipital lobes: Brodmann areas 19 and 37 in reported cases of fixation sensitivity occipital spiking (Iannetti et al., 2002; Avesani, 2008/b) or the left occipital lobe in cases of cryptogenic and symptomatic (cortical malformation) occipital epilepsy (Salek-Haddadi et al., 2006). In our patient, an analogous BOLD activation was elicited by the NKH. Hyperglycemia may induce paroxysmal activity in brain areas more susceptible to metabolic changes – the occipital lobe in this case - with an analogous pattern of activation of self-sustained focal discharges. Neuroimaging, in this case fMRI-EEG co-registration, pointed to a change in blood volume in the involved posterior areas.

In the patient (P7) in whom fMRI revealed BOLD activation in the left frontal region (Brodmann area 6), standard EEG showed a left fronto-temporal irritative focus characterized by frequent slow-spiked waves. A recent polygraphic study (recorded during stage I and II non-rapid-eye-movement [NREM] sleep) showed polymorphic slow waves (theta-delta) in the left frontal regions, with phase inversion at F7 and without spread. These findings suggested that the patient was a good candidate for an EEG-fMRI study. During the EEG-fMRI sessions, we confirmed the fMRI activation area within the precentral gyrus.

Patient no. 11, a young woman, illustrates an interesting case of frontal lobe epilepsy characterized by focal seizures, with speech arrest and right arm clonus followed by generalization (Borelli, 2010), where, as reported elsewhere (So, 1998; Westmoreland, 1998), scalp EEG is often ambiguous because it is poorly sensitive to deep generators on the mesial surface of the frontal lobe. Also in this instance, EEG-fMRI effectively identified the interictal focus.

According to a detailed account by relatives, the events took the form of sudden episodes of speech arrest lasting from a few seconds up to several minutes, without any warning sensation. The patient reported she was able to move, understand and write properly during the ictal phase (sometimes writing a note to her husband that she was unable to speak). No clonic movements or orofacial automatisms were experienced at this early stage. Usually, an event did not progress any further and the patient was able to fully recollect the episode. Sometimes an episode was followed by clonic jerking over the right side of the face and arms with occasional, generalized tonic-clonic seizures. The seizure frequency was weekly despite polytherapy. The 3T MRI was normal. She reported no febrile seizures nor having sustained significant head injuries. Pregnancy, delivery and developmental milestones were unremarkable, as was the remainder of her medical history. Trials with various antiepileptic drugs (first with dintoine, then carbamazepine, and then fenobarbital) were unsuccessful. She was admitted to an intensive care unit for a status epilepticus and begun on valproate and lamotrigine.

Interictal scalp EEG showed frequent generalized high-amplitude (2 to 3 Hz) spiked slow-wave discharges. There was an inconstant, mild amplitude prevalence over the left hemisphere electrodes (F7-T3).

During a conventional scalp EEG recording, she complained of a brief episode of speech arrest associated with an EEG pattern characterized by diffuse spike and wave discharges (fig. 15). This event was witnessed by a neurologist from our ward who was aware of the patient's clinical history. He noted that the patient had a brief inability to speak (a few seconds) during which she waved her hands to attract his attention. There were no clonic movements, and after regaining speech, she accurately described the event. Three-hour video-EEG monitoring during a day of seizure clustering recorded no usual events. On the basis of these elements, a diagnosis of generalized epilepsy was also made in another hospital.

The clinical syndrome suggested involvement of the left supplementary motor area (SMA) with spread to the primary motor area. EEG -fMRI recording session confirmed the same pattern EEG identified by standard EEG (fig. 16) and following analysis showed prominent BOLD activation over the left SMA during the high-amplitude spiked slow-wave discharges compared to the rest state (Fig. 17). According to the Duncan criteria, such an activation pattern is reproducible since it was present in two contiguous slices (Duncan, 1999). The statistical significance of the activation was $p < 0.0028$ even after FDR correction. More activations were found in the contralateral SMA and homolateral motor strip as well. No significant deactivation areas or thalamic involvement (activation or deactivation) were found. The patient was referred to a level II epilepsy surgery center for presurgical work-up, including long-term video-EEG monitoring, but she refused further testing.

The speech arrest noted in this patient is an epileptic feature usually related to involvement of the supplementary motor cortex over either the dominant or the non-dominant hemisphere. A bilateral spike and wave discharge pattern (secondary bilateral synchrony) is often detected in frontal-lobe epilepsy, particularly if the generator is deep, for instance, over the mesial surface of the frontal lobe (So, 1998; Westmoreland, 1998). In the presurgical work-up for epilepsy surgery, such a scalp EEG pattern certainly raises questions about the origin of the focal epilepsy especially when conventional MRI is negative. In the latter case, more investigations are usually obtained to guide depth electrode placement for invasive EEG. Ictal SPECT and interictal PET are commonly used for this purpose, but they are expensive, difficult to interpret, and usually provide regional rather than local data. In addition, if the ictal event is

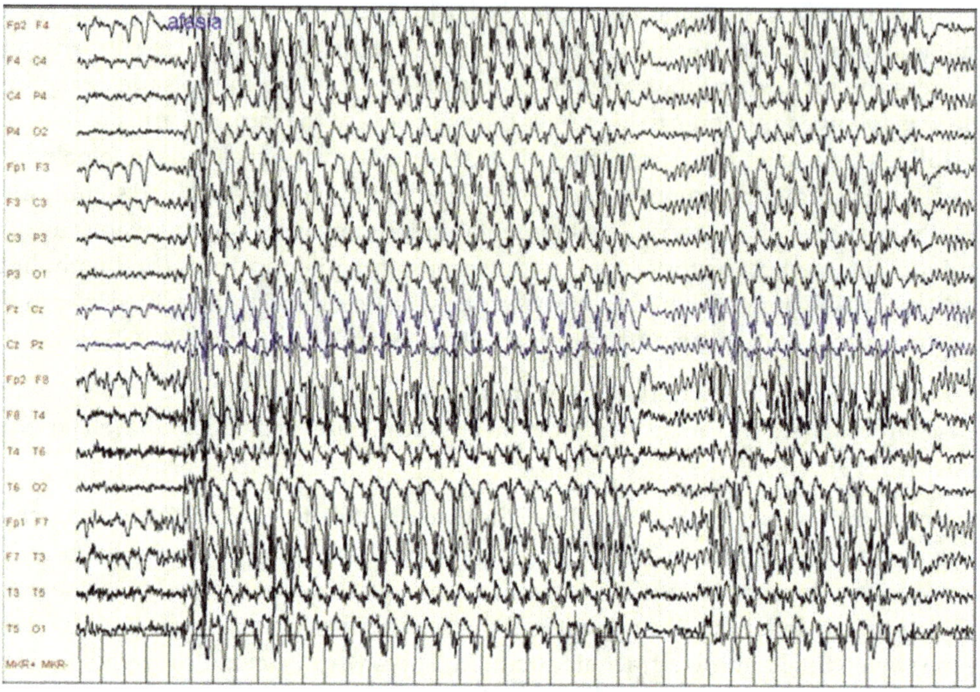


**Figure 15.** Patient n. 11. Ictal EEG during a brief speech arrest episode ("Afasia" marks the beginning of the speech impairment).

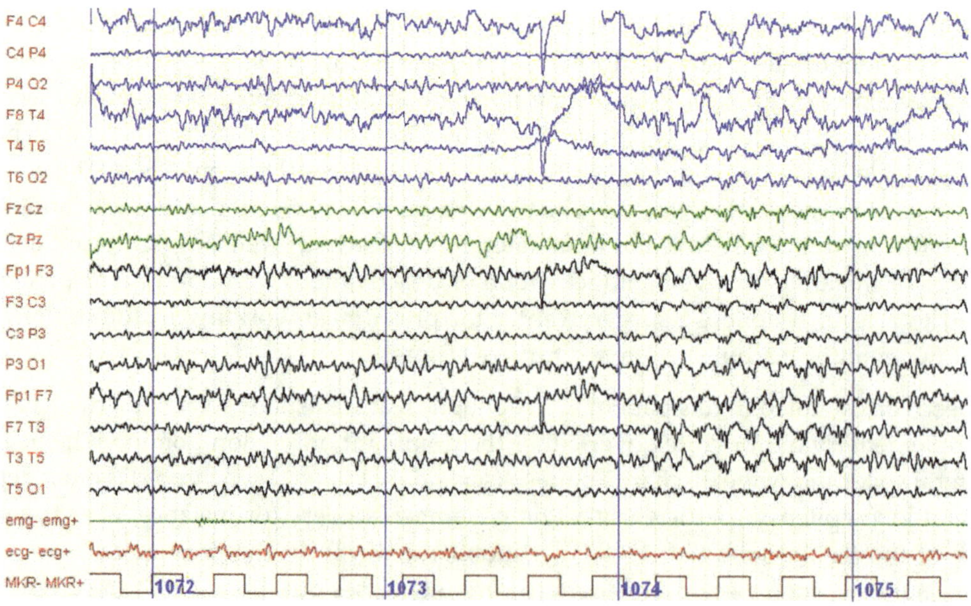


**Figure 16.** Patient n.11. EEG recorded during the fMRI acquisition showing generalized high amplitude spiked slow wave discharges, prevalent on left fronto-temporal regions.

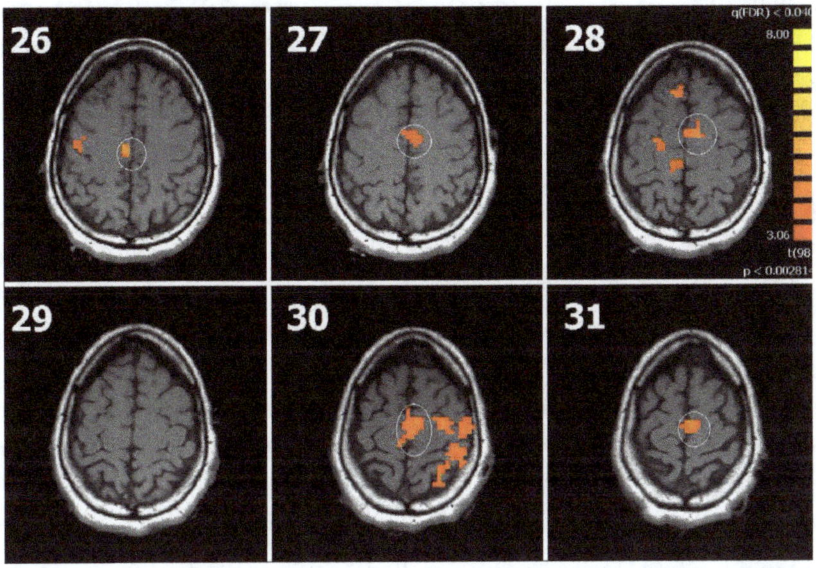


**Figure 17.** Patient n. 11. The EEG-fMRI shows a clear-cut activation of the left (radiological convention) Supplementary Motor Area (SMA) and on the contralateral SMA on a lesser degree. Spread over the left motor strip is also evident.

brief, SPECT may yield false negatives due to incorrect timing of the tracer injection (Salmenpera, 2005; Devous, 1998). The use of radioactive substances also raises safety issues.

A relatively new tool to obtain localizing data on the basis of EEG changes, EEG-fMRI is safe for the patient and relatively inexpensive (Al Asmi, 2003; Di Bonaventura, 2006). As our knowledge about the technique increases, it is gaining acceptance in the study of focal nonlesional epilepsy and presurgical work-up, as reported by Moeller et al. and Zijlmans et al. (Devous, 1998; Moeller, 2009). Nonetheless, few studies to date have applied EEG-fMRI in patients with secondary bilateral synchrony, except for one by Aghakhani (Aghakhani, 2006) involving 11 patients with such an EEG pattern, with a variable activation-deactivation pattern including thalamic involvement in 6 out of 11 (55%). The clinical seizure pattern and the MRI findings were variable.

In our patient, EEG-fMRI revealed the origin of the epileptiform discharges, including the spread over the homolateral motor strip, which was highly consistent with the patient's clinical features (speech arrest followed by clonic jerks over right half of the face and right arm), whereas 3T MRI and conventional interictal scalp EEG were useless in this regard. Some involvement of the contralateral SMA was also detected but its significance is less clear: it may have been the result of a transcallosal spread from the left SMA or simply an imperfect spatial resolution of the technique. In contrast with Aghakhani (Aghakhani, 2006) in our case no thalamic changes were seen.

Unfortunately, our localizing hypothesis could not be proved by invasive EEG and postsurgical outcome since the patient refused surgical treatment. Nonetheless, this patient suggests that, in the presurgical work up for epilepsy, EEG-fMRI may be considered a useful tool to generate a localizing hypothesis to be tested with invasive recording also in patients with focal epilepsy and bilateral slow spiked-wave discharges on EEG (secondary bilateral synchrony) and negative MRI. The recording of ictal EEG demonstrates that the slow waves we triggered in our study were irritative and not lesional.

## 7. Conclusions

The main finding in our EEG-fMRI study of patients with partial epilepsy is that the focal interictal slow-wave activity was invariably associated with increased focal fMRI-BOLD activation responses in a spatially related brain area. Our study extends current knowledge on epileptic foci localization and confirms previous reports suggesting that EEG-fMRI BOLD activation associated with modeled slow activity might have a role in localizing the epileptogenic region, even in the absence of clear interictal spikes (Laufs, 2006; Avesani, 2008/a).

All the patients with partial epilepsy we enrolled in this study had frequent interictal focal slow-wave activity on standard EEG. In all continuous EEG-fMRI recording sessions, after fMRI artifact removal, we obtained good quality EEG that allowed us to detect spontaneous IEDs and analyze the related fMRI BOLD activation. The EEG recording left the quality of the fMRI data almost undistorted, and the focal activity seen in the concurrent EEG was associated, in 15 of 16 patients enrolled, with a focal increase in the MRI signal in all patients. In their focal distribution, these BOLD activations resembled the focal IEDs seen on routine scalp EEG and EEG recorded during EEG-fMRI sessions.

An interesting finding came from the patients with lesional epilepsy. These patients, whose standard MRI documented a lesion and whose standard EEG identified an irritative focus, are ideal candidates for verifying a possible spatial relationship between the epileptogenic and the irritative focus (Ebersole, 1991; Benbadis, 1996).

In the patient who had undergone surgery to remove a cavernoma (P3), the EEG-fMRI study, by localizing the irritative focus and linking it to fMRI as an "active state", showed a significant BOLD activation signal closely related to the poro-encephalic cavity (a residual of previous treatment). Although this focal BOLD activation presumably arose from a blood vessel (residual cavernoma), it was undoubtedly obtained by a protocol study linking an active fMRI state to IEDs on EEG. To clarify the relationship, we decided to progressively test the specificity to a very high level ($p < 0.0001$), as demonstrated in the iconography. Even with these high specificity values, the BOLD activation in that site persisted.

Another new finding is the BOLD activation we detected on fMRI in the patients with MTS. In contrast to others who studied a series of patients with MTS (5 studied with continuous co-registration) (Al Asmi, 2003) and found no significant activation, we detected significant BOLD activation in 4 patients (P1, P4, P9 and P10). These results suggest a possible role of simultaneous EEG-fMRI in disclosing focal activation in the mesial temporal cortex. This cortical area is notoriously difficult to study with standard methods because the deep localization of the irritative area often makes spikes smoother and therefore harder to recognize on recordings from standard EEG scalp electrodes than in SEEG. Hence, IEDs presenting as slow-wave discharges could be useful in determining significant BOLD activation in a corresponding area, as previously suggested by Laufs et al. (Laufs, 2006).

Useful information that may help us to understand BOLD responses in various forms of epilepsy came also from studying activation in extratemporal IEDs. In the patients with extratemporal discharges (P5, P7, P11, and P12), we noted a good correlation between the clinical polygraphic data and BOLD activation during fMRI. No significant difference was found between activation in the frontal or the occipital lobe. In both regions, BOLD activation increased after focal IEDs. One patient (P11) demonstrated the usefulness of EEG-fMRI, especially when scalp EEG is ambiguous because it is poorly sensitive to detect deep generators on the mesial surface of the frontal lobe, and confirmed that the slow waves were irritative and not lesional.

The reason for such good results (15/16 activations -- significant concordance between EEG and fMRI data) is open to question. The most plausible reason is that during enrolment, to obtain the largest possible percentage of activations, patients were explicitly selected whose standard EEGs showed a high IED firing rate confirmed on EEG during the scanning session. The mean frequency of IEDs in the 15 patients was about 2/min, considerably higher than the 1 IED per minute Duncan considered as the minimum to obtain a focal BOLD activation (Krakow, 1999). Collectively, these findings confirm the importance of IED firing rates in EEG-fMRI.

Perhaps the most interesting finding in this study was that morphology seemed less important than IED firing rates in triggering EEG-fMRI-BOLD activation: 8 of the 16 patients had pure slow waves on standard EEG (4 with high amplitude and 4 with a normal voltage) and 7 had slow spike-wave discharges (4 with high amplitude and 3 with normal voltage); 1 patient (P10) had a focus of normal amplitude, sometimes pure, sometimes with spiked morphology. There were no differences in BOLD activation between the two groups.

Although these slow spike-wave discharges might have originated from a spike focus smoothed by filtering (unlikely because EEG detected the same IEDs before the patients entered the magnet room), there was no difference in the statistical significance of BOLD activation between the two groups. Specifically, slow spike-wave IEDs were no more efficient than slow-wave IEDs in eliciting significant BOLD activation. Hence, it was agreed as previously suggested (Laufs, 2006/a; Avesani, 2008/a) that slow-wave IEDs, like spikes, could elicit a significant increase in cerebral blood flow in a spatially related brain area.

The study also suggests that voltage might have a minor role in determining BOLD activation: in this small study sample there were no differences in BOLD activations between IEDs with high-amplitude (9 patients) and those with normal amplitude slow waves (7 patients).

The significant concordance between EEG and fMRI data, and the absence of multiple activation areas in particular, depended on the high specificity threshold the study design envisaged. In designing this study, only the single activation with the strongest specificity was maintained so that we could verify whether this activation, and this activation alone, coincided with the epileptic focus previously documented by standard EEG and used as a paradigm for the activation-state during the fMRI analysis.

Given the criticism raised against the use of EEG-fMRI instead of other techniques such as EEG-source analysis in the presurgical work-up (Elshoff, 2012), a possible objection to the conclusions we draw could derive from our decision to include only a well-defined sample of patients, all characterized by a focus with a high firing rate, without evidence of the same result in other patients with low firing rate foci (being the most frequent among patients affected by focal drug-resistant epilepsy of surgical interest. We reply that this study was the first approach to investigating interictal slow-wave foci. This will be addressed in a future study in order to validate the technique in patients with slow-wave interictal activity with a low firing rate focus.

At the moment, the complete EEG-fMRI concordance achieved in this study suggests that slow-wave IEDs, even without spikes, may be useful in activating fMRI BOLD responses during the presurgical, noninvasive evaluation of patients with partial drug-resistant seizures.

## Acknowledgements

The authors wish to thank:

- Prof. Bernardo Dalla Bernardina, Dp of Life and Reproduction Sciences, University of Verona
- Dr. Giuseppe Moretto and Dr. Tiziano Zanoni, Dp of Neurological Sciences, Civil Hospital of Verona, Dp of Neurological Sciences, Civil Hospital of Verona
- Prof. Nicolò Rizzuto, Dp of Neurological, Neuropsychological, Morphological and Movement Sciences, University of Verona
- Dr. Paolo Manganotti, Dr. Luigi Giuseppe Bongiovanni, Dr. Paolo Borelli, Dr. Alessandra Del Felice, dott. Emanuela Formaggio, dott. Silvia Francesca Storti, Dp of Neurological, Neuropsychological, Morphological and Movement Sciences, University of Verona, Dp of Neurological, Neuropsychological, Morphological and Movement Sciences, University of Verona for their collaboration
- Prof. Roberto Pozzi Mucelli, Dr.ssa Anna Gasparini and Dr. Roberto Cerini , Dp of Radiology University of Verona

## Author details

Mirko Avesani[1], Silvia Giacopuzzi[2] and Antonio Fiaschi[1]

1 University of Verona, Department of Neurological, Neuropsychological, Morphological and Movement Sciences, Italy

2 University of Verona, Department of Life and Reproduction Sciences, Italy

## References

[1] Aghakhani et al. fMRI activation during spike wave discharges in idiopatic generalized epilepsy. Brain, 2004; 127: 1127-1144

[2] Aghakhani et al. The role of periventricular nodular heterotopia in epileptogenesis. Brain, 2005; 128: 641-651

[3] Aghakhani et al. Cortical and thalamic fMRI responses in partial epilepsy with focal and bilateral synchronous spikes. Clin Neurophysiol 2006;117:177–91.

[4] Archer et al. fMRI "deactivation" of the posterior cingulate during generalized spike and wave. Neuroimage. 2003;20:1915–1922.

[5] Al-Asmi et al. fMRI activation in continuous and spike-triggered EEG-fMRI studies of epileptic spikes. Epilepsia, 2003; 44: 1328-1339.

[6] Allen et al. Identification of EEG events in the MR scanner: the problem of pulse artifact and a method for its subtraction. Neuroimage, 1998; 8: 229-239.

[7] Allen et al. A method for removing imaging artefact from continuous EEG recorded during functional MRI. Neuroimage, 2000; 12:230-239.

[8] Archer et al. fMRI "deactivation" of the posterior cingulate during generalized spike and wave. Neuroimage. 2003;20:1915–1922.

[9] Archer et al. Spike-triggered fMRI in reading epilepsy: involvement of left frontal cortex working memory areas. Neurology, 2003; 60: 415-421

[10] Avesani et al. Continuous EEG-fMRI in pre surgical evaluation of a patient affected by symptomatic seizures: BOLD activation linked to interictal epileptiform discharges caused by cavernoma. The Neuroradiology Journal, 2008/a; 21: 183-191.

[11] Avesani et al. fMRI in epilepsy with spike and wave activity evoked by eye closure: different BOLD activation in a patient with idiopathic partial epilepsy with occipital spikes and a control group. Neuroradiol. J., 2008/b; 21:159—165.

[12] Bagshaw et al. EEG-fMRI of focal epileptic spikes: analysis with multiple haemodyamic functions and comparision with gadolinium-enhanced MR angiograms. Human Brain Mapping, 2004; 22: 179-192

[13] Bagshaw et al. Correspondence between EEG-fMRI and EEG dipole localization of interictal discharges in focal epilepsy. Neuroimage, 2006; 30: 417-425

[14] Benar et al. Quality of EEG in simultaneous EEG-fMRI for epilepsy. Clin Neurophysiol, 2003; 114: 569-580.

[15] Benar et al. EEG-fMRI of epileptic spikes. Concordance with EEG source localization and intracranial EEG. Neuroimage, 2006; 30: 1161-1170

[16] Berns. Functional neuroimaging. Life Sci. 1999; 65: 2531-2540.

[17] Bernasconi et al. Proton magnetic resonance spectroscopic imaging suggests progressive neuronal damage in human temporal lobe epilepsy. Prog. Brain Res, 2002; 135: 297-304

[18] Binder et al. Determination of language dominance using functional MRI: a comparision with Wada test. Neurology, 1996; 46: 978-984

[19] Boly et al. Intrinsic brain activity in altered states of consciousness: how conscious is the default mode of brain function? Ann N Y Acad Sci. 2008;1129:119–129.

[20] Boor et al. EEG-related functional MRI in beningn childhood epilepsy with centrotemporal spikes. Epilepsia, 2003; 44: 688-692

[21] Borelli et al. EEG-fMRI as an useful tool to detect epileptic foci associated with secondary

[22] bilateral synchrony. Seizure, 2010; 19:605-608.

[23] Cavanna. The precuneuos and consciousness. CNS Spectr. 2007;12:545–552.

[24] Cavanna et al . The precuneus: a review of its functional anatomy and behavioural correlates. Brain. 2006;129:564–583.

[25] David et al. Identifying neural drivers with functional MRI: an electrophysiological validation. PLoS Biol. 2008;23:2683–2697.

[26] Del Felice et al. EEG-fMRI coregistration in non ketotic hyperglicemic occipital seizures. Epilepsy Research, 2009;85(2-3):321-324

[27] De Tiège et al. Impact of interictal epileptic activity on normal brain function in epileptic encephalopathy: an EEG-fMRI study. Epilepsy Behav. 2007;11:460–465.

[28] Devous et al. SPECT brain imaging in epilepsy: a meta-analysis. J Nucl Med 1998;39:285–93.

[29] Devous et al. Single-photon emission computed tomography in neurotherapeutic. NeuroRx 2005, 2: 237-249

[30] Di Bonaventura. EEG/fMRI study of ictal and interictal epileptic activity: methodological issues and future perspectives in clinical practice. Epilepsia, 2006; 47, Suppl. 5: 52-58.

[31] Duncan et al. Imaging and epilepsy. Brain 1997; 120: 339-377

[32] Dupon et al. Bilateral hemispheric alteration of memory processes in right medial temporal lobe epilepsy. J Neurol Neurosurg Psych, 2002; 73: 478-485

[33] Elshoff et al. The value of EEG-fMRI and EEG source analysis in the presurgical setup of children with refractory focal epilepsy. Epilepsia, 2012; 53: 1597-1606.

[34] Engel et al. Comparative localization of epileptic foci in partial epilepsy by PCT and EEG. Ann Neurol 1982; 12: 529-537.

[35] Engel et al. Local cerebral metabolism during partial seizures. Neurology, 1983; 33: 400-413

[36] Faymonville et al. Functional neuroanatomy of the hypnotic state. J Physiol Paris. 2006;99:463–469.

[37] Frackowiak RSJ, Friston KJ, Frith CD, Dolan RJ, Mazziotta JC, editors. San Diego: Academic Press; 1997. Human brain function.

[38] Friston et al. Statistical parametric maps in functional imaging: a general linear approach. Hum Brain Mapp, 1995; 2: 173-181.

[39] Friston et al. Event-related fMRI: characterizing differential responses. Neuroimage, 1998; 7: 30-40

[40] Fransson et al. The precuneus/posterior cingulate cortex plays a pivotal role in the default mode network: Evidence from a partial correlation network analysis. Neuroimage. 2008;42:1178–1184.

[41] Gonçalves,et al. Correlating the alpha rhythm to BOLD using simultaneous EEG-fMRI: inter-subject variability. Neuroimage, 2006; 30: 203-213;

[42] Gotman et al. Combining EEG and fMRI in epilepsy: methodological challenges and clinical results. I Clin Neurophysiol, 2004; 21: 229-240

[43] Gotman et al. Generalized epileptic discharges show thalamocortical activation and the suspension of the default state of the brain. PNAS, 2005; 142: 15236-15240

[44] Gotman et al. Epileptic networks studied with EEG-fMRI. Epilepsia, 2008; 49 Suppl 3:42-51.

[45] Gusnard et al. Medial prefrontal cortex and self-referential mental activity: relation to a default mode of brain function. Proc Natl Acad Sci USA. 2001;98:4259–4264.

[46] Gusnard et al. Searching for a baseline: functional imaging and the resting human brain. Nat Rev Neurosci. 2001;2:685–694.

[47] Hamandi et al. EEG-fMRI of Generalized Spike-Wave Activity. Neuroimage. 2006;31:1700–1710.

[48] Hamandi et al. BOLD and perfusion changes during epileptic generalised spike wave activity. Neuroimage. 2008;39:608–618.

[49] Hammers et al. Abnormalities of grey and white matter [11C] flumazenil binding in temporal lobe epilepsy with normal MRI. Brain 2002; 125: 2257-2271

[50] Henry et al. Positron emission tomography. In: J. Engel, Jr. (Ed.), Surgical Treatment of Epilepsies, 2nd edn, Raven Press, New York, 1993: pp. 211-232

[51] Hill et al. Haemodynamic and metabolic aspects of photosensitive epilepsy revealled by functional magnetic resonance imaging and magnetic resonance spectroscopy. Epilepsia. 1999;40:912–920.

[52] Holmes et al. Are "generalized" seizures truly generalized? Evidence of localized mesial frontal and frontopolar discharges in absence. Epilepsia. 2004;45:1568–1579.

[53] Huggs et al. Normalization of controlateral metabolic function following temporal lobectomy demonstrated by 1H magnetic resonance spectroscopic imaging. Ann Neurol 1996; 40: 236-239

[54] Iannetti et al. fMRI/EEG in paroxysmal activity elicited by elimination of central vision and fixation. Neurology, 2002; 58: 976—979.

[55] Ives et al. Monitoring the patient's EEG during echo planar MRI. EEG and Clin Neurophysiol, 1993; 87: 417-420

[56] Kobayashi et al. Intrisic epileptogenicity in polymicrogyric cortex suggested by EEG-fMRI BOLD responses. Neurology, 2005; 64: 1263-1266

[57] Kobayashi et al. Grey matter heterotopia: what EEG-fMRI can tell us about epileptogenicity of neuronal migration disorder. Brain, 2006; 129: 366-374

[58] Kobayashi et al. Widespread and intense BOLD changes during brief focal electrographic seizures. Neurology, 2006; 66: 1049-1055

[59] Kobayashi et al. Negative BOLD responses to epileptic spikes. Human Brain Mapping, 2006; 27: 488-497

[60] Kobayashi et al.Temporal and extratemporal BOLD responses to temporal lobe interictal spikes. Epilepsia, 2006; 47: 343-354

[61] Kokkinos et al. "Epileptogenic networks in two patients with hypothalamic hamartoma." Brain Topogr. 2012;25(3):327-31.

[62] Krakow et al. EEG-fMRI of interictal epileptiform activity in patients with partial seizures. Brain, 1999; 122: 1679-1688

[63] Krakow et al. Spatio-temporal imaging of focal interictal epileptiform activity using EEG-triggered functional MRI. Epileptic Disord, 2001; 3: 67-74

[64] Kuzniecky et al.Cortical dysplasia in temporal lobe epilepsy: magnetic resonance imaging correlations. Ann. Neurol, 1991; 29: 293-298

[65] Krausz et al. Brain SPECT imaging in temporal lobe epilepsy. Neuroradiol 1991; 33: 274-276.

[66] Labate et al. Typical childhood absence seizures are associated with thalamic activation. Epileptic Disord. 2005;7:373–377.

[67] Laufs et al. EEG-fMRI mapping of asymmetrical delta activity in a patient with refractory epilepsy is concordant with the epileptogenic region determined by intracranial EEG. Magnetic Resonance Imaging, 2006/a; 24: 367-371

[68] Laufs et al. linking generalized spike-and wave discharges and resting state brain activity by using EEG-fMRI in a patient with absence seizures. Epilepsia, 2006; 47: 444-448

[69] Laufs et al. Linking Generalized Spike-and-Wave Discharges and Resting State Brain Activity by Using EEG-fMRI in a Patient with Absence Seizures. Epilepsia. 2006;47:444–448.

[70] Laufs et al. Electroencephalography/functional MRI in human epilepsy: what it currently can and cannot do. Curr Opin Neurol. 2007;20:417–423.

[71] Laureys et al. Brain function in coma, vegetative state, and related disorders. Lancet Neurol. 2004;3:537–546.

[72] Lazeyras et al. Functional MRI with simultaneous EEG recording: feasibility and application to motor and visual activation. J Magn Reson Imaging, 2001; 13: 943-948

[73] Lee et al. Single Photon emission computed tomography (SPECT) brain imaging using N,N,NI-trimethyl-N-(2 hydroxy-3-methyl-5-123-iodobenzyl)-1,3-propanediamine 2 HCl (HIPDM): intractable complex partial seizures. Neurology 1986; 36:1471-1477

[74] Leiderman et al. The dynamic of metabolic change following seizures ad measured by positron emission tomography with fludeoxyglucose F 18. Arch Neurol, 1994; 51: 932-936

[75] Lemieux et al. Event-related fMRI with simultaneous and continuous EEG: description of the method and initial case report. Neuroimage, 2001; 1: 780-787

[76] Liu et al. EEG-fMRI study of the interictal epileptic activity in patients with partial epilepsy. J Neurol Sci, 2008; 268: 117-123

[77] Logothetis et al. Neurophysiological investigation of the basis of the fMRI signal. Nature, 2001; 412: 150-157

[78] Manganotti et al. Continuous EEG-fMRI in patients with partial epilepsy and focal interictal slow-wave discharges on EEG. Magn Res Imaging, 2008; 26: 1089-1100.

[79] Marks et al. Localization of extra-temporal epileptic foci during single photon emission computed tomography. Ann Neurol 1992; 31:250-255

[80] Meeren et al. Cortical focus drives widespread corticothalamic networks during spontaneous absence seizures in rats. J Neurosci. 2002;22:1480–1495.

[81] Meeren et al. Evolving concepts on the pathophysiology of absence seizures: the cortical focus theory. Arch Neurol. 2005;62:371–376.

[82] Menon et al. Imaging function in the working brain with fMRI. Curr Op Neurobiol, 2001; 11:630-636.

[83] Moeller et al. EEG-fMRI: adding to standard evaluations of patients with nonlesional frontal lobe epilepsy. Neurology 2009;73:2023–30.

[84] Newton et al. SPECT in the localisation of extra-temporale and temporal seizure foci. J Neurol Neurosurg Psychiatry, 1995; 59: 26-30

[85] Ogawa et al. Brain Magnetic Resonance Imaging with contrast dependent on blood oxygenation. Proc Natl Acad Sci, 1990; 87: 9868-9872

[86] Petroff et al. GABA and glutamate in the human brain. Neuroscientist, 2002; 8: 562-573

[87] Polack et al. Deep Layer Somatosensory Cortical Neurons Initiate Spike and Wave Discharges in a Genetic Model of Absence Seizures. J Neurosci. 2007; 27:6590–6599.

[88] Prichard et al. Fuctional study of the brain by NMR. J Cereb Blood Metab, 1994; 14: 365-372

[89] Puce et al. Functional Magnetic Resonance Imaging of sensory and motor cortex: comparision with electrophysiological localisations. I Neurosurg, 1995; 83: 262-270

[90] Ruben et al. Neuroimaging of epilepsy: therapeutic implications. Neurorx, 2005; 2: 384-393

[91] Salek-Haddadi. Functional magnetic resonance imaging of human absence seizures. Ann Neurol, 2003; 53: 663-667

[92] Salek-Haddadi et al. Hemodynamic correlates of epileptiform discharges: an EEG-fMRI study of 63 patients with focal epilepsy. Brain Research, 2006; 1088: 148-166

[93] Salmenpera TM, Duncan JS. Imaging in epilepsy J. Neurol Neurosurg Psychiatry 2005;76:2–10.

[94] So. Mesial frontal epilepsy. Epilepsia, 1998; 39(Suppl 4):S49–61.

[95] Steriade et al. Spike-Wave Complexes and Fast Components of Cortically Generated Seizures. I. Role of Neocortex and Thalamus. J Neurophysiol. 1998;80:1439–1455.

[96] Tai et al. Applications of positron emission tomography (PET) in Neurology. J. Neurol Neurosurg Psych, 2004; 75: 669-676.

[97] Thorton et al. EEG correlated functional MRI and postoperative outcome in focal epilepsy. J Neurol Neurosurg Psychiatry,2010; 81:922-927.

[98] Tucker et al. Discharges in ventromedial frontal cortex during absence spells. Epilepsy Behav. 2007;11:546–557.

[99] Vaudano. Causal hierarchy within the thalamo-cortical network in spike and wave discharges. PLoS One, 2009; 4(8):e6475

9

# Brain Mapping of Language Processing Using Functional MRI Connectivity and Diffusion Tensor Imaging

Todd L. Richards and Virginia W. Berninger

## 1. Introduction

Because the brain's language systems have no end organs for interacting directly with the external world, language systems work with sensory (ears or eyes) and motor (mouth and hands) systems, which are the only brain systems with direct links to external environment. Liberman contributed to understanding of how the language by ear (listening) and language by mouth (reading) systems work together at the behavioral level and also become integrated to support acquisition of language by eye (reading) [1]. Berninger and colleagues extended the work of Liberman and colleagues at the Haskins Laboratory to language by hand (writing), which is not just a motor skill as many assume [2]. This University of Washington research team also showed that Language by Ear, Language by Mouth, Language by Eye, and Language by Hand are separate, but interacting functional language systems, which draw on common as well as unique processes at the behavioral [3] and brain levels of analysis [4]. Moreover, each of the functional language systems has different levels of organization, ranging from subword, to word, to syntax, to text, and has connections with other brain systems such as working memory, attention and executive functions, and cognitive.

The emerging work on the complex functional language systems that connect with other brain systems illustrates the need for brain imaging methods that not only assess localized brain areas or functions but also their structural and functional connections. First, we discuss how the modern imaging techniques have confirmed knowledge of localized structures and functions first acquired in autopsy studies with patients. Second, we discuss how advances in imaging techniques are adding knowledge about the structural and functional connections among specific functional language systems.

### 1.1. Localized structures and functions

In early work in neurolinguistics researchers studied people with brain lesions and discovered relationships between the patient's specific language deficit and the location of the lesion. In this way, they discovered that two areas in the brain are involved in language processing: Wernicke's area located in the posterior section of the superior temporal gyrus in the dominant cerebral hemisphere. People with a lesion in this area of the brain develop receptive aphasia, a condition in which there is a major language comprehension impairment, but the capability for speech production remains intact. The other area is Broca's area located in the posterior inferior frontal gyrus of the dominant hemisphere. Patients with a lesion to this area develop expressive aphasia and are unable to produce speech even though they are able to understand other's that they hear [4].

Neurolinguist researchers have adopted non-invasive brain imaging techniques such as functional magnetic resonance imaging and electrophysiology to study language processing in individuals without impairments [5]. For example, in the study of phonological processing, the receptive processing of phonemes in heard words has been localized to Wernicke's area (posterior Brodmann's Area [BA] 22) and BA 40 [6] [7-11], and expressive production of phonemes during speech has been localized to the posterior Broca's area (BAs 44 and 6) [11-15]. Thus, research using these newly developed brain imaging techniques has confirmed what was was classically thought based on patient studies for right-handed individuals: The two major language areas are Broca's area for production of language by mouth [16] and Wernicke's area for comprehension of language by ear [17], which receives input from the ear through the auditory cortex. The arcuate fasciculus, a fiber pathway that originates in the temporal lobe and curves in an anterior/posterior direction to project to the frontal lobe [18], was thought to connect these 2 areas.

Figure 1 that follows shows these important language processing areas of the brain superimposed on a side/surface view of the brain based on more recent non-invasive brain imaging methods. These areas may also play a role in production of language by hand (writing) and comprehension of language by eye (reading), via related processing in angular gyrus and supramarginal gyrus [4].

## 2. Brain's structural and functional connectivity

In 2010 the US National Institute of Health (NIH) announced the Human Connectome Project:

"Knowledge of human brain connectivity will transform human neuroscience by providing not only a qualitatively novel class of data, but also by providing the basic framework necessary to synthesize diverse data and, ultimately, elucidate how our brains work in health, illness, youth, and old age." Included in this connectome is the study of language-related neural connections which enable the brain to perform written and oral language.

Mullen [19] has on online manual that defines several important terms used in research about structural and functional networks.

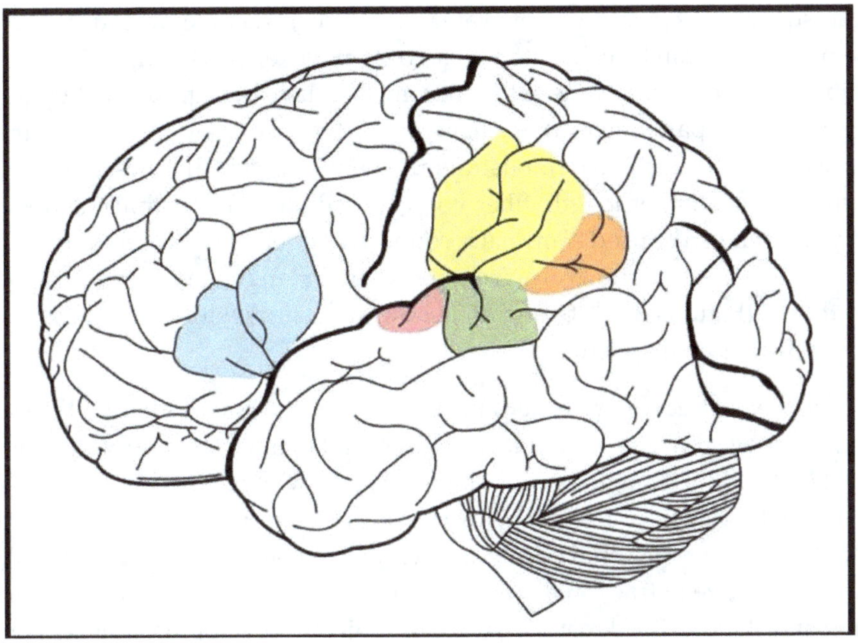

**Figure 1.** Brain regions important for language. Broca's area (blue), auditory cortex (pink), Wernicke's area (green), Supramarginal gyrus (yellow), angular gyus (orange). (Figure from the wikipedia website http://en.wikipedia.org/wiki/File:Brain_Surface_Gyri.SVG).

The study of human brain connectivity generally falls under one or more of three categories: structural, functional, and effective [20].

### 2.1. DTI structural connectivity studies of brain

Structural connectivity denotes networks of anatomical (e.g., axonal) links) for which the primary goal is to understand what brain structures are capable of influencing each other via direct or indirect axonal connections. Structural connectivity might be studied in vivo using invasive axonal labeling techniques or noninvasive MRI-based diffusion weighted imaging (DWI/DTI) methods. These methods cannot measure individual axons but can measure the water diffusion signal from a group of axons that have parallel geometric properties within a fiber bundle. DTI connectivity is influenced by the number of axons and the amount of myelination within the fiber bundle.

Diffusion Tensor Imaging (DTI) tractography is a neuroimaging technique that allows for the virtual dissection of fiber tracts in the living brain based on the directionally biased diffusion of water in white matter [21]. DTI analysis provides several parameters that quantify the properties of the fiber bundle: fractional anisotropy ( a measure of the amount of anisotropy of water diffusion between the primary fiber direction and the perpendicular to the primary fiber direction); axial water diffusion diffusivity ( the amount of water diffusion along the primary direction of the fiber bundle); radial diffusivity ( the amount the water diffusion perpendicular to the primary direction of the fiber bundle); mean diffusivity (characterizes the overall mean-squared displacement of water molecules); relative anisotropy; and volume ratio. These parameters can be calculated on a voxel by voxel basis within the DTI image The exact equations used to calculate these DTI parameters have been published by LeBihan et al [22]. Other important parameters that characterize the fiber bundle are the tractography analysis which is a procedure to demonstrate the neural tracts[23]. These neural tracts have properties such as mean fiber length, fiber volume, and mean FA within the fiber tract. This tractography analysis can be used to measure connectivity between specific regions of the brain such as between Broca's area and Wernicke's area or other language-related brain regions. The figures that follow (Figures 2 A, 2B, and 2C) show an example of fibers tract4s connected to Broca's area in the left hemisphere.

DTI [24-27] has been used to study language connections. For example, DTI studies have identified association between variation in white matter microstructure and differences in reading skill [28] [29] [30]. Klingberg et al [30] found that white matter diffusion anisotropy in the temporo-parietal region of the left hemisphere was significantly correlated with reading scores within the reading-impaired adults and within the control group. Nioqi et al [28] found strong correlation between fractional anisotropy (FA) values in a left temporo-parietal white matter region and standardized reading scores of typically developing children. Deutsch et al [29] found that white matter structure (as measured by fractional anisotropy) and coherence index (CI) significantly correlated with behavioral measurements of reading, spelling, and rapid naming performance in children. Glasser et al used Diffusion Tensor Imaging (DTI) tractography to detect leftward asymmetries in the arcuate fasciculus [31]. The arcuate fasciclus is a pathway that links temporal and inferior frontal language cortices and is divided into 2 segments with different hypothesized functions, one terminating in the posterior superior temporal gyrus (STG) and another terminating in the middle temporal gyrus (MTG). STG terminations were strongly left lateralized and overlapped with phonological activations in the left but not the right hemisphere, suggesting that only the left hemisphere phonological cortex is directly connected with the frontal lobe via the arcuate fasciculus. MTG terminations were also strongly left lateralized, overlapping with left lateralized lexical--semantic activations. Smaller right hemisphere MTG terminations overlapped with right lateralized prosodic activations. They used a recent model of brain language processing to explain 6 aphasia syndromes [31].These studies demonstrate the potential for using DTI to measure white matter structural changes in dyslexia.

### 2.2. Brain studies of functional and effective connectivity

Functional connectivity denotes symmetrical correlations in activity between brain regions during information processing. Here the primary goal is to understand which regions are functionally related through correlations in their activity, as measured by some imaging technique. Functional connectivity is a powerful noninvasive technique used to investigate the distribution of neural networks in healthy participants and affected subjects, which can be characterized by low-frequency fluctuations in the BOLD signal when the subject is performing a task [32, 33]. The BOLD response of a continuous task leads to coherent signal changes in anatomically different, but functionally connected, brain structures and thus implies the

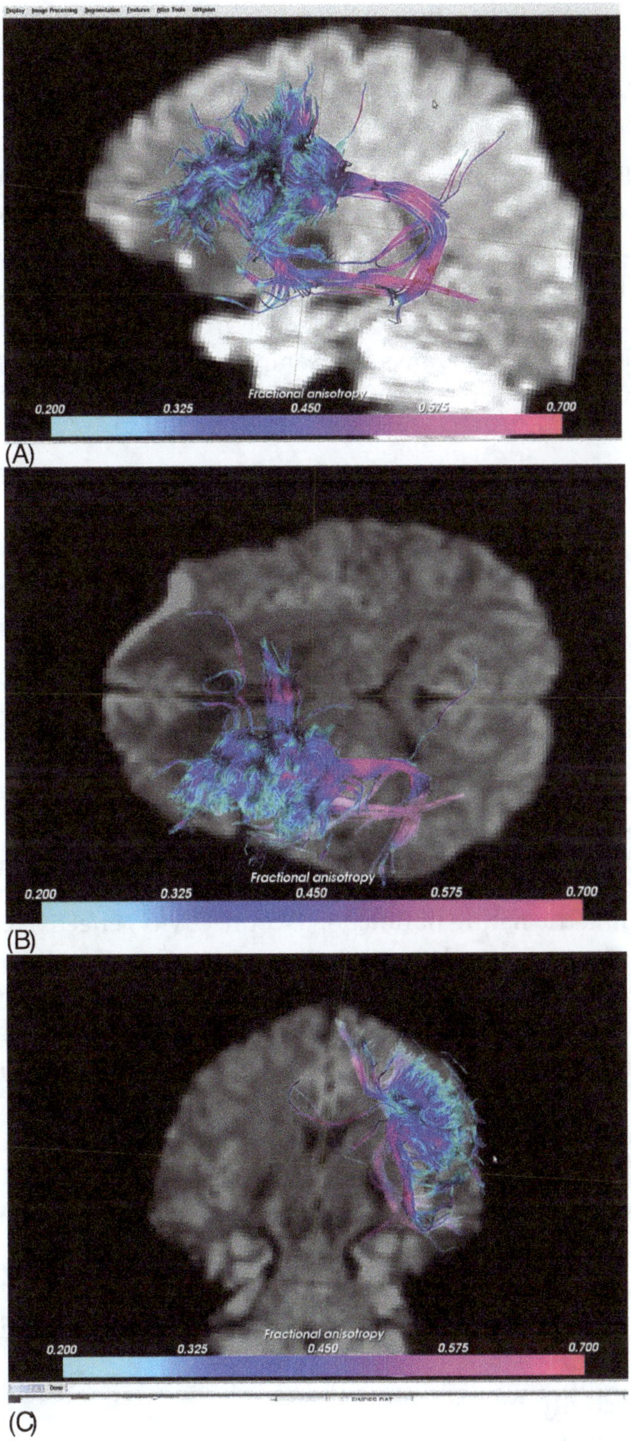


**Figure 2.** DTI fiber tracts connected to Broca's area. Sagittal view (part A), axial view (part B), and coronal view (part C) showing fibers in the frontal and temporal lobe. The color coding of the fibers is related to the amplitude of the fractional anisotropy within the fiber. A color scale bar is shown at the bottom.

existence of neuronal connections between these regions. Coherent signal changes in anatomically different brain structures imply the existence of neuronal connections between these regions. Exploratory data analysis methods have the attractive feature of being model free and thus allowing unbiased studies of brain signal responses.

Examples in fMRI/PET include principal component analysis (PCA), independent component analysis (ICA), and cluster analysis. There are also model-free analyses of interregional connectivity [34-41]. A popular form of functional connectivity analysis using functional magnetic resonance imaging (fMRI) has been to compute the pairwise correlation (or partial correlation) in BOLD activity for a large number of voxels or regions of interest within the brain volume. The figure 3 below shows an example pair of BOLD signals that have a high degree of correlation. For example functional MRI connectivity can be used to study the functional signal correlations between Broca's area and Wernicke's area.

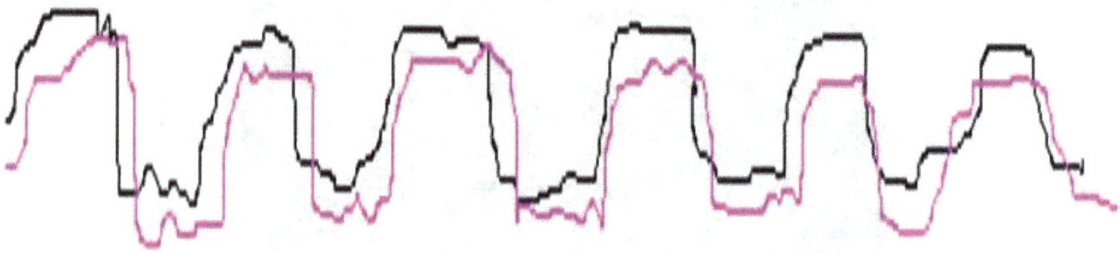

**Figure 3.** Example of the time course of fMRI signals from two different brain regions which are functionally connected. Notice that the two signals (black and red lines) are closely correlated but not exactly the same.

In contrast to the symmetric nature of functional connectivity, effective connectivity denotes asymmetric or causal dependencies between brain regions. Here the primary goal is to identify which brain structures in a functional network are causally influencing other elements of the network during some stage or form of information processing. Often the term "information flow" is used to indicate directionally specific (although not necessarily causal) effective connectivity between neuronal structures. Popular effective connectivity methods, applied to fMRI and/or electrophysiological (EEG, iEEG, MEG) imaging data, include dynamic causal modeling, structural equation modeling, transfer entropy, and Granger-causal methods. An example of fMRI connectivity using Broca's area as a seed region is shown below in Figure 4.

## 3. Connectivity imaging studies of specific learning disabilities

### 3.1. Functional connectivity studies

Currently, imaging research studies of dyslexia are moving away from simply localizing task-related activation to regions of interest (ROI) to analyzing functional connectivity among different brain regions in specific task environments [42] or resting states [43]. Previous functional connectivity studies of dyslexia were mostly focused on the angular gyrus. Asyn-

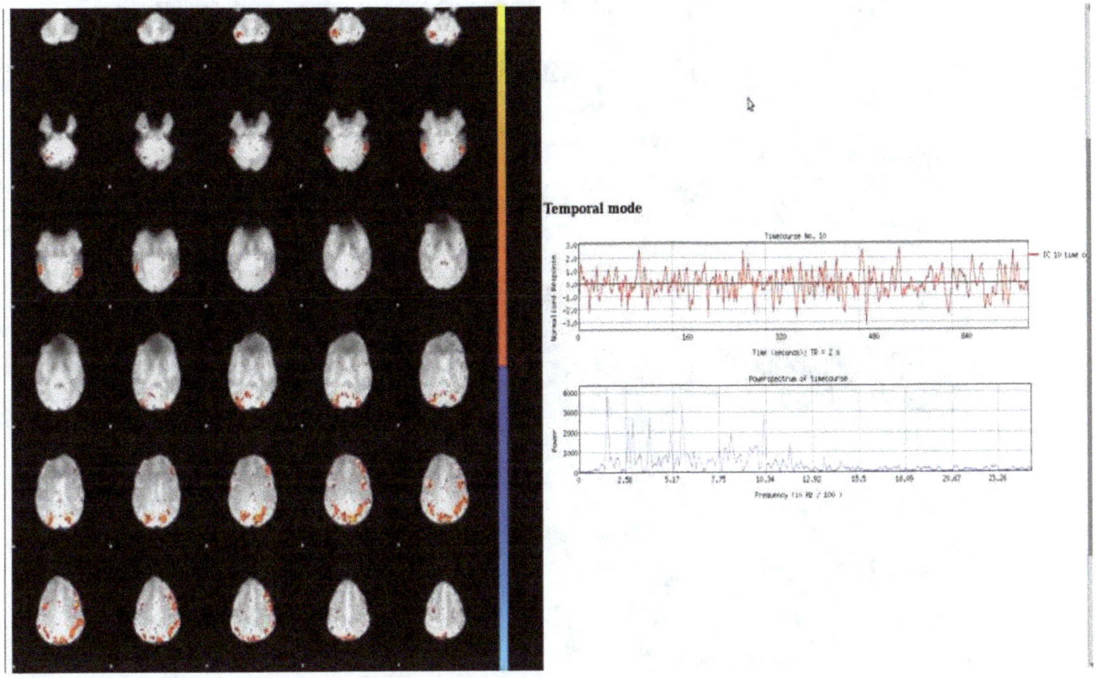


**Figure 4.** FMRI connectivity analysis related to left-sided Broca's area using FSL's Independent Component Analysis software Melodic combined with UW software. The red plot shows the time course of this ICA component and the plot in blue shows the frequency spectrum. Notice that there are several anatomical regions of the brain that are involved in this component including the left frontal lobe (which includes Broca's area), left and right parietal lobe, left and right temporal lobe.

chrony of regional cerebral blood flow changes in the angular gyrus and extrastriate occipital/temporal lobe regions suggested functional disconnection during single word reading [44]. Pugh et al [45] showed functional disconnections between the angular gyrus and temporal and occipital areas (namely, lateral extrastriate, medial extrastriate, and primary visual cortex) in the left hemisphere specific to the phonological processing. Shaywitz et al. [46] found functional connections between the occipitotemporal region and inferior frontal gyrus in the left hemisphere in normal readers under a real-word reading condition. Poor readers, in contrast, exhibited more functional connections between the left occipitotemporal region and right middle and inferior frontal gyri [46].

Shaywitz et al documented that the important difference between compensated young adults with a history of dyslexia and young adults who are good readers without a history of dyslexia lies in connectivity among regions rather than in regions of activation per se [46]. Milne et al. [47] reported that an individual with developmental dyslexia showed increased activation, as the phonological processing demands increased, in the left inferior frontal gyrus, right parietal cortex, right occipital cortex, and cerebellum. Both the Shaywitz et al. [46] and Milne et al. [47] studies had shown the importance of connectivity between posterior and anterior language systems in supporting the reading process. Betan et al, [48] have recently used fMRI connectivity to examine task-specific modulations of effective connectivity within a left-hemisphere

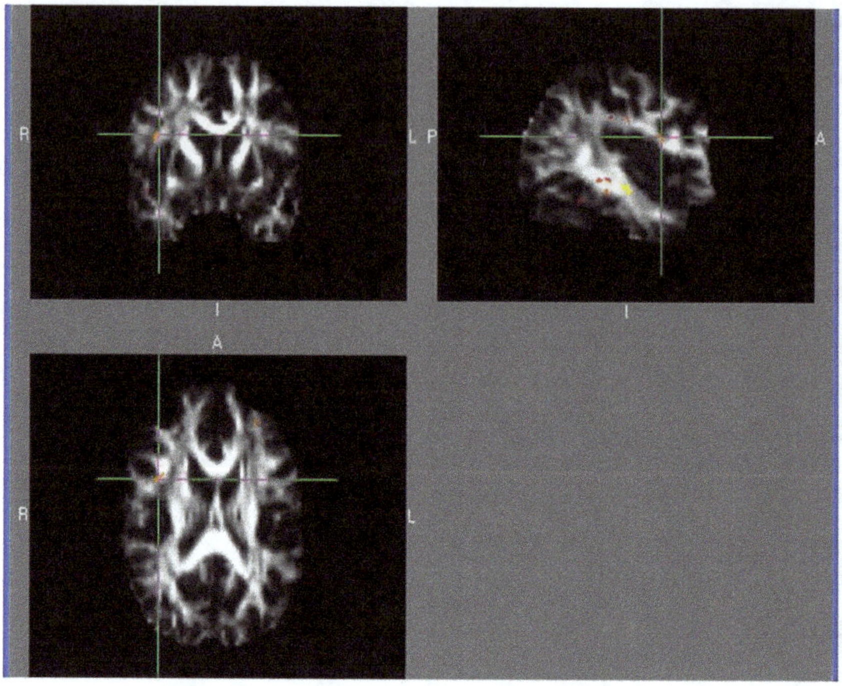


**Figure 5.** Group differences for controls > dyslexics in analysis of fractional anisotropy with FSL-based TBSS software. Crosshair on a significant cluster near R inf. frontal gyrus.

language network during spelling and rhyming judgments on visually presented words. They used dynamic causal modeling to show that each task preferentially strengthened modulatory influences converging on its task-specific site (LTC for rhyming, IPS for spelling). Their findings also showed that switching tasks led to changes in the target area influenced by the IFG, suggesting that the IFG may play a pivotal role in setting the cognitive context for each task [48].

### 3.2. Converging fMRI and DTI Imaging findings

Our first DTI Study [49] identified differences between adults with and without dyslexia (which is also a writing disorder, [50]) in the right inferior gyrus (See Figure 5). This is one of the same regions where structural differences were found between dyslexics and good readers in an MRI structural study (Eckert et al., 2003) [51] and the same region where functional differences were found in an fMRI orthographic task contrast before but not after orthographic treatment (Richards et al., 2006a) [52]. Trends towards less activation in right inferior frontal gyrus were associated with improved phonological decoding following treatment (Richards et al., 2006b) [53].

Trends towards less activation in right inferior frontal gyrus were associated with improved phonological decoding following treatment [53]. These findings suggest that right inferior frontal gyrus plays a role in orthographic coding, a process which our behavioral studies for nearly two decades have shown contributes uniquely to handwriting, spelling, and composi-

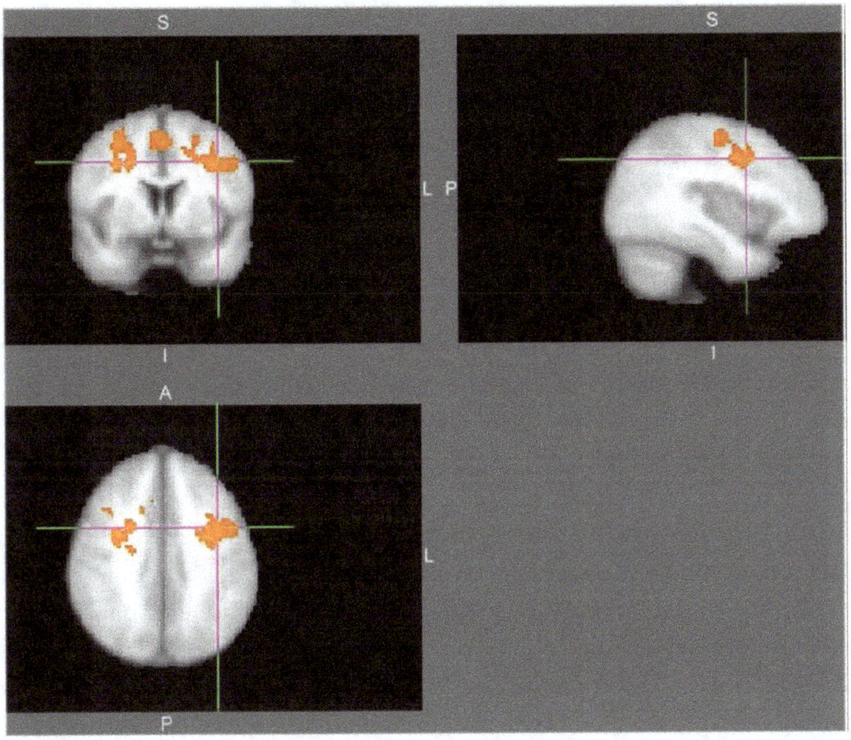


**Figure 6.** Group difference map for dyslexics greater than controls. The individual maps used in this analysis were correlation maps created when the seed ROI in the left inferior frontal gyrus was compared to the rest of the brain voxels.

tion[54]. Thus, we predict that in studies in progress children with handwriting disabilities will differ from good writers in the right inferior frontal gyrus.

Differences in functional connectivity were also found between children with and without dyslexia before but not after treatment on a phonological spelling task (phoneme mapping—deciding whether letter(s) in pair of pronounceable nonwords could stand for the same sound[55]. These data were analyzed with a seed point correlational method for functional connectivity from four seed points based on prior studies: inferior frontal gyrus, middle frontal gyrus, the occipital region, and cerebellum. Before treatment, there was a significant difference in fMRI connectivity between children with dyslexia and normal reading controls in the degree of connectivity between left inferior frontal gyrus and the following regions: right and left middle frontal gyrus, right and left supplemental motor area, left precentral gyrus, and right superior frontal gyrus. There were no significant differences when seed regions were placed in the middle frontal gyrus, occipital gyrus or cerebellum. Children with dyslexia had greater functional connectivity from the left inferior frontal gyrus seed point to the right inferior frontal gyrus than did the children without dyslexia as shown in Figure 6.

The children with dyslexia then participated in a 3-week instructional program that provided explicit instruction in linguistic awareness, alphabetic principle (taught in a way to maximize temporal contiguity of grapheme–phoneme associations and to train both phonological and orthographic loops), decoding and spelling. At Time2, the treated children with did not differ from the children without dyslexia in any of the clusters in the group. The main result was that children with dyslexia had greater functional connectivity from the left inferior frontal gyrus seed point to the right inferior frontal gyrus than did the children without dyslexia before but not after treatment [55]. Thus, the structural and functional connectivity studies provided converging evidence for abnormalities related to inferior frontal gyrus (on right or left) in children with dyslexia.

### 3.3. Stanberry model of fMRI connectivity in dyslexia

Stanberry et al [35] developed a model of fMRI connectivity based on earlier results that predicts that for normal readers there will be functional connectivity among 5 major reading-related brain regions: (a) frontal lobe (including the inferior frontal gyrus and middle frontal gyrus); (b) parietal lobe (including the angular gyrus); (c) visual processing areas (including occipitotemporal region); (d) fusiform/lingual word form region; and (e) the cerebellum. This model is generally consistent with that reported by other research groups for normal reading [46]; it is also consistent with phonological loop in verbal working memory as a deficit in dyslexia [56, 57]. We predicted that individual dyslexics may have impaired connectivity in any one or a combination of these major circuits. In our first fMRI connectivity study, we investigated differences in cortical networks used by adult controls compared to adult dyslexics during the previously described Phoneme Mapping. By definition, functional connectivity refers to a correlation or synchronization between the time courses of activation of two brain regions. We hypothesized that two brain regions that work together have similar temporal response profiles [58]. A model-independent method was used to analyze the time-synchronized activations induced by the phoneme mapping paradigm (adapted from [59]) presented during a continuous task presentation. A standard fMRI acquisition and analysis of the on-off block design was also performed using Phoneme Mapping. Native English speakers ranging in age from 30 to 45 years participated in the connectivity study: 10 healthy right-handed control males (fathers from the family genetics study who did not meet research criteria for dyslexia on tests and also did not have a history of reading problems) and 13 right-handed, otherwise healthy, adult males who did meet the research criteria for dyslexia and had a history of reading and writing problems. The two groups did not differ significantly in mean Verbal IQ [dyslexics, M=113.8 (SD = 10.3); controls, M=107.7 (SD=11.1), but the dyslexics were significantly lower than the control fathers on each of the reading, spelling, and RAN measures.

Structural and functional MR images were collected in accordance with institutional regulations (IRB approval) on a commercial 1.5T MR scanner (General Electric, Waukesha, WI) equipped with echo-speed gradients and a standard birdcage head coil. Functional images were acquired using an echo-planar sequence with imaging parameters set as follows:
"On-Off" task: 20 axial slices, FOV 24cm x 24cm, BW +/- 62.5 kHz, TR 2000ms, TE 40ms, Flip 82 deg, slice thickness 6mm, gap 1mm, resolution 64x64, 162 time points; Continuous task: 20 axial slices, FOV 24cm x 24cm, BW +/- 62.5 kHz, TR 2000ms, TE 40 ms, Flip 82 deg, slice thickness 6mm, gap 1mm, resolution 64x64, 483 time points.

Cardiac and respiratory rates were digitally recorded with a pulse oximeter and a flexible belt, respectively, using a sampling frequency of 100Hz. Three different seed regions were used for connectivity analysis – right and left inferior frontal gyrus and cerebellum.

For the standard block fMRI acquisition and analysis of controls, fMRI brain activation was detected in the following brain regions: for the right side - inferior frontal gyrus, middle frontal gyrus, cerebellum crus I, cerebellum crus II, occipital gyrus, superior parietal gyrus, inferior parietal gyrus, angular gyrus, lingual gyrus, and fusiform gyrus; for the left side – superior parietal gyrus, angular, occipital gyrus, cerebellum crus I, cerebellum crus II, lingual.

For the fMRI connectivity analysis of the continuous phoneme mapping paradigm, we narrowed the five region model above to a focus on three regions based on structural MRI differences in dyslexics from a family genetics study [51]. Results showed that (a) when the right IFG was chosen as the seed region, significant differences ($p<.05$) were found between dyslexics and controls in right inferior frontal triangularis, bilateral fusiform, bilateral middle and inferior occipital gyri, right angular gyrus, bilateral ITG and cerebellum; (b) when the left IFG was chosen as the seed region, significant differences ($p<.05$) were found between dyslexics and controls in the following brain regions: right inferior frontal triangularis, right middle occipital gyrus, right inferior occipital gyrus, and right cerebellum (VI); and (c) when the cerebellum was chosen as the seed region, significant differences ($p<.05$) were found between dyslexics and controls in the following brain regions: bilateral superior frontal gyrus, left middle frontal gyrus, right angular gyrus, and right middle occipital gyrus. Adult dyslexics, when compared to controls, had impaired cortical connections in brain regions important for phonological processing. The abnormality in functional connectivity from cerebellum in dyslexics may be related to Klingberg et al.'s [30] finding, based on DTI, that white matter diffusion anisotropy in the temporo-parietal region of the left hemisphere is significantly correlated with reading in normal and dyslexic readers. Insufficient myelination of the axonal pathways is one possible explanation for the low anisotropy index values observed in poor readers [60]. Structural abnormalities in white matter pathways could interfere with neuronal transmission, which will directly affect the synchrony of the BOLD signal. Of most importance, functional disconnections were also observed when seed regions were set in bilateral IFG. Bilateral IFG and right cerebellum were found to be abnormal in child dyslexics compared to normal controls ascertained using the same research criteria in our structural MRI studies [51]. Also see Berninger, Raskind, Richards et al. [50].

## 4. Future perspectives

One of the great potential techniques in this area of language connectivity analysis is the integration of both functional and structural connectivity as shown by Morgan et al [61]. They measured connections between Wernicke's (WA), Broca's (BA) and supplementary motor area (SMA). Along the path between BA and SMA, they showed that fibers tracked measured from DTI generally formed a single bundle and the mean radius of the bundle was positively correlated with functional connectivity. They concluded that the insights gained from this work offers a useful guidance for non-invasive means to evaluate brain network integrity in vivo for use in diagnosing and determining disease progression and recovery [61]. The concept of integrating information across brain imaging modalities will allow the study of human language network as a systems approach. Another futuristic concept has been described by Rota et al [62] where they discuss the mechanisms of cortical reorganization underlying the enhancement of speech. They were able to measure changes in functional and effective connectivity induced in subjects who learned to deliberately increase activation in the right inferior frontal gyrus [62]. Also, see [63] for a model of the four multi-leveled functional language systems, which provides the conceptual framework for testing a model that differentiates among typical oral and written language learners (OWLs), dysgraphia, dyslexia, and OWL LD at the behavioral (phenotype and response to instruction) and brain levels of analysis.

## 5. Conclusions

The language connectivity findings discussed in this chapter suggest that structural and functional connectivity are adding and will continue to add to our understanding of language and language learning. There are specific language pathways and connections that are crucial for language acquisition and function. The integrity of these connections can be tested using structural DTI and functional MRI connectivity imaging. Individuals with learning and language disabilities have been reported to have different fMRI and DTI measurable connections than those with normal language functions. Once the techniques have been fully tested and developed, the application of language connectivity techniques to the individual assessment, treatment design, and response to treatment would also have enormous practical applications in the clinic and schools.

## Acknowledgements

This project received support from the NIH/NICHD Grant 1P50HD071764 (overall PI Virginia Berninger, PI of project 3 Todd Richards).

## Author details

Todd L. Richards[1*] and Virginia W. Berninger[2]

*Address all correspondence to: toddr@u.washington.edu

1 Department of Radiology, University of Washington Medical Center, Seattle, WA, USA

2 Department of Educational Psychology, University of Washington, Seattle, WA, USA

## References


[1] Liberman A. The reading researcher and the reading teacher need the right theory of speech. Scientific Studies of Reading 1999;3:95-111.

[2] Berninger V, Graham S. Language by hand: A synthesis of a decade of research on handwriting. Handwriting Review 1998;12:11-25.

[3] Berninger V. Development of language by hand and its connections to language by ear, mouth, and eye. Topics in Language Disorders, 20, 65-84 2000;20:65-84.

[4] Trask RL. Language: The Basics. New York: Routledge; 1999.

[5] Lesser R. Language in the Brain: Neurolinguistics, An Encyclopedia of Language. New York: Routledge; 1989.

[6] Binder JR, Frost JA, Hammeke TA, Cox RW, Rao SM, Prieto T. Human brain language areas identified by functional magnetic resonance imaging. J Neurosci 1997;17:353-362.

[7] Binder JR, Frost JA, Hammeke TA, Bellgowan PS, Springer JA, Kaufman JN, et al. Human temporal lobe activation by speech and nonspeech sounds. Cereb Cortex 2000;10(5):512-28.

[8] Cannestra AF, Bookheimer SY, Pouratian N, O'Farrell A, Sicotte N, Martin NA, et al. Temporal and topographical characterization of language cortices using intraoperative optical intrinsic signals. Neuroimage 2000;12(1):41-54.

[9] Castillo EM, Simos PG, Davis RN, Breier J, Fitzgerald ME, Papanicolaou AC. Levels of word processing and incidental memory: dissociable mechanisms in the temporal lobe. Neuroreport 2001;12(16):3561-6.

[10] Jancke L, Wustenberg T, Scheich H, Heinze HJ. Phonetic perception and the temporal cortex. Neuroimage 2002;15(4):733-46.

[11] McDermott KB, Petersen SE, Watson JM, Ojemann JG. A procedure for identifying regions preferentially activated by attention to semantic and phonological relations using functional magnetic resonance imaging. Neuropsychologia 2003;41(3):293-303.

[12] Bookheimer S. Functional MRI of language: new approaches to understanding the cortical organization of semantic processing. Annu Rev Neurosci 2002;25:151-88.

[13] Hickok G, Poeppel D. Dorsal and ventral streams: a framework for understanding aspects of the functional anatomy of language. Cognition 2004;92(1-2):67-99.

[14] Price CJ, Mummery CJ, Moore CJ, Frakowiak RS, Friston KJ. Delineating necessary and sufficient neural systems with functional imaging studies of neuropsychological patients. J Cogn Neurosci 1999;11(4):371-82.

[15] Paulesu E, Goldacre B, Scifo P, Cappa SF, Gilardi MC, Castiglioni I, et al. Functional heterogeneity of left inferior frontal cortex as revealed by fMRI. Neuroreport 1997;8(8):2011-7.

[16] Broca P. Nouvelle observation d'aphemie produite par une lesion de la troisieme circonvolution frontale. Bulletins de la Societe anatomie (Paris), 2e serie 1861;6:398-407.

[17] Wernicke C. The symptom complex of aphasia (1874). Reprinted in English in Proc. Boston Colloq. Philos. Sci. 1874;4:34-97.

[18] Dejerine J. Anatomy of central nervous system. Paris: Masson; 1895.

[19] Mullen T. SIFT Online Handbook and User Manual. http://sccn.ucsd.edu/wiki/SIFT 2010.

[20] Bullmore E, Sporns O. Complex brain networks: graph theoretical analysis of structural and functional systems. Nat Rev Neurosci 2009;10(3):186-98.

[21] Beaulieu C. The basis of anisotropic water diffusion in the nervous system - a technical review. NMR Biomed 2002;15(7-8):435-55.

[22] Le Bihan D, Mangin JF, Poupon C, Clark CA, Pappata S, Molko N, et al. Diffusion tensor imaging: concepts and applications. Journal of magnetic resonance imaging: JMRI 2001;13(4):534-546.

[23] Filler AI. The History, Development and Impact of Computed Imaging in Neurological Diagnosis and Neurosurgery: CT, MRI, and DTI. Internet Journal of Neurosurgery 2010;7(1).

[24] Catani M, Mesulam M. The arcuate fasciculus and the disconnection theme in language and aphasia: history and current state. Cortex 2008;44(8):953-61.

[25] Nucifora PG, Verma R, Melhem ER, Gur RE, Gur RC. Leftward asymmetry in relative fiber density of the arcuate fasciculus. Neuroreport 2005;16(8):791-4.

[26] Parker GJ, Luzzi S, Alexander DC, Wheeler-Kingshott CA, Ciccarelli O, Lambon Ralph MA. Lateralization of ventral and dorsal auditory-language pathways in the human brain. Neuroimage 2005;24(3):656-66.

[27] Powell HW, Parker GJ, Alexander DC, Symms MR, Boulby PA, Wheeler-Kingshott CA, et al. Hemispheric asymmetries in language-related pathways: a combined functional MRI and tractography study. Neuroimage 2006;32(1):388-99.

[28] Niogi SN, McCandliss BD. Left lateralized white matter microstructure accounts for individual differences in reading ability and disability. Neuropsychologia 2006;44: 2178-2188.

[29] Deutsch GK, Dougherty RF, Bammer R, Siok WT, Gabrieli JD, Wandell B. Children's reading performance is correlated with white matter structure measured by diffusion tensor imaging. Cortex 2005;41:354-363.

[30] Klingberg T, Hedehus M, Temple E, Salz T, Gabrieli JD, Moseley ME, et al. Microstructure of temporo-parietal white matter as a basis for reading ability: evidence from diffusion tensor magnetic resonance imaging [see comments]. Neuron 2000;25(2):493-500.

[31] Glasser MF, Rilling JK. DTI tractography of the human brain's language pathways. Cereb Cortex 2008;18(11):2471-82.

[32] Hampson M, Peterson B, Skudlarski P., Gatenby J, Gore J. Detection of functional connectivity using temporal correlations in MR images. Human Brain Mapping 2002;15:247-262.

[33] Lowe M, Mock B, Sorenson J. Functional connectivity in single and multislice echo-planar imaging using resting-state fluctuations. Neuroimage 1998;7:119-132.

[34] Stanberry L, Nandy R, Cordes D. Cluster analysis of fMRI Data using Dendrogram Sharpening. Human Brain Mapping 2003;20:201-219.

[35] Stanberry LI, Richards T, Berninger VW, Stock P, Nandy RR, Aylward E, et al. Low Frequency Signal Changes Reflect Differences in Functional Connectivity between Good Readers and Dyslexics during Continuous Phoneme Mapping. Magnetic Resonance Imaging 2006;24:217-229.

[36] Nandy R, Cordes D. Improving the spatial specificity of canonical correlation analysis in fMRI. Magn Reson Med 2004;52(4):947-52.

[37] Nandy RR, Cordes D. Novel nonparametric approach to canonical correlation analysis with applications to low CNR functional MRI data. Magn Reson Med 2003;50(2): 354-65.

[38] Nandy RR, Cordes D. Novel ROC-type method for testing the efficiency of multivariate statistical methods in fMRI. Magn Reson Med 2003;49(6):1152-62.

[39] Cordes D, Haughton V, Carew JD, Arfanakis K, Maravilla K. Hierarchical clustering to measure connectivity in fMRI resting-state data. Magn Reson Imaging 2002;20(4): 305-17.

[40] Cordes D, Haughton VM, Arfanakis K, Carew JD, Turski PA, Moritz CH, et al. Frequencies contributing to functional connectivity in the cerebral cortex in "resting-state" data. AJNR Am J Neuroradiol 2001;22(7):1326-33.

[41] Cordes D, Haughton VM, Arfanakis K, Wendt GJ, Turski PA, Moritz CH, et al. Mapping functionally related regions of brain with functional connectivity MR imaging [In Process Citation]. AJNR Am J Neuroradiol 2000;21(9):1636-44.

[42] Büchel C, Coull, J., Friston, K. The predictive value of changes in effective connectivity for human learning. Science 1999;283:1538-1540.

[43] Cordes D, Haughton VM, Arfanakis K, Wendt GJ, Turski PA, Moritz CH, et al. Mapping functionally related regions of brain with functional connectivity MR imaging. AJNR Am J Neuroradiol 2000;21(9):1636-44.

[44] Horwitz B, Rumsey JM, Donohue BC. Functional connectivity of the angular gyrus in normal reading and dyslexia. Proc Natl Acad Sci U S A 1998;95(15):8939-44.

[45] Pugh K, Mencl, W., Shaywitz, B., Shaywitz, S., Fulbright, R., Constable, R., Skudlarski, P., Marchione, K., Jenner, A., Fletcher, J., Liberman, A., Shankweiler, D., Katz, L., Lacadie, C., Gore,J. The angular gyrus in developmental dyslexia: Task-specific differences in functional connectivity within posterior cortex. Psychological Science 2000;11:51-56.

[46] Shaywitz SE, Shaywitz BA, Fulbright RK, Skudlarski P, Mencl WE, Constable RT, et al. Neural systems for compensation and persistence: young adult outcome of childhood reading disability. Biol Psychiatry 2003;54(1):25-33.

[47] Milne D, Syngeniotis A, Jackson G, Corballis M. Mixed lateralization of phonological assembly in developmental dyslexia. Neurocase 2002;8:205-209.

[48] Bitan T, Booth JR, Choy J, Burman DD, Gitelman DR, Mesulam MM. Shifts of effective connectivity within a language network during rhyming and spelling. J Neurosci 2005;25(22):5397-403.

[49] Richards T, Stevenson J, Crouch J, Johnson LC, Maravilla K, Stock P, et al. Tract-based spatial statistics of diffusion tensor imaging in adults with dyslexia. AJNR Am J Neuroradiol 2008;29(6):1134-9.

[50] Berninger VW, Raskind W, Richards T, Abbott R, Stock P. A multidisciplinary approach to understanding developmental dyslexia within working-memory architecture: genotypes, phenotypes, brain, and instruction. Dev Neuropsychol 2008;33(6): 707-44.

[51] Eckert MA, Leonard CM, Richards TL, Aylward EH, Thomson J, Berninger VW. Anatomical correlates of dyslexia: frontal and cerebellar findings. Brain 2003;126(Pt 2): 482-494.

[52] Richards T, Aylward E, Berninger V, Field K, Parsons A, Richards A, et al. Individual fMRI activation in orthographic mapping and morpheme mapping after orthographic or morphological spelling treatment in child dyslexics. Journal of Neurolinguistics 2006;19:56-86.

[53] Richards T, Aylward E, Raskind W, Abbott R, Field K, Parsons A, et al. Converging evidence for triple word form theory in child dyslexia. Special Issue on Brain Imaging in Developmental Neuropsychology 2006;in press.

[54] Berninger V, Richards T. Inter-relationships among behavioral markers, genes, brain and treatment in dyslexia and dysgraphia. Future Neurol 2011;5(4):597-617.

[55] Richards TL, Berninger VW. Abnormal fMRI Connectivity in Children with Dyslexia During a Phoneme Task: Before But Not After Treatment. J Neurolinguistics 2008;21(4):294-304.

[56] Heilman KM, Voeller K, Alexander AW. Developmental dyslexia: a motor-articulatory feedback hypothesis. Ann Neurol 1996;39(3):407-12.

[57] Chen SH, Desmond JE. Cerebrocerebellar networks during articulatory rehearsal and verbal working memory tasks. Neuroimage 2005;24:332-338.

[58] Koshino H, Carpenter PA, Minshew NJ, Cherkassky VL, Keller TA, Just MA. Functional connectivity in an fMRI working memory task in high-functioning autism. Neuroimage 2005;24(3):810-21.

[59] Aylward EH, Richards TL, Berninger VW, Nagy WE, Field KM, Grimme AC, et al. Instructional treatment associated with changes in brain activation in children with dyslexia. Neurology 2003;61(2):212-9.

[60] Wimberger DM, Roberts TP, Barkovich AJ, Prayer LM, Moseley ME, Kucharczyk J. Identification of 'premyelination" by diffusion-weighted MRI. J Comput Assist Tomogr 1995;19:28-33.

[61] Morgan VL, Mishra A, Newton AT, Gore JC, Ding Z. Integrating functional and diffusion magnetic resonance imaging for analysis of structure-function relationship in the human language network. PLoS One 2009;4(8):e6660.

[62] Rota G, Handjaras G, Sitaram R, Birbaumer N, Dogil G. Reorganization of functional and effective connectivity during real-time fMRI-BCI modulation of prosody processing. Brain Lang 2011;117(3):123-32.

[63] Berninger V, Niedo J. Individualizing instruction for students with oral and written language difficulties. In: Mascolo J, Flanagan D, Alfonso V, editors. Essentials of planning, selecting and tailoring intervention: Addressing the needs of unique learners. New York: Wiley; 2013. In Press

# 10

# FDG-PET Imaging in Neurodegenerative Brain Diseases

L. K. Teune, A. L. Bartels and K. L. Leenders

## 1. Introduction

### 1.1. Cerebral glucose metabolism

Increases and decreases of synaptic activity in the brain are accompanied by proportional changes in capillary perfusion and local glucose consumption. These changes in glucose consumption are the effect of changed activity or density of the afferent nerve terminals in that region. Loss of neurons may result in decreased glucose consumption in distant brain regions by deafferentiation, while also increased regional glucose consumption by increased activation of afferent neurons can occur. The PET tracer [$^{18}$F]fluorodeoxyglucose (FDG) allows the measurement of glucose consumption. FDG is a glucose analog with physiological aspects almost identical to glucose. It is transported from the blood to the brain by a carrier-mediated diffusion mechanism. FDG and glucose are phosphorylated by hexokinase as the first step of the glycolytic process. FDG differs from glucose in that a hydrogen atom replaced the hydroxyl group at the second carbon atom of the molecule. Glucose is then phosphorylated to glucose-6-$PO_4$, and continues along the glycolytic pathway for energy production. However, FDG is phosphorylated to FDG-6-$PO_4$, which is not a substrate for further metabolism and trapped in tissues. As glucose is the only source of energy for the brain it reflects the neuronal integrity of underlying brain pathology. Since FDG is a competitive substrate with glucose for both transport and phosphorylation, it is important for tracer uptake to avoid high blood glucose levels during an FDG-PET scan in subjects with diabetes.

In neurodegenerative brain diseases, specific brain regions degenerate and specific patterns of metabolic brain activity develop. This happens before clear structural changes can be detected with imaging techniques.

Measurement of glucose consumption with FDG PET imaging thus allows us to identify disease-specific cerebral metabolic brain patterns in several neurodegenerative brain diseases at an early disease stage. Since the first FDG PET study in man in 1979 (Reivich, et al. 1979) regional differences in cerebral glucose metabolism have been reported in various neurodegenerative brain diseases including parkinsonian syndromes.

## 2. Disease-specific metabolic brain patterns: Methods

Univariate methods like voxel-based statistical parametric mapping (SPM) analyses have been used to identify group differences between patients with neurodegenerative brain diseases and controls. (Eckert, et al. 2005, Juh, et al. 2004, Yong, et al. 2007).

At the University Medical Center Groningen, The Netherlands we have performed a retrospective study (Teune, et al. 2010) selecting typical patients with 7 different neurodegenerative brain diseases who had had a clinical FDG brain scan at a time point when their diagnosis was not sure yet. These patients developed in the following years the mentioned typical disease states. Images of each of the seven patient groups were separately compared to controls using a two-sample t test. At those early scans, already typical differences between patient - and control groups were found for each disease.

However, Scaled Subprofile modelling/principal component analysis (SSM/PCA), a multivariate method, not only identifies group differences, but is also able to identify relationships in relatively increased and decreased metabolic activity between different brain regions in combined samples of patients and control scans (Eidelberg. 2009, Moeller, et al. 1987). Covariance analysis techniques are considered appropriate methods to explore network activity. In the SSM, a threshold of the whole-brain maximum can be applied to remove out-of-brain voxels, followed by a log transformation. A threshold of 35% is used by the Eidelberg research group resulting in a mask of mainly grey matter (Spetsieris and Eidelberg. 2010). After removing between-subject and between-region averages, a principal component analysis (PCA) can be applied. PCA transformes a set of correlated variables into a new set of orthogonal uncorrelated variables that are called the principal components. Voxels participating in each principal component (PC) may have either a positive or a negative loading. The loadings express the covariance structure (i.e. the strength of the interaction) between the voxels that participate in the PC. They are ordered in terms of the variability they represent. That is, the first principal components represents for a single dimension (variable) the greatest amount of variability in the original dataset. Each succeeding orthogonal component accounts for as much of the remaining variability as possible. They can be very helpful in determining how many of the components are really significant and how much the data can be reduced.

In most studies, the components that together describe at least 50% of the variance are used for further analysis, but this is an arbitrary limit. To identify a covariance pattern that best discriminates a patient group from a control group, each subject's expression of the selected principal components with the lowest AIC (Akaike information criterion) value (Akaike. 1974) are entered into a stepwise regression procedure. This regression results in a linear combination of the PCs that best discriminated the two groups and is designated as the disease-specific metabolic covariance pattern.

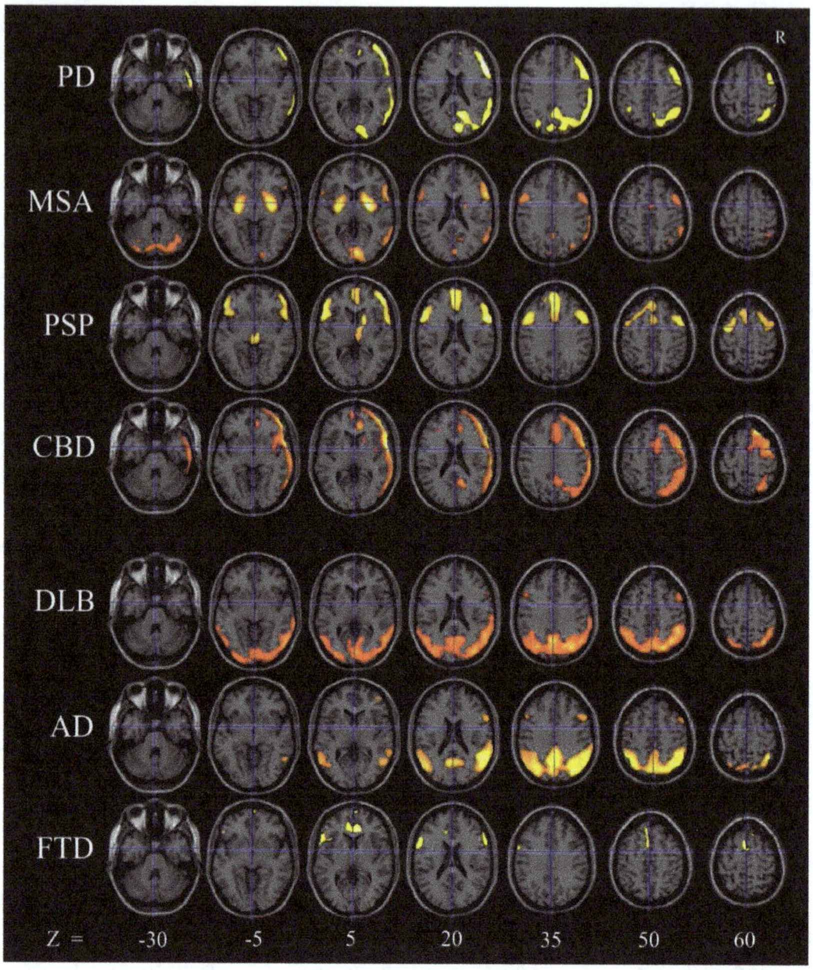


**Figure 1.** Typical cerebral metabolic patterns in neurodegenerative brain diseases. SPM (t) maps of decreased metabolic activity were overlaid on a T1 MR template thresholded at P< 0.001 with cluster cutoff of 20 voxels. Patient groups are indicated on the vertical axis and on the horizontal axis, seven transversal slices through the brain are shown. PD = Parkinson's disease: decreased metabolic activity in the contralateral to the most affected body side parieto-occipital and frontal regions; MSA = multiple system atrophy: decreased metabolic activity in bilateral putamen and cerebellum; PSP = progressive supranuclear palsy: decreased metabolic activity in the prefrontal cortex, caudate nucleus, thalamus and mesencephalon; CBD = corticobasal degeneration: decreased metabolic activity in the contralateral to the most affected body side cortical regions; DLB = dementia with Lewy bodies: decreased metabolic activity in the occipital and parieto-temporal regions. AD = Alzheimer's Disease: decreased metabolic activity in the angular gyrus and other parieto-temporal regions including precuneus extending to the posterior- and middle cingulate gyrus. FTD = frontotemporal dementia: decreased metabolic activity in the superior and inferior frontal gyrus, anterior cingulate gyrus, SMA, sensorimotor area and middle temporal gyrus. Adapted from: Teune et al. (2010) Typical cerebral metabolic patterns in neurodegenerative brain diseases. Movement Disorders. 2010;25:2395-404.

Important for its use in clinical practice is that this metabolic covariance pattern can then be applied to individual patients to test whether they express the pattern or not. Every voxel value in a subject scan is multiplied by the corresponding voxel weight in the covariance pattern, with a subsequent summation over the whole brain volume. The resulting subject score captures to what extent a subject expresses the covariance pattern.

## 3. Disease-specific metabolic brain patterns in patients with parkinsonism

### 3.1. Parkinson's disease

Parkinson's disease (PD) is characterized by bradykinesia, rigidity, sometimes rest tremor and postural instability. A disturbed $\alpha$-synuclein protein forming so-called Lewy bodies seems to play a causal role, which was a reason to designate PD as a $\alpha$-synucleinopathy. The main pathophysiological changes result from degeneration of catecholaminergic, especially dopaminergic cells in brainstem regions.

A characteristic metabolic covariance pattern has been identified in PD patients (PD-related pattern, PDRP) showing regionally relatively increased metabolism in the globus pallidus and putamen, thalamus, pons and cerebellum and relatively decreased metabolism in the lateral frontal, premotor and parietal association areas (Ma, et al. 2007) Network expression in PD patients also increases linearly with disease progression(Huang, et al. 2007b). Tang et al. tried to study network changes in the PD-related motor pattern before symptom onset by studying 15 hemiparkinsonian patients and focusing mainly on the "presymptomatic" hemisphere. They conclude that abnormal PDRP activity antecedes the appearance of motor signs by approximately 2 years (Tang, et al. 2010a). However, this needs to be proven in future research in true presymptomatic patients.

### 3.2. Parkinson's disease and metabolic brain patterns related to specific symptoms

In addition to motor symptoms, cognitive dysfunction is also common in PD, especially executive and visuospatial dysfunction. FDG-PET studies have been performed to study these specific symptoms and their relations with neural network pathophysiology. The Eidelberg research group has shown PD subclassifications related to specific symptoms. Network analysis with the SSM/PCA approach detected a significant covariance pattern in non-demented PD patients that correlated with memory and executive functioning tasks. The expression of this PD-related cognitive pattern (PDCP) in individual patients correlated with severity of cognitive dysfunction(Huang, et al. 2007a).

Alterations in neuropsychological test results in advanced PD were found to correlate with decreases in glucose metabolism in the dorsolateral prefrontal cortex (DLPFC), lateral orbitofrontal cortex (LOFC) ventral and dorsal cingulum (v/dACC) and in Broca area (Kalbe, et al. 2009). In the study of Kalbe et al, PD patients with deep brain stimulation in the subthalamic nucleus (STN-DBS) showed cognitive decline that correlated with decrease in glucose metabolism in these areas. In another study in STN-DBS treated patients, STN DBS was found to activate glucose metabolism in the frontal limbic and associative territory (Hilker, et al. 2004). Interestingly, cortical areas that show hypometabolism in patients with depression (Mayberg HS. 1994) are similar to the regions that show restored glucose metabolism after STN DBS. This finding agrees with the clinical observation that PD-related depression tends to improve after STN DBS.

Mure et al. identified a spatial covariance pattern associated with Parkinson tremor which was characterized by covarying increases in the cerebellum/dentate nucleus and primary cortex and to a minor degree in the caudate/putamen (Mure, et al. 2011).

Hallucinations in PD have been related to relative frontal hypermetabolism compared to PD patients without hallucinations(Nagano-Saito, et al. 2004). However, another study showed hypometabolism in occipitotemporoparietal regions in PD patients with hallucinations, sparing the occipital pole, while no significant increase in regional glucose metabolism was detected (Boecker, et al. 2007). Interestingly, in patients with dementia with Lewy bodies (DLB), who also suffer from hallucinations, glucose metabolism was also decreased in occipitoparietal regions, however without sparing of the occipital pole (see DLB section).

### 3.3. Multiple system atrophy

Multiple system atrophy is a sporadic neurodegenerative brain disease which affects both men and women and generally starts in the sixth decade of life. The main clinical features are parkinsonism, autonomic failure, cerebellar ataxia, and pyramidal signs in any combination. However, two major motor presentations can be distinguished. Parkinsonian features predominate in 80% of patients (MSA-P subtype) and cerebellar ataxia is the main motor feature in 20% of patients (MSA-C subtype) ((Gilman, et al. 2008, Wenning, et al. 1997)

In MSA-P the striatonigral system is the main site of pathology but less severe degeneration can be widespread and normally includes the olivopontocerebellar system. In MSA-C pathological changes are mainly seen in the olivopontocerebellar system and involvement of striatum and substantia nigra are less severe (Wenning, et al. 1997). The discovery of glial cytoplasmic inclusions in MSA brains highlighted the unique glial pathology as biological hallmark of the disease. Their distribution selectively involves basal ganglia, supplementary and primary motor cortex, the reticular formation and pontocerebellar system. Glial cytoplasmic inclusions contain besides classical cytoskeletal antigens also $\alpha$-synuclein, which is a presynaptic protein present in Lewy Bodies, and this accumulation seems to play a central part not only in MSA but also in other $\alpha$-synucleinopathies such as PD and DLB.

Disease-related metabolic patterns were also present in MSA consisting of hypometabolism in putamen and cerebellum in MSA (Eckert, et al. 2008). Poston et al. found that differences in expression of the MSA-related pattern correlated with clinical disability (Poston, et al. 2012).

### 3.4. Progressive supranuclear palsy

The clinical picture of progressive supranuclear palsy (PSP) has been first described by Steele, Richardson and Olszewski (Steele JC, Richardson J,Olszewski J. 1964) and is characterized by progressive parkinsonism, early gait and balance impairment, vertical gaze palsy and more profound frontal cognitive disturbances. PSP is one of several neurodegenerative diseases characterised by accumulation of hyperphosphorylated tau (tauopathy), forming abnormal filamentous inclusions in neurons and glia in the precentral and postcentral cortical areas but also in the thalamus, subthalamic nucleus, red nucleus and substantia nigra. Other neurodegenerative brain diseases which show disturbances in tau protein handling are corticobasal degeneration (CBD) and frontotemporal dementia (FTD) but there is also overlap in pathology with Alzheimer's disease (AD).

However the metabolic brain patterns in these tauopathies are quite different. The covariance pattern of PSP consists of decreased metabolism in the prefrontal cortex, frontal eye fields, caudate nuclei, medial thalamus and upper brainstem (Eckert, et al. 2008). Brain stem atrophy and atrophy of the medial frontal cortical regions have also been reported in histopathological studies (Hauw, et al. 1994).

### 3.5. Corticobasal degeneration

The most striking features of patients with corticobasal degeneration (CBD) include marked asymmetrical parkinsonism and apraxia but also postural instability, limb dystonia, cortical sensory loss, dementia and the alien limb phenomenon. CBD is one of the tauopathies and clinical diagnosis is complicated by both the variability of presentation of true CBD and the syndromes that look alike but are caused by other tauopathies with parkinsonism like PSP or FTD (Josephs, et al. 2006). However with functional neuroimaging a clear distinction can be made. In CBD a typical pattern of hypometabolism is seen in cortical regions contralateral to the affected body side, including parieto-temporal regions, prefrontal cortex and motor cortex. Furthermore, a decrease can be found in the contralateral caudate nucleus, putamen and thalamus (Eckert, et al. 2005, Teune, et al. 2010). No covariance pattern has been described using the SSM/PCA technique in CBD.

## 4. Disease-specific metabolic brain patterns in the differential diagnosis of individual patients with parkinsonism

Interestingly, Tang and co-workers studied the potential role of FDG PET in the individual diagnosis of 167 patients who had parkinsonian features but uncertain clinical diagnosis (Tang, et al. 2010b) After FDG PET imaging, patients were assessed by blinded movement disorders specialists for a mean of 2.6 years before a final clinical diagnosis was made (gold standard). SSM/PCA analysis can quantify the expression of an obtained covariance pattern in each subject which allows assessing the expression of a given pattern on a single case basis. Using this automated image-based classification procedure and the previously defined disease related covariance patterns in PD, MSA and PSP, individual patients were differentiated with high specificity.

However, blinded, prospective imaging studies (ideally involving multiple centers, a larger validation group, repeat imaging, and more extensive post-mortem confirmation) are needed to establish the accuracy and precision of this pattern-based categorisation procedure. These studies are currently undertaken.

For routine clinical practice, this knowledge of disease specific patterns of regional metabolic activity in neurodegenerative brain diseases can be a valuable aid in the differential diagnosis of individual patients, especially at an early disease stage.

# 5. Disease-specific metabolic brain patterns in dementia

## 5.1. Alzheimer's disease

Alzheimer's disease (AD) is a progressive neurodegenerative brain disease accounting for 50-60% of cases of dementia. AD is characterized by a severe decline in episodic memory together with general cognitive symptoms such as impaired judgement, decision making and orientation (McKhann, et al. 1984). A correct clinical diagnosis can be difficult, especially in early disease stages or in patients with for example comorbid depression, high education or young age (Bohnen, et al. 2012). FDG-PET imaging can be used to assist in the differential diagnosis, because for different dementia syndromes, a separate pattern of hypometabolism can be found. In Alzheimer's disease (AD), decline of FDG uptake in posterior cingulate, temporoparietal and prefrontal association cortex was related to dementia severity (Herholz, et al. 2002). Foster et al used visual interpretation of an automated three-dimensional stereotactic surface projection technique of patients with AD and FTD. They showed that visual interpretation of FDG-PET scans after training is more reliable and accurate in distinguishing FTD from AD than clinical methods alone (Foster, et al. 2007).

Although multivariate analytical techniques might identify diagnostic patterns that are not captured by univariate methods, they have rarely been used to study neural correlates of Alzheimer's Disease or cognitive impairment. Because cognitive processes are the result of integrated activity in networks rather than activity of any one area in isolation, functional connectivity can be better captured by multivariate methods. A study from Habeck et al. examined the efficacy of multivariate and univariate analytical methods and concluded that multivariate analysis might be more sensitive than univariate analysis for the diagnosis of early Alzheimer's disease (Habeck, et al. 2008).

Scarmeas et al. were the first to derive an AD related covariance pattern using $H_2{}^{15}O$ to measure brain perfusion (Scarmeas, et al. 2004). It consisted of relatively increased perfusion in the bilateral insula, lingual gyri and cuneus with bilaterally decreased flow in bilateral inferior parietal lobule and cingulate in AD patients. However, using this PET tracer they found a sensitivity of 76-94% and a specificity of 63-81% with considerable overlap in pattern expression among AD patients and controls. Therefore they concluded that the derived $H_2{}^{15}O$ pattern cannot be used as a sufficient diagnostic test in clinical settings. Specific FDG covariance patterns to distinguish early AD-related cognitive decline using multivariate methods have yet to be specified.

## 5.2. Frontotemporal dementia

Frontotemporal dementia (FTD) is one of the neurodegenerative diseases commonly mistaken for AD. FTD patients do not have a true amnestic syndrome but can present with either gradual and progressive changes in behaviour, or gradual and progressive language dysfunction. Gross examination of the post-mortem brain from a patient with FTD usually reveals frontal or temporal lobar atrophy or both, but the distribution or severity of brain atrophy are not specific for a particular neurodegenerative brain disease. Jeong et al. and Diehl-Schmid et al.

analysed FDG-PET scans of FTD patients on a voxel-by-voxel basis using Statistical Parametric Mapping (SPM). They found hypometabolism depending on disease stage in the frontal lobe, parietal and temporal cortices (Diehl-Schmid, et al. 2007, Jeong, et al. 2005).

### 5.3. Dementia with Lewy Bodies

The clinical overlap of dementia and parkinsonism is highlighted in Dementia with Lewy Bodies (DLB). These patients show besides dementia extrapyramidal motor symptoms and marked neuropsychiatric disturbances including visual hallucinations, depression, variability in arousal and attention (McKeith. 2006). Consistent observation of a metabolic reduction in the medial occipital cortex in DLB patients (Minoshima, et al. 2001, Teune, et al. 2010) using FDG-PET imaging suggests the use of FDG-PET in the differential diagnosis of AD and DLB and of PD and DLB. Minoshima et al. found that the presence of occipital hypometabolism distinguished DLB from AD with 90% sensitivity and 80% specificity when using post-mortem diagnosis as the gold standard diagnosis (Minoshima, et al. 2001).

## 6. Disease-specific metabolic brain patterns in hyperkinetic movement disorders

### 6.1. Huntington's disease

Huntington's disease (HD) is characterized by progressive dementia and chorea, starting around 30-40 years of age. HD is caused by a dominantly inherited CAG repeat expansion mutation that generates lengthening of the protein huntingtin, with size-dependent neuro-toxicity. Several PET studies have shown hypometabolism in the caudate nucleus, both in symptomatic and asymptomatic mutation carriers (Grafton, et al. 1992) (Antonini A., et al. 1996) In asymptomatic carriers, metabolic decreases were also significantly associated with the CAG repeat number (Antonini A., et al. 1996). Furthermore, it was found that FDG uptake in the caudate nucleus provided a predictive measure for time of onset of the disease, in addition to the mutation size (Ciarmiello A., et al. 2012).

Another study applied network analysis of FDG-PET scans in presymptomatic mutation carriers (Feigin, et al. 2001). They found a HD related metabolic covariance pattern (HDRP) characterized by caudate and putamenal hypometabolism, but also including mediotemporal reductions as well as relative increases in occipital regions. Disturbances of these striatotem-poral projections may underlie aspects of the psychiatric and cognitive abnormalities that occur in the earliest stages of HD, before the onset of motor signs (Cummings JL. 1995).

### 6.2. Dystonia

Dystonia is a movement disorder characterized by involuntary, sustained muscle contractions causing twisting movements and abnormal postures. The most common forms of primary torsion dystonia (PTD) are DYT1 and DYT6, both caused by autosomal inherited mutations with a reduced penetrance.

Functional neuroimaging techniques have been applied in different dystonic disorders including primary generalized dystonia, mainly DYT1 and DYT6 and dopa-responsive dystonia, as well as focal dystonic syndromes such as torticollis, writer's cramp and blepharospasm. A common finding is abnormality of the basal ganglia, cerebellum and associated outflow pathways to sensorimotor cortex and other regions involved with motor performance. However, controversial results have been found in imaging dystonias, partly attributed to methodological differences but also to the heterogeneity of the dystonias. Using the SSM/PCA approach a reproducible pattern of abnormal regional glucose utilization in two independent cohorts of DYT1 carriers have been found (Eidelberg D. 1998)(Trost M., et al. 2002).

This torsion-dystonia related metabolic pattern is characterized by increases in the posterior putamen/globus pallidus, cerebellum and SMA. Interestingly, also in clinically non-manifesting mutation carriers this pattern was found, suggesting a cerebral "vulnerability to develop dystonia" network change. Also in manifesting and non-manifesting DYT 6 carriers abnormal network activity has been identified. A difference between DYT1 and DYT6 metabolic patterns can be seen in the putamen, where glucose metabolism is increased in DYT1 and decreased in DYT6, possibly do to cell loss in DYT6. Furthermore, the cerebellum shows increased activity in DYT1 and normal activity in DYT6 (Carbon M., et al. 2004).

The TDRP network is not expressed in patients with Dopa-responsive dystonia (DRD) (Trost M., et al. 2002).

DRD is characterized by an early onset of dystonic symptoms and later appearance of parkinsonian symptoms. A defining feature is a marked and sustained response to low doses of levodopa, suggesting that the lesion may be functional in the presynaptic dopaminergic system rather than anatomical. The DRD related metabolic pattern is characterized by relative increases in the dorsal midbrain, cerebellar vermis,and SMA, assiocated with covarying decreases in putamen, lateral premotor and motor cortical regions (Asanuma, et al. 2005b). This DRD related pattern is not apparent in DYT 1 and 6 carriers supporting the hypothesis that the pathophysiology of DRD differs from that of other forms of dystonia. They also found that the Parkinson-related metabolic pattern is not apparent in DRD patients. Thus FDG-PET can be useful to distinguish PD related dystonia from dopa-responsive dystonia with parkinsonism (Asanuma, et al. 2005a).

### 6.3. Gilles de la Tourette

Tourette syndrome is characterized by the presence of chronic motor and vocal tics that develop before the age of 18. Comorbid behavioural abnormalities are common in Tourette syndrome, most notably obsessive-compulsive disorder and attention deficit/hyperactivity disorder (Lebowitz, et al. 2012). The neurophysiology remains poorly understood with varying and inconsistent neuropathological and neuroimaging findings, possibly due to the clinical heterogeneity of the disorder. Pourfar et al. identified a Tourette syndrome related pattern characterized by reduced metabolic activity of the striatum and orbitofrontal cortex associated with relatively increased metabolic activity in the premotor cortex and cerebellum. A second metabolic brain pattern was found in patients with Tourette syndrome and obsessive compulsive disorder characterized by reduced activity in the anterior cingulate and dorsolateral prefrontal cortex and relative increases in primary motor cortex and precuneus. Subject expression correlated with symptom severity. These findings suggest that the different clinical manifestations of the Tourette syndrome are associated with different abnormal brain networks (Pourfar, et al. 2011).

## 7. Conclusion

FDG-PET imaging is increasingly available for routine clinical practice and has remained the only available radiotracer to detect accurately and reliably the cerebral glucose metabolism. As glucose is the only source of energy for the brain it reflects the energy needs of underlying brain neuronal systems. The SSM/PCA method can identify relationships in relatively increased and decreased metabolic activity between different brain regions in combined samples of patients and controls. The expression of an obtained covariance pattern can be quantified in an individual patient and this resulting subject score captures to what extent a patient expresses the covariance patterns. The disease-related metabolic brain patterns can therefore be a valuable aid in the early differential diagnosis of individual patients with neurodegenerative brain diseases.

## Author details

L. K. Teune, A. L. Bartels* and K. L. Leenders

*Address all correspondence to: a.l.bartels@umcg.nl

Department of Neurology, University Medical Center Groningen, The Netherlands

## References

[1] Akaike, H. A new look at the statistical model identification. A New Look at the Statistical Model Identification (1974)., 1974, 716-23.

[2] Antonini, A, Leenders, K. L, Spiegel, R, Meier, D, Vontobel, P, Weigell-weber, M, et al. Striatal glucose metabolism and dopamine D2 receptor binding in asymptomatic gene carriers and patients with huntington's disease. (1996).

[3] Asanuma, K, Carbon-correll, M, & Eidelberg, D. Neuroimaging in human dystonia. (2005a).

[4] Asanuma, K, Ma, Y, Huang, C, Carbon-correll, M, Edwards, C, Raymond, D, et al. The metabolic pathology of dopa-responsive dystonia. (2005b).

[5] Boecker, H, Ceballos-baumann, A. O, Volk, D, Conrad, B, Forstl, H, & Haussermann, P. Metabolic alterations in patients with parkinson disease and visual hallucinations. Arch Neurol (2007)., 64, 984-8.

[6] Bohnen, N. I. Djang DSW, Herholz K, Anzai Y, Minoshima S. Effectiveness and safety of 18F-FDG PET in the evaluation of dementia: A review of the recent literature. Journal of Nuclear Medicine (2012)., 53, 59-71.

[7] Carbon, M, Trost, M, Ghilardi, M. F, & Eidelberg, D. Abnormal brain networks in primary torsion dystonia. (2004).

[8] Ciarmiello, A, Giovacchini, G, Orobello, S, Bruselli, L, Elifani, F, & Squitieri, F. F-FDG PET uptake in the pre-huntington disease caudate affects the time-to-onset independently of CAG expansion size. (2012).

[9] Cummings, J. L. Behavioral and psychiatric symptoms associated with huntington's disease. (1995).

[10] Diehl-schmid, J, Grimmer, T, Drzezga, A, Bornschein, S, Riemenschneider, M, Forstl, H, et al. Decline of cerebral glucose metabolism in frontotemporal dementia: A longitudinal 18F-FDG-PET-study. Neurobiol Aging (2007)., 28, 42-50.

[11] Eckert, T, Barnes, A, Dhawan, V, Frucht, S, Gordon, M. F, Feigin, A. S, et al. FDG PET in the differential diagnosis of parkinsonian disorders. Neuroimage (2005). , 26, 912-21.

[12] Eckert, T, Tang, C, Ma, Y, Brown, N, Lin, T, Frucht, S, et al. Abnormal metabolic networks in atypical parkinsonism. Mov Disord (2008).

[13] Eidelberg, D. Abnormal brain networks in DYT1 dystonia. (1998).

[14] Eidelberg, D. Metabolic brain networks in neurodegenerative disorders: A functional imaging approach. Trends Neurosci (2009)., 32, 548-57.

[15] Feigin, A, Leenders, K. L, Moeller, J. R, Missimer, J, Kuenig, G, Spetsieris, P, et al. Metabolic network abnormalities in early huntington's disease: An [(18)F]FDG PET study. J Nucl Med (2001)., 42, 1591-5.

[16] Foster, N. L, Heidebrink, J. L, Clark, C. M, Jagust, W. J, Arnold, S. E, Barbas, N. R, et al. FDG-PET improves accuracy in distinguishing frontotemporal dementia and alzheimer's disease. Brain (2007)., 130, 2616-35.

[17] Gilman, S, Wenning, G. K, Low, P. A, Brooks, D. J, Mathias, C. J, Trojanowski, J. Q, et al. Second consensus statement on the diagnosis of multiple system atrophy. Neurology (2008)., 71, 670-6.

[18] Grafton, S. T, Mazziotta, J. C, & Pahl, J. J. St George-Hyslop P, Haines JL, Gusella J, et al. Serial changes of cerebral glucose metabolism and caudate size in persons at risk for huntington's disease. (1992).

[19] Habeck, C, Foster, N. L, Perneczky, R, Kurz, A, Alexopoulos, P, Koeppe, R. A, et al. Multivariate and univariate neuroimaging biomarkers of alzheimer's disease. Neuroimage (2008)., 40, 1503-15.

[20] Hauw, J. J, Daniel, S. E, Dickson, D, Horoupian, D. S, Jellinger, K, Lantos, P. L, et al. Preliminary NINDS neuropathologic criteria for steele-richardson-olszewski syndrome (progressive supranuclear palsy). Neurology (1994)., 44, 2015-9.

[21] Herholz, K, Salmon, E, Perani, D, Baron, J. C, Holthoff, V, Frolich, L, et al. Discrimination between alzheimer dementia and controls by automated analysis of multicenter FDG PET. Neuroimage (2002)., 17, 302-16.

[22] Hilker, R, Voges, J, Weisenbach, S, Kalbe, E, Burghaus, L, Ghaemi, M, et al. Subthalamic nucleus stimulation restores glucose metabolism in associative and limbic cortices and in cerebellum: Evidence from a FDG-PET study in advanced parkinson's disease. J Cereb Blood Flow Metab (2004)., 24, 7-16.

[23] Huang, C, Eidelberg, D, Habeck, C, Moeller, J, Svensson, L, Tarabula, T, et al. Imaging markers of mild cognitive impairment: Multivariate analysis of CBF SPECT. Neurobiol Aging (2007a)., 28, 1062-9.

[24] Huang, C, Tang, C, Feigin, A, Lesser, M, Ma, Y, Pourfar, M, et al. Changes in network activity with the progression of parkinson's disease. Brain (2007b)., 130, 1834-46.

[25] Jeong, Y, Cho, S. S, Park, J. M, Kang, S. J, Lee, J. S, Kang, E, et al. F-FDG PET findings in frontotemporal dementia: An SPM analysis of 29 patients. J Nucl Med (2005)., 46, 233-9.

[26] Josephs, K. A, Petersen, R. C, Knopman, D. S, Boeve, B. F, Whitwell, J. L, Duffy, J. R, et al. Clinicopathologic analysis of frontotemporal and corticobasal degenerations and PSP. Neurology (2006)., 66, 41-8.

[27] Juh, R, Kim, J, Moon, D, Choe, B, & Suh, T. Different metabolic patterns analysis of parkinsonism on the 18F-FDG PET. Eur J Radiol (2004)., 51, 223-33.

[28] Kalbe, E, Voges, J, Weber, T, Haarer, M, Baudrexel, S, Klein, J. C, et al. Frontal FDG-PET activity correlates with cognitive outcome after STN-DBS in parkinson disease. Neurology (2009)., 72, 42-9.

[29] Lebowitz, E. R, Motlagh, M. G, Katsovich, L, King, R. A, Lombroso, P. J, Grantz, H, et al. Tourette syndrome in youth with and without obsessive compulsive disorder and attention deficit hyperactivity disorder. (2012).

[30] Ma, Y, Tang, C, Spetsieris, P. G, Dhawan, V, & Eidelberg, D. Abnormal metabolic network activity in parkinson's disease: Test-retest reproducibility. Journal of cerebral blood flow and metabolism : official journal of the International Society of Cerebral Blood Flow and Metabolism (2007)., 27, 597-605.

[31] Mayberg, H. S. Frontal lobe dysfunction in secondary depression. (1994).

[32] Mckeith, I. G. Consensus guidelines for the clinical and pathologic diagnosis of dementia with lewy bodies (DLB): Report of the consortium on DLB international workshop. J Alzheimers Dis (2006)., 9, 417-23.

[33] Mckhann, G, Drachman, D, Folstein, M, Katzman, R, Price, D, & Stadlan, E. M. Clinical diagnosis of alzheimer's disease: Report of the NINCDS-ADRDA work group under the auspices of department of health and human services task force on alzheimer's disease 35. Neurology (1984)., 34, 939-44.

[34] Minoshima, S, Foster, N. L, Sima, A. A, Frey, K. A, Albin, R. L, & Kuhl, D. E. Alzheimer's disease versus dementia with lewy bodies: Cerebral metabolic distinction with autopsy confirmation. Ann Neurol (2001)., 50, 358-65.

[35] Moeller, J. R, Strother, S. C, Sidtis, J. J, & Rottenberg, D. A. Scaled subprofile model: A statistical approach to the analysis of functional patterns in positron emission tomographic data. J Cereb Blood Flow Metab (1987)., 7, 649-58.

[36] Mure, H, Hirano, S, Tang, C. C, Isaias, I. U, Antonini, A, Ma, Y, et al. Parkinson's disease tremor-related metabolic network: Characterization, progression, and treatment effects. Neuroimage (2011)., 54, 1244-53.

[37] Nagano-saito, A, Washimi, Y, Arahata, Y, Iwai, K, Kawatsu, S, Ito, K, et al. Visual hallucination in parkinson's disease with FDG PET. Mov Disord (2004)., 19, 801-6.

[38] Poston, K. L, Tang, C. C, Eckert, T, Dhawan, V, Frucht, S, Vonsattel, J, et al. Network correlates of disease severity in multiple system atrophy. Neurology (2012). , 78, 1237-44.

[39] Pourfar, M, Feigin, A, Tang, C. C, Carbon-correll, M, Bussa, M, Budman, C, et al. Abnormal metabolic brain networks in tourette syndrome. Neurology (2011). , 76, 944-52.

[40] Reivich, M, Kuhl, D, Wolf, A, Greenberg, J, Phelps, M, Ido, T, et al. The [18F]fluorodeoxyglucose method for the measurement of local cerebral glucose utilization in man. Circ Res (1979)., 44, 127-37.

[41] Scarmeas, N, Habeck, C. G, Zarahn, E, Anderson, K. E, Park, A, Hilton, J, et al. Covariance PET patterns in early alzheimer's disease and subjects with cognitive impairment but no dementia: Utility in group discrimination and correlations with functional performance. Neuroimage (2004)., 23, 35-45.

[42] Spetsieris, P. G, & Eidelberg, D. Scaled subprofile modeling of resting state imaging data in parkinson's disease: Methodological issues. Neuroimage (2010).

[43] Steele, J. C, Richardson, J, & Olszewski, J. Progressive supranuclear palsy: A heterogeneous degeneration involving the brain stem, basal ganglia and cerebellum with vertical gaze and pseudobulbar palsy, nuchal dystonia and dementia. Archives of Neurology (1964)., 10, 333-59.

[44] Tang, C. C, Poston, K. L, Dhawan, V, & Eidelberg, D. Abnormalities in metabolic network activity precede the onset of motor symptoms in parkinson's disease. J Neurosci (2010a)., 30, 1049-56.

[45] Tang, C. C, Poston, K. L, Eckert, T, Feigin, A, Frucht, S, Gudesblatt, M, et al. Differential diagnosis of parkinsonism: A metabolic imaging study using pattern analysis. Lancet Neurol (2010b)., 9, 149-58.

[46] Teune, L. K, Bartels, A. L, De Jong, B. M, Willemsen, A. T, Eshuis, S. A, De Vries, J. J, et al. Typical cerebral metabolic patterns in neurodegenerative brain diseases. Mov Disord (2010)., 25, 2395-404.

[47] Trost, M, Carbon, M, Edwards, C, Ma, Y, Raymond, D, Mentis, M. J, et al. Primary dystonia: Is abnormal functional brain architecture linked to genotype? (2002).

[48] Wenning, G. K, & Tison, F. Ben Shlomo Y, Daniel SE, Quinn NP. Multiple system atrophy: A review of 203 pathologically proven cases. Mov Disord (1997). , 12, 133-47.

[49] Yong, S. W, Yoon, J. K, An, Y. S, & Lee, P. H. A comparison of cerebral glucose metabolism in parkinson's disease, parkinson's disease dementia and dementia with lewy bodies. Eur J Neurol (2007)., 14, 1357-62.

# Permissions

All chapters in this book were first published by InTech Open; hereby published with permission under the Creative Commons Attribution License or equivalent. Every chapter published in this book has been scrutinized by our experts. Their significance has been extensively debated. The topics covered herein carry significant findings which will fuel the growth of the discipline. They may even be implemented as practical applications or may be referred to as a beginning point for another development.

The contributors of this book come from diverse backgrounds, making this book a truly international effort. This book will bring forth new frontiers with its revolutionizing research information and detailed analysis of the nascent developments around the world.

We would like to thank all the contributing authors for lending their expertise to make the book truly unique. They have played a crucial role in the development of this book. Without their invaluable contributions this book wouldn't have been possible. They have made vital efforts to compile up to date information on the varied aspects of this subject to make this book a valuable addition to the collection of many professionals and students.

This book was conceptualized with the vision of imparting up-to-date information and advanced data in this field. To ensure the same, a matchless editorial board was set up. Every individual on the board went through rigorous rounds of assessment to prove their worth. After which they invested a large part of their time researching and compiling the most relevant data for our readers.

The editorial board has been involved in producing this book since its inception. They have spent rigorous hours researching and exploring the diverse topics which have resulted in the successful publishing of this book. They have passed on their knowledge of decades through this book. To expedite this challenging task, the publisher supported the team at every step. A small team of assistant editors was also appointed to further simplify the editing procedure and attain best results for the readers.

Apart from the editorial board, the designing team has also invested a significant amount of their time in understanding the subject and creating the most relevant covers. They scrutinized every image to scout for the most suitable representation of the subject and create an appropriate cover for the book.

The publishing team has been an ardent support to the editorial, designing and production team. Their endless efforts to recruit the best for this project, has resulted in the accomplishment of this book. They are a veteran in the field of academics and their pool of knowledge is as vast as their experience in printing. Their expertise and guidance has proved useful at every step. Their uncompromising quality standards have made this book an exceptional effort. Their encouragement from time to time has been an inspiration for everyone.

The publisher and the editorial board hope that this book will prove to be a valuable piece of knowledge for researchers, students, practitioners and scholars across the globe.

# List of Contributors

**P. Read Montague, Ann H. Harvey and Ulrich Kirk**
Virginia Tech Carilion Research Institute, Virginia, USA

**Vincent Lai**
The University of Hong Kong, Hong Kong

**D.Y. Phua**
Nanyang Business School, Nanyang Technological University, Singapore
Culture Science Institute, Nanyang Technological University, Singapore

**G.I. Christopoulos**
Nanyang Business School, Nanyang Technological University, Singapore
Culture Science Institute, Nanyang Technological University, Singapore
Virginia Tech Carilion Research Institute, VA, USA

**Richard S. Pond, Jr., Stephanie B. Richman, David S. Chester and C. Nathan DeWall**
University of Kentucky, United States of America

**Kirsten G. Volz**
Werner Reichardt Centre for Integrative Neuroscience, Tuebingen, Germany

**Gerd Gigerenzer**
Max Planck Institute for Human Development, Berlin, Germany

**Victoria A.L. Mosher and Bradley G. Goodyear**
University of Calgary, Canada

**Einat Liebenthal**
University of Calgary, Canada
Medical College of Wisconsin, USA

**Long Jiang Zhang**
Department of Medical Imaging, Nanjing University College of Clinical Medicine, Nanjing, China

**Guang Ming Lu and Hui Mao**
Department of Radiology, Emory University School of Medicine, Atlanta, Georgia, USA

**Mirko Avesani and Antonio Fiaschi**
University of Verona, Department of Neurological, Neuropsychological, Morphological and Movement Sciences, Italy

**Silvia Giacopuzzi**
University of Verona, Department of Life and Reproduction Sciences, Italy

**Todd L. Richards**
Department of Radiology, University of Washington Medical Center, Seattle, WA, USA

**Virginia W. Berninger**
Department of Educational Psychology, University of Washington, Seattle, WA, USA

**L. K. Teune, A. L. Bartels and K. L. Leenders**
Department of Neurology, University Medical Center Groningen, The Netherlands

# Index


**A**

Acute Ischemia, 15-17, 166

Acute Stroke Imaging, 15, 20-21, 166

Allais Paradox, 98-101, 120-121

Altruism, 47-48, 63-64

Amygdala, 35-36, 43-44, 51-56, 69-74, 79-80, 85-88, 106-107, 116-117

Analgesic Effect, 67-68

Angular Gyrus, 127-130, 139-140, 158-161, 204, 208-209, 212-213, 218, 222

Anterior Insula, 61-62, 69-70, 73-82, 108-109

Arterial Blood, 16-17

Arterial Protons, 18-19

Arterial Spin Labeling, 16-19, 22-23

**B**

Basal Skull, 16-17

Bayesian Decision Theory, 96-97, 102-103, 110-111

Behavioral Economics, 2-3, 93, 96-97, 100-105, 112-115

Bilateral Caudate, 2-3

Biological Motion, 35-38, 55-56

Brain Mechanisms, 1, 45-46, 83-84

Brain Pathology, 135-136, 220

Brain Tumor, 124-126, 147-148, 164-165

Bulk-blood Correction, 22-23

**C**

Cardiac Pain, 65-66

Cerebral Blood Flow, 20-21, 26-33, 168-169, 171, 174-175, 195, 209

Cerebral Blood Volume, 18-21

Chronic Pain, 65-66, 83-84, 89-92

Chronic Stroke, 20-21

Cognitive Functions, 34, 124-126, 135-136, 141-142, 170

Cognitive Neuroscience, 49-58, 87-88, 93-97, 104-105, 110-111, 116-123

Computed Tomography, 15, 24-25, 166, 168, 188-189, 198, 201

**D**

Diffusion Pulse, 16-17

Diffusion Tensor Imaging, 133-134, 147-148, 152-155, 160-165, 203, 205-206, 216, 218

Dorsal Portion, 71-72

Dorsolateral Prefrontal Cortex, 8-11, 223, 229

**E**

Echo-planar Imaging, 18-19, 30-31

Endogenous Method, 16-17

Epilepsy, 124-128, 135-148, 160-161, 167-175, 177-178, 180, 182, 185, 188, 190-191, 193-202

Epileptic Foci, 137-138, 194, 198-199, 201

**F**

Functional Brain Imaging, 4-5, 81-82, 145-146

Functional Mapping, 124-126, 141-142

Functional Neuroimaging, 67-72, 81-82, 118-119, 141-142, 147-148, 167, 198, 225, 228

Fusiform Gyrus, 67-68, 127-128, 213

**G**

Glial Cell, 16-17, 156-157

Glioma, 127-128, 131-132, 137-138

Glutamate, 149, 154-157, 164-165, 202

Glutamine, 149, 154-157, 164-165

**H**

Hemodynamic State, 16-17

Hepatic Encephalopathy, 15, 149-152, 154, 156, 158-166

**I**

Intracarotid Injection, 125-126, 147-148

Intracerebral Hemorrhage, 15, 26-29, 166

Intracranial Hemorrhage, 15, 166

Ischemic Brain Tissue, 18-19

Ischemic Infarction, 15, 166

**L**

Language Asymmetry, 125-128

Language Processing, 135-140, 203-204, 206

Lateralization Indices, 127-130

## M

Magnetic Resonance Imaging, 14-15, 24-34, 55-58, 60, 67-68, 81-82, 87-90, 116-117, 124, 141-149, 152, 156, 158-160, 162-166, 171, 200-202, 204, 208, 215-217, 219

Mean Transit Time, 18-21, 28-29

Membrane Ionic Homeostasis, 16-17

Middle Temporal Gyrus, 127-128, 181, 187, 206, 222

Motor Cortex, 125-126, 135-138, 141-144, 180, 188, 191, 202, 224-225, 229

## N

Neural Mechanisms, 4-5, 37-38, 51-58, 69-70, 79-80, 89-90, 122-123, 158-159

Neurologic Deficit, 20-21

Neuronal Activity, 135-136, 147-148, 158-159, 172-173

Neuroscience, 1, 34-37, 39, 41-59, 67-68, 83-90, 93-99, 102-105, 110-123, 204

## P

Parahippocampal Gyrus, 2-3, 181

Penumbral Flow, 20-23, 32-33

Penumbral Tissue, 16-17

Perfusion Parameters, 18-21

Perfusion Pressures, 15, 166

Perfusion-weighted Imaging, 15-17, 20-21, 30-31, 166

Periaqueductal Gray, 65-66

Positron Emission Tomography, 20-21, 30-33, 124, 169, 199, 201-202

Presurgical Mapping, 124-127, 129, 131, 133, 135-137, 139, 141, 143-147

## R

Recognition Heuristic, 96-97

Recognition Memory, 53-54, 65-66

Retrosplenial Cortex, 2-3

## S

Semantic Word Decision, 127-132

Silent Word Generation, 127-132, 139-140

## T

Theory Of Mind, 39-40, 53-54, 57-58

Tissue Signal, 18-19, 22-23

Transient Ischemic Attack, 22-23, 26-27

Trier Social Stress Test, 79-80, 87-88

## U

Unsalvageable Tissue, 16-19

## V

Ventromedial Prefrontal Cortex, 2-5, 8-13, 49-50, 67-68, 108-109

Visual Cognition, 38

www.ingramcontent.com/pod-product-compliance
Lightning Source LLC
LaVergne TN
LVHW080623210926
848485LV00003B/206